VASCULAR HEMODYNAMICS

BIOENGINEERING AND CLINICAL PERSPECTIVES

Edited by

Peter J. Yim
Department of Radiology
UMDNJ—Robert Wood Johnson Medical School

⟨W⟩WILEY-BLACKWELL

A John Wiley & Sons, Inc., Publication

Wiley-Blackwell is an imprint of John Wiley & Sons, formed by the merger of Wiley's global Scientific, Technical, and Medical business with Blackwell Publishing.

Published by John Wiley & Sons, Inc., Hoboken, New Jersey
Published simultaneously in Canada

For general information on our other products and services or for technical support, please contact our Customer Care Department within the United States at 877-762-2974, outside the United States at 317-572-3993 or fax 317-572-4002.

Wiley also publishes its books in a variety of electronic formats. Some content that appears in print may not be available in electronic formats. For more information about Wiley products, visit our web site at www.wiley.com.

Library of Congress Cataloging-in-Publication Data:

Vascular hemodynamics: bioengineering and clinical perspectives /
[edited by] Peter J. Yim.
    p. ; cm.
  Includes bibliographical references.
  ISBN 978-0-470-08947-7 (cloth)
  1.   Blood circulation disorders. 2.   Hemodynamics–Research–Methodology.   I.
Yim, Peter J.
  [DNLM: 1.   Cardiovascular Diseases–physiopathology. 2.   Diagnostic Imaging.
3.   Diagnostic Techniques, Cardiovascular. 4.   Models, Cardiovascular. WG 120
V3315 2008]
  RB144.V37 2008
  616.1'3–dc22

                                           2007039339

Printed in the United States of America

10 9 8 7 6 5 4 3 2 1

CONTENTS

PREFACE

Hemodynamic characterization of the vasculature has grown increasingly sophisticated in recent years. Significant developments have been taking place in the areas of modeling, intrumentation, and experimentation. As such, the study of hemodynamics continues to play an essential role in advancing our understanding of normal vascular function and vascular disease processes. In a more recent development, a clinical component of this field has begun to emerge with the goal of improving the management of patients with vascular disease and circulatory dysfunction. This book addresses the full scope of this field with representative contributions on a wide range of both technical and investigative topics.

The order of the chapters in the book reflects the intent to convey some sense of continuity. The earlier chapters focus primarily on either normal vascular function or the role of blood flow in vascular disease processes.

In Chapter 1, a dimensionless scaling model of the circulatory system is presented by Dawson in which the overall behavior of the circulatory system, from one species to another, can be understood in terms of a relatively small number of characteristics of the circulatory system.

The role of shear stress in the atherosclerotic disease process has been under intensive investigation since early observations of the coincidence of disturbed flow at the location in the carotid artery at which atherosclerosis most commonly occurs. In Chapter 2, Reneman, Arts, and Hoeks present methodology for in vivo measurement of wall shear stress and observations from clinical studies involving his methodology.

The role of hemodynamic factors in the progression of cerebral aneurismal disease has also been hypothesized. This hypothesis has investigated in the clinical setting. Methodology for the study of the hemodynamics of this disease and early clinical investigations using this methodology are described by Cebral and Putman in Chapter 3.

Systemic arterial stiffening is believed to be a very insidious process and has long been a focus of hemodynamics-based and other investigations. In Chapter 4, Hansen, Jeppesen, and Torp-Pedersen present clinical studies involving the aortic pulsed-wave velocity, a metric of arterial stiffness, and its relationship to cardiovascular events.

Characterization of the bahavior of the vascular system as a whole and the interaction between the vascular system and the heart has been at the core of the field of hemodynamics since its inception. In Chapter 5, Lucas, Cole, and Yoganathan trace the development of systemic hemodynamic models to their current state, which includes modeling of surgically created circulations.

Accurate assessment of arterial wall properties presents considerable technical challenges. In Chapter 6, Hoeks, Hermeling, and Reneman discuss the mechanics of wall motion and describe methodologies that offer the potential for the in vivo assessment of arterial wall properties.

The process that leads to the rupture of atherosclerotic plaque, and its often devastating consequences, is the subject of considerable investigation. Mechanical conditions within atherosclerotic plaque have been hypothesized to play a role in plaque destabilization. In Chapter 7, Li presents work based on this hypothesis including early work on the development of methodology for in vivo assessment of stress patterns within the plaque.

The later chapters focus, in large part, on the hemodynamics of ischemia and infarction. In Chapter 8, I review developments in the emerging field of noninvasive estimation of the hemodynamic significance of arterial stenoses.

Phase contrast magnetic resonance imaging offers the potential for making direct measurement of blood flow and even velocity distributions in large arteries, which are certainly key hemodynamic features. In Chapter 9, Nezafat and Thompson provide background and insights into this rapidly developing methodology, including the demonstration of a number of potential applications.

Accurate evaluation of the brain tissue in the acute phases of stroke has considerable importance for patient care. Very promising imaging techniques have emerged for performing this evaluation. In Chapter 10, Calamante provides a technical perspective on one of these techniques, cerebral perfusion magnetic resonance imaging, with insights on both image acquisition and on perfusion modeling.

In Chapter 11, Wintermark makes the case, from the clinical perspective, for rapid adaption of the related technique of cerebral perfusion computed tomography in the evaluation of acute stroke patients.

The study of the intracranial circulation, through measurements of cerebrovascular reactivity, is beginning to yield important insights into stroke mechanisms and risk factors. In Chapter 12, Bornstein and Gur address the topic of changes in cerebrovascular reactivity with carotid artery stenosis and the possibly very significant clinical implications of this hemodynamic measurement.

In Chapter 13, Sierra addresses the relationship between hypertension and increased risk of stroke with a focus on the role of cerebrovascular reactivity.

PETER J. YIM

■■■■ CONTRIBUTORS

Theo Arts, PhD Department of Biophysics, Cardiovascular Research Institute Maastricht, Maastricht University, 6200 MD Maastricht, The Netherlands

Natan M. Bornstein, MD Stroke Unit, Department of Neurology, Tel Aviv Sourasky Medical Center, Sackler Faculty of Medicine, 6 Weizmann Street, Tel Aiv University, Tel Aviv, Israel [email: strokeun@tasmc.health.gov.il]

Fernando Calamante, PhD Brain Research Institute, Austin Health, Neurosciences Building, Banksia Street, Victoria 3081, Australia [email: fercala@brain.org.au]

Juan R. Cebral, PhD Center for Computational Fluid Dynamics, George Mason University, 4400 University Drive, Fairfax, VA 22030 [email: jcebral@gmu.edu]

Randal Cole, PhD Department of Biomedical Engineering, University of North Carolina at Chapel Hill, Chapel Hill, NC

Thomas H. Dawson, PhD United States Naval Academy, Annapolis, MD 21409 [email: dawson@usna.edu]

Alexander Y. Gur, MD, PhD Stroke Unit, Department of Neurology, Tel Aviv Sourasky Medical Center, Sackler Faculty of Medicine, 6 Weizmann Street, Tel Aiv University, Tel Aviv, Israel

Tine Willum Hansen, MD, PhD Department of Clinical Physiology, Hvidovre Hospital, University of Copenhagen, DK-2650 Hvidovre, Denmark [email: tw@heart.dk]

Evelien Hermeling, MSc Department of Biophysics, Cardiovascular Research Institute Maastricht, University of Maastricht, 6200 MD Maastricht, The Netherlands

Arnold P. G. Hoeks, PhD Departments of Biophysics, Cardiovascular Research Institute Maastricht, University of Maastricht, 6200 MD Maastricht, The Netherlands [email: a.hoeks@bf.unimaas.nl]

Jorgen Jeppesen, MD, DMSc Department of Medicine, Glostrup University Hospital, Ndr. Ringvej, DK-2600 Glostrup, Denmark

*Zhi-Yong Li, PhD   Departments of Radiology and Engineering, Cambridge University Hospitals NHS Foundation Trust, Addenbrooke's Hospital, Cambridge CB2 2QQ, UK [email: zyl22@cam.ac.uk]

*Carol L. Lucas, PhD   Department of Biomedical Engineering, Surgery, and Applied Sciences, University of North Carolina at Chapel Hill, 152 MacNider Hall, Chapel Hill, NC 27599 [email: clucas@bme.unc.edu]

*Reza Nezafat, PhD   Harvard-Thorndlike Laboratory of the Department of Medicine, Division of Cardiology, Beth Israel Deaconess Medical Center and Harvard Medical School, Boston, MA [email: rnezafat@bidmc.harvard.edu]

Christian Torp-Pedersen, MD   Department of Cardiology, Bispebjerg University Hospital, DK-2400, Copenhagen, Denmark

Christopher M. Putman, PhD   Interventional Neuroradiology, Inova Fairfax Hospital, 3300 Gallows Road, Falls Church, VA 22042

*Robert S. Reneman, MD, PhD   Department of Physiology, Cardiovascular Research Institute Maastricht, University of Maastricht, 6200 MD Maastricht, The Netherlands [email: reneman@fys.unimaas.nl]

*Christina Sierra, MD, PhD   Hypertension and Geriatrics Units, Department of Internal Medicine, Hospital Clinic of Barcelona, University of barcelona, Barcelona 08036 Spain [email: csierra@clinic.ub.es]

Richard B. Thompson, PhD   Department of Biomedical Engineering, University of Alberta, Canada

*Max Wintermark, MD   Department of Radiology, Neuroradiology Section, University of California, San Francisco, 505 Parnassus Avenue, San Francisco, CA 94143 [email: max.wintermark@radiology.ucsf.edu]

*Peter J. Yim, PhD   Department of Radiology, UMDNJ—Robert Wood Johnson Medical School, New Brunswick, NJ 08903 [email: yimpj@umdnj.edu]

Ajit Yoganathan, PhD   Department of Biomedical Engineering, Georgia Institute of Technology, Atlanta, GA

*Corresponding author.

CHAPTER 1

Modeling the Vascular System and Its Capillary Networks

THOMAS H. DAWSON

United States Naval Academy, Annapolis, Maryland

Abstract. Modeling of the vascular system and its capillary networks is considered within the context of associated scaling laws relating measurements of cardiovascular variables of mammals ranging in size from the mouse to the human and onward to the elephant. Topics include competing effects of viscous and inertial resistances to blood flow in the system and their appropriate separation for modeling purposes. Adequacy of the separation is confirmed by the demonstrated success of the scaling theory in consolidating size-dependent measurements into a single underlying description. Applications of the work include scaling of form and function for different-size systems directly to the human for confirmation of physiological descriptions and for practical matters such as the projection of safe drug dosage from small mammals to humans. Specific topics of form include discussion of detailed scaling laws for radius and length of arterial and venous vessel and for the radius, length, and number of capillary vessels. Topics of function include discussion of underlying physiological processes responsible for heart rate, ventricular outflow, blood circulation time, and kidney operation. The scaling of therapeutic drug concentrations from mouse to human is considered as an illustration of practical matters of interest.

1.1. INTRODUCTION

The vascular system of the body consists of the piping system of arteries and veins and the various capillary networks that it serves. The piping system is responsible for directing blood to the various capillary networks spread throughout the body and for returning it to the heart for further circulation. The capillaries themselves are responsible for transfer of life-sustaining substances between the blood and surrounding tissues. When considering the subject in physiological studies, attention is usually focused on the vascular system of humans. However, there exists a strong similarity between the vascular system of the human and other mammals, and this similarity allows study of the system with greater perspective than would otherwise be possible.

This chapter is concerned with modeling the vascular system and its capillary networks for the purpose of interpreting related measurements on mammals ranging in size from the mouse to the elephant. With such modeling theory, data on form and function for these different-size systems can be scaled directly to the human system for increased understanding and for application, as, for example, in drug therapy studies. The theory can also be used to establish important physical aspects of the operation of the vascular system and its parent cardiovascular system through their dependence on scale. The work described here is based on earlier work of the author [1–4], although some new perspectives and results are presented regarding theory and experimental support from existing measurements.

1.2. SOME BACKGROUND ON SCALING LAWS

Scaling laws for a physical system generally involve relations connecting measurable variables when *all* length measures of the system (e.g., lengths and diameters of pipes in a piping system) are increased or decreased by the same factor. Such scaling is referred to as *uniform scaling*. Relations for physiological variables based on this concept were provided many years ago by Lambert and Teissier [5]. When applied to vascular hemodynamics, they are, however, inadequate because of competing effects of inertial and viscous forces [6].

For perspective purposes, this inadequacy may be illustrated by considering the volume of ventricular blood V_S forced into the vascular system during each heartbeat, and its possible uniform scaling with mammal size. This quantity can be expected to depend on the volume V of the ventricle, representative lengths of the system l_1 and l_2 (among several), the contractile force F_0 of the ventricle per unit of wall area, a *constant* elastic modulus E with the same units as the contractile force, the heart rate ω, and the viscous and inertial resistances to blood flow as represented, respectively, by the coefficient of viscosity μ and density ρ of the blood. Each of these variables has, of course, fundamental measuring units (or dimensions) associated with it. In the simplest cases, V_S and V have units of length cubed and l_1 and l_2 have units of length. Correspondingly, consistent with their definitions, F_0 and E both have units of force divided by length squared, ω has units of reciprocal time, μ has units of force times time divided by length squared, and ρ has units of mass divided by length cubed.

Now, the governing equation connecting these variables must be expressible in terms of dimensionless ratios in order to be independent of particular units employed (meters or feet, newtons or pounds, etc.). With m-dimensional variables and n fundamental units, there will, in fact, generally be $m - n$ independent dimensionless ratios that can be formed. In the present case, there are nine variables and four units involved: those of length, time, force, and mass. However, the units of force are also the units of mass times acceleration (mass times length divided by time squared) so that there are only three fundamental units involved. Accordingly, there are six independent dimensionless ratios to be considered. A set of the required independent ratios can readily be formed by inspection, and the governing relation for the problem thus written as

$$\frac{V_S}{V} = f\left(\frac{\rho l_1^2 \omega^2}{E}, \frac{\mu\omega}{E}, \frac{F_0}{E}, \frac{l_2}{l_1}, \frac{V}{l_1^3}\right) \tag{1.1}$$

where $f(\ )$ denotes an unspecified function.

That each term in this equation is indeed dimensionless can be verified by direct examination of the units involved. For example, the first term on the right side can be written as $\rho l_1 \times l_1\omega^2/E$, which has units of mass per length squared (ρl_1) times acceleration $(l_1\omega^2)$, divided by force per length squared (E). Since mass times acceleration has dimensions of force, the numerator has equivalent units of force per length squared, like the denominator, so that all units cancel and leave the ratio in the required dimensionless form.

As to physical interpretation, this first term can be regarded as the ratio of inertial resistance to elastic restoring force of the ventricle and the second, as the ratio of viscous resistance to this same elastic force. Similarly, the third term can be regarded as the ratio of ventricular contractile force to the elastic restoring force and the last two terms regarded simply as variables representing explicit dependence on size.

As to scaling requirements, the term on the left side of this equation represents the ratio of two volumes and hence will be constant (or fixed) in uniform scaling from one mammal to another. The independent ratios on the right side must then also be fixed if scaling is to be possible. The last two terms in the equation are automatically fixed because of the geometric similarity that exists with uniform scaling. The third from last term can be fixed when the contractile force F_0 per unit of ventricular wall area is scale-independent. However, a problem arises with the first two terms that are required to be fixed in uniform scaling. For scale-invariant density and viscosity coefficient, as assumed here and as generally considered appropriate [6], the first requires that heart rate vary inversely with the length scale, while the second requires invariant heart rate among mammals. Thus, with these contradictory requirements, no scaling laws are possible under the restriction of uniform scaling.

In the presently described work, the general requirement of uniform scaling is replaced with more restrictive conditions where the viscosity coefficient and density are combined appropriately with the linear dimensions of the separate vessels in which viscous and inertial effects dominate. This leads to non-uniform scaling laws for the length and radius of these vessels and to scaling laws for related physiological variables that are free of contradictions and consistent with measurements. In developing this subject, considerably more insight into vascular hemodynamics is required than in the case of uniform scaling. Background material and related developments are thus considered here in some detail before taking up the development of the scaling laws.

1.3. THE VASCULAR SYSTEM

It has long been known that the vascular system consists of two main parts: the systemic part, associated with transport of blood to the main body for exchange of oxygen and other products; and the pulmonary part, associated with transport of blood to the lungs for discharge of unwanted gaseous products and recharge of oxygen. Discussion here will be directed mainly toward the systemic part of the circulation, but similar remarks will apply to the pulmonary part, and some reference will be made to it when possible.

A simplified representation of the various vessels of the systemic circulation is illustrated in Figure 1.1. Estimates of the size and number of these vessels for the complete systemic vascular system of the human are summarized in Table 1.1. These are projections of corresponding estimates for the dog by Green [7]. The scaling laws of the author [1] were used as a guide in making the projections. The (unspecified) body mass of the dog was assumed equal to 14 kg, based on Green's values for the aortic radius (5 mm) and length (40 cm) and associated empirical relations of Holt et al. [8]. Some minor adjustments and rounding of values have been made in forming the estimates for the human (assumed body mass of 70 kg). For example, the aortic radius has been increased by 20% to allow for vessel distension under mean blood pressure, and the radius and length of the small arteries and veins have been chosen as the weighted averages of the scaled values for the main and terminal branches of the original work. Noteworthy, for example, is the fact that the total volume of the vessels

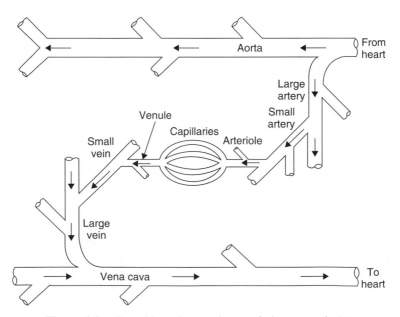

Figure 1.1.   Branching of systemic vessels in mammals [1].

TABLE 1.1. Estimated Measures of Systemic Vascular Vessels of Humans

Vessel	Radius (mm)	Length (mm)	Number	Volume (mL)
Aorta	11	600	1	228
Large arteries	3	300	40	339
Small arteries	1	50	2400	377
Arterioles	0.01	3	1.1×10^8	104
Capillaries	0.005	1	3.3×10^9	259
Venules	0.02	3	2.2×10^8	829
Small veins	1	50	2400	377
Large veins	5	300	40	943
Venae cavae	11	500, 100	1	228

is equal to 3700 mL, which represents about 75% of the volume of the entire (systemic and pulmonary) vascular system and heart chambers and is consistent with generally accepted estimates.

1.4. IDEALIZED VASCULAR HEMODYNAMICS

In addition to the size and number of the vessels, a further important characterization can be made regarding resistance to blood flow during the cardiac cycle. This resistance may be divided into two parts: the inertial resistance associated with acceleration of the blood in the vessels and the viscous resistance associated with velocity of the blood through the vessels. Of interest are the relative importance of these two resistances in the individual vessels and the general mathematical forms that can be used to describe them. These matters will be investigated here using an idealized version of vascular hemodynamics based on average blood flow in the vessels at any instant rather than on the actual flow. Detailed variations of the blood flow in the arteries, arising from vessel distension and resulting wave propagation, will thus be neglected, as will the irregular intermittent blood flow in the individual capillary networks. The adequacy of results from the simplified description will be checked initially in terms of blood pressure predictions and then later in terms of scaling predictions derived using the description.

With the latter idealization, the inertial resistance f_I (in units of pressure) provided by any one set of the parallel vessels listed in Table 1.1 may be estimated using the basic force–acceleration equation in the form

$$f_I = \beta \, \frac{\rho L}{\pi R^2} \frac{Q_r}{N} \tag{1.2}$$

where ρ denotes mass density of the blood; L and R denote, respectively, the length and radius of the individual vessel; N denotes the number of similar parallel vessels; and Q_r denotes the average blood acceleration (rate of change of blood flow) in the set of vessels under consideration at any instant that results from the periodic cardiac contractions. Also, the coefficient β denotes a factor that takes into account branching of vessels from the vessels under consideration. For all except the nonbranching capillaries, its value may be estimated as one-half, corresponding to uniform branching with average flowrate equal to Q_r/N at the vessel entrance and equal to zero at its far end. For the capillaries, the value of the coefficient is, of course, unity.

The viscous resistance f_V (in units of pressure) for flow through any one set of vessels may similarly be estimated using the standard Hagen–Poiseuille equation in the form

$$f_V = \beta \, \frac{8 \, \mu L}{\pi R^4} \frac{Q}{N} \tag{1.3}$$

where μ denotes viscosity coefficient of the blood and Q denotes the average flow of the blood in the set of vessels at any instant. An implicit assumption involved in the use of this equation is that sufficient time exists in the interval of interest to allow flow development from its initiation to fully viscous conditions.

In forming estimates with these equations, measured values of ventricular flowrate and flow will be used for the average flow conditions in the vessels. Well-known outflow characteristics of the left ventricle (measured in the ascending aorta) are indicated in Figure 1.2 for humans, together with corresponding values of aortic blood pressure. Interest in the present work is in the initial stage (0.21–0.26 s) where extreme conditions exist, with an essentially constant flowrate of 11,000 mL/s^2 and flow increasing from zero to a maximum of about 550 mL/s.

The inertial and viscous resistances to blood flow at the ventricle arise from the respective sums of the inertial and viscous resistances of each class of vessels. The resistive pressure at the far end of the system, where the blood empties into the right atrium, is essentially zero, so that the total resistance at the ventricle is that involved in overcoming the flow resistances in the individual vessels. In applying equations (1.2) and (1.3) for calculating these resistances, the mass density of the blood may be taken as 1.05 g/cm^3 and the value for the viscosity coefficient as 0.03 dyn·s/cm^2. The latter is appropriate for blood flow in macroscale arterial and venous vessels. However, within the small microscale vessels of the capillary networks, its value is less because of the nonhomogenous nature of the blood (plasma, components, and red blood cells) on this small scale. The actual value is unknown, and an approximate value of 0.02 dyn·s/cm^2, about midway between that of the plasma and the nominal value, will be used here.

Resulting calculations of the resistances for each vessel category are given in Table 1.2. A flow acceleration of 11,000 mL/s^2 and a mean flow of 275 mL/s have been assumed, consistent with the early part of the ventricular data shown in Figure 1.2a. It can be seen that the inertial resistance in macroscale arterial vessels is essentially 100% of the total inertial resistance and that the viscous resistance in microscale vessels is essentially 100% of the total viscous resistance.

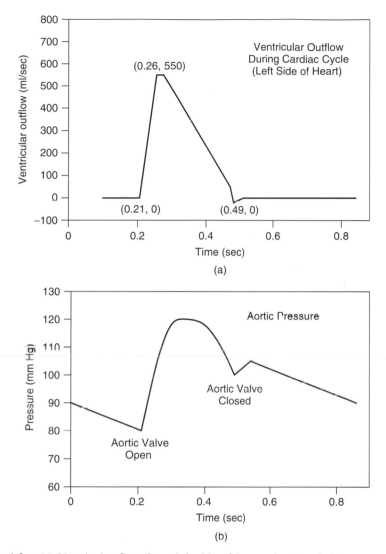

Figure 1.2. (a) Ventricular flow from left side of human heart and (b) corresponding blood pressures. (Data source: Selkurt and Bullard [9].)

Vessel dimensions alone limit the inertial resistance in the capillary networks, and calculated inertial resistances in the veins are ignored since measurements indicate the absence of accelerated flow in these vessels (presumably because of viscous damping in the capillary networks).

The total calculated resistance to the blood flow is 135,500 dyn/cm^2 (102 mmHg) as determined with the average flow of 275 mL/s. When the viscous resistance is greatest (for blood flow of 550 mL/s), the total calculated resistance

TABLE 1.2. Estimated Inertial and Viscous Resistances (dyn/cm^2) in Systemic Vessels of Humans

Vessel	Inertial	Viscous	Vessel Class
Aorta	91,200	430	Macroscale
Large arteries	15,300	970	Macroscale
Small arteries	380	220	Macroscale
Arterioles	5.0	19,100	Microscale
Capillaries	0.4	6,790	Microscale
Venules	0.6	600	Microscale
Small veins	—	220	Macroscale
Large veins	—	130	Macroscale
Venae cavae	—	110	Macroscale

is 164,000 dyn/cm^2 (123 mmHg) and when the viscous resistance is zero (for blood flow of zero) at the beginning of the ventricular contraction, the total resistance is 106,900 dyn/cm^2 (80 mmHg). These calculated values are in excellent agreement with the known systolic (120 mmHg) and diastolic (80 mmHg) blood pressures of healthy humans, as indicated in Figure 1.2b, and this suggests a possibly wider application of the simple theory and vessel characterization than might otherwise be expected.

An interesting consequence of this division between arterial and viscous resistances, perhaps worthy of note in passing, is that a reduction in the flow area of the large arteries will increase the lower blood pressure and cause in turn the maximum and mean pressures to increase by the same amount. In contrast, a reduction in the flow area of the arterioles will leave the lower blood pressure unchanged but will cause an increase in the maximum pressure equal to twice the increase of the mean pressure.

1.5. IDEALIZED VESSEL CATEGORIES

The preceding results suggest for modeling purposes that the vascular system may be divided broadly into the categories of a connecting vessel between the left side of the heart and the systemic capillary system where inertial resistance is dominant, and the systemic capillary system itself, where viscous resistance is dominant. In addition, it may also be considered to consist of a connecting vessel between the systemic capillaries and the right side of the heart, where viscous resistance also dominates. A similar idealized arrangement can be assumed applicable to the pulmonary side, with a connecting vessel between the right side of the heart and the pulmonary capillary system, and a connecting vessel from these capillaries to the left side of the heart. This idealization is illustrated in Figure 1.3.

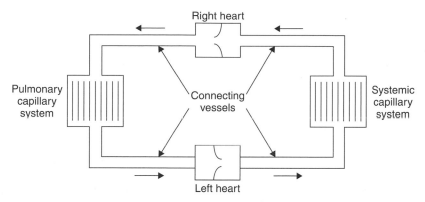

Figure 1.3. Idealized description of the vascular system of mammals indicating collective systemic and pulmonary capillary networks and connecting vessels [1].

A diagram like that in Figure 1.3 has often been used to illustrate the series connection of the left and right sides of the heart in terms of pumping action [10]. In the present work, it has added meaning in illustrating the division of the flow characteristics of the blood, with inertial resistance dominating in the arterial connecting vessels from the left and right sides of the heart and viscous resistance dominating in the capillaries and in the venous connecting vessels to the left and right sides.

1.6. THEORETICAL SCALING LAWS

Similar to earlier work of the writer, the conceptual model shown in Figure 1.3 will be used to derive scaling laws that relate the dimensions of the arterial and venous vessels and the dimensions and number of vessels in the capillary networks for mammals of vastly different sizes [1]. The theoretical presentation here will be a simplified treatment of the early work and will be based on the necessary requirement that any physical equation be independent of particular units employed and hence must be expressible in dimensionless form.

Resting conditions will be assumed as the basic conditions governing the sizing of the vascular system of different mammals, consistent with results from earlier work. As in the previous discussion of idealized vascular hemodynamics and associated blood pressure calculations, average flow in the blood vessels at any instant will be assumed to be representative of the actual complex flows insofar as scaling matters are concerned.

A typical dependent variable of the cardiovascular system, considered previously in connection with equation (1.1), is the stroke volume of the left side of the heart, that is, the total volume of blood ejected into the systemic vascular system during each contraction of the left ventricle. In a more restrictive sense than earlier, this can now be expected to depend on the volume of the ventricle

V, a typical length dimension l of the ventricle, the contractile force F_0 per unit area of the ventricular wall (measuring the strength of the contraction), a scale-independent constant E (in units of force per unit area) associated with the general relation between fractional volume change of the ventricle and contractile force in the absence of restraint from blood flow, the heart rate ω, and the inertial and viscous resistances to blood flow in the vascular system, as represented, respectively, by equations (1.2) and (1.3), with constant blood density ρ and constant viscosity coefficients μ_c and μ_v associated with blood flow in the microscopic capillary vessels and macroscopic venous vessels, respectively.

Now, from equations (1.2) and (1.3), it can be seen that the expression for the inertial resistance to blood flow has both the density of blood ρ and the ratio L/NR^2 appearing together as a product and that for the viscous resistance has both the blood viscosity μ and the ratio L/NR^4 appearing as a product. Thus, the stroke volume can be expected to depend not on the blood density and viscosity by themselves, but rather as they appear in these two products. Considering independent dimensionless ratios of the variables, the stroke volume V_S may accordingly be expressed in general mathematical form as

$$\frac{V_S}{V} = f\left(\frac{\rho L_a \omega^2 V}{R_a^2 E}, \frac{\mu_c L_c \omega V}{N_c R_c^4 E}, \frac{\mu_v L_v \omega V}{R_v^4 E}, \frac{F_0}{E}, \frac{V}{l^3}\right) \qquad (1.4)$$

where $f(\ )$ denotes an undefined function of the indicated variables and R_a and L_a denote the radius and length of the connecting arterial vessel, respectively; R_c, L_c, and N_c denote the radius, length, and number of the characteristic capillaries; respectively; and R_v and L_v denote, respectively, the radius and length of the venous connecting vessel. Consistent with the earlier discussion, single arterial and venous connecting vessels have been assumed so that N_a and N_v are both equal to 1 in the conceptual model.

The physical interpretation of the terms in this equation is similar to that discussed earlier in connection with equation (1.1). The first term represents the ratio of inertial resistance in the arteries to the elastic ventricular restoring force, and the second and third terms represent the ratios of viscous forces in the capillaries and veins to this same force. Similarly, the fourth term represents the ratio of ventricular force to elastic restoring force, and the last term represents the ratio of ventricular volume to the cube of any of its linear length measures. As will be seen below, the explicit inclusion of separate measures for the arteries, capillaries, and veins in this equation now allow scaling relations to be developed without the contradictions associated with equation (1.1).

Measurements of Holt et al. [11] have shown that the ratio of stroke volume to ventricular volume, denoted by the left side of equation (1.4), is constant for mammals ranging in size from the rat to the horse, consistent with the idea of similitude in mechanical systems having different sizes. This condition is illustrated in Figure 1.4 for typical mammals. The implication is that the dimensionless variables on the right side of equation (1.4) are also constant under change of scale. These ratios provide the conditions needed for similarity and scale modeling of the system.

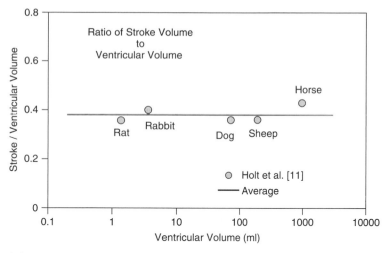

Figure 1.4. Measurements (circles) showing that the ratio of stroke volume to ventricle volume is essentially constant for mammals ranging from rats to horses.

The ventricular volume V represented in equation (1.4) is known from the work of Holt et al. [11] to vary directly with mammal mass M under change of scale so that the condition for the first three terms on the right side to remain fixed for different mammals may be written as

$$\frac{L_a\omega^2}{R_a^2} \propto M^{-1}, \quad \frac{L_c\omega}{N_c R_c^4} \propto M^{-1}, \quad \frac{L_v\omega}{R_v^4} \propto M^{-1} \qquad (1.5)$$

where the symbol $\propto$ denotes proportionality under change of scale and where the density and viscosity coefficient of the blood are assumed scale-independent. The fourth term in equation (1.4) requires also that the contractile force F_0 per unit area of ventricular wall remain fixed under scale change, and the fifth term requires that all important length dimensions of the ventricle vary in the same way, as ventricular volume raised to the one-third power. Since ventricular volume varies directly with mammal mass, the last condition also means that these length dimensions must vary as mammal mass raised to the one-third power.

In addition to relations (1.5), three other relations may be written associated with the fact that the total blood volume in mammals is known to vary directly with mammal mass [12]. As parts of the whole, the blood volumes in the connecting vessels and the capillary system can therefore similarly be considered to vary in this manner. The following additional relations represent this requirement:

$$R_a^2 L_a \propto M, \quad N_c R_c^2 L_c \propto M, \quad R_v^2 L_v \propto M \qquad (1.6)$$

Relations (1.5) and (1.6) provide six relations between the eight variables involved, that is, the seven variables associated directly with the vascular system and the heart rate. Two additional relations are thus needed for determining their variations with mammal mass. A theoretical approach involving basic cardiac cell processes was taken in the first work of the author [1] in order to obtain these needed relations and an empirical one in later works [2,3]. Here, attention will be directed again to the theoretical approach, with perhaps some further clarification.

The main idea behind the theoretical development of the needed additional relations is that the scaling relations for the variables associated with the characteristic capillary system can be expected to apply (in the resting state) to the capillaries of any organ of the body. Thus, the number of capillaries in the heart can be considered to be proportional under scale change to the number of capillaries N_c referred to in relations (1.5) and (1.6). The number of cardiac cells in the heart can also be considered to be proportional to the number of capillaries supplying them. Thus, tissue volume of the heart can be considered proportional under scale change to the product of capillary number and the volume of a single cell. Since tissue volume of the heart and heart mass are proportional, the latter can also be substituted for the former in this last relation. Moreover, heart mass and body mass are known to be proportional [12] under scale change, so that, on inverting the tissue–volume relation and using this last condition, the volume of a single cardiac cell is predicted from these arguments to be proportional to the ratio M/N_c.

This last relation provides the connection between cardiac-cell size and variables already present in the discussion, and this in turn allows further description in terms of fundamental processes. For this purpose, it is convenient to use a simple length measure of a cell. Assuming all lengths of the cells scale in the same way, the cell volume must then be proportional to the cube of any length measure, and a characteristic length d of a cell can therefore be expressed simply as

$$d \propto \left(\frac{M}{N_c} \right)^{1/3} \tag{1.7}$$

Insofar as application is concerned, this last relation has significance because cardiac tissue is known to consist mainly of cardiac fibers which, when excited, contract and provide the pumping action of the heart. These fibers are also known to consist of series connections of cardiac cells. The diameter of the cells and hence that of the fibers can thus be expected to be proportional under change of scale to the characteristic dimension d defined by relation (1.7).

With respect to operation, it is known that resting cardiac fibers, like all muscle fiber, have an excess of positive ions immediately outside, relative to their interiors. Contraction is initiated in the upper heart by the relatively slow movement of positive ions into specialized fibers until the inside potential is raised to a critical value needed for rapid influx of additional ions under the electrical attraction existing. This sudden increase generates a voltage pulse (or action potential), which then propagates across the heart, causing contraction and pumping action. At the same time, the newly arrived positive ions in the fibers are forced out by a metabolic energy source and the potential at the initiation site is returned to its initial value. The process repeats itself periodically to provide the heartbeat and cyclic pumping action.

On the basis of this brief description, two issues can be considered for obtaining the additional relations needed to complete the scaling description of the vascular system: (1) the initial cyclic slow influx of ions into the fibers at the initiation region of the heart and (2) propagation of the contraction signal over the heart fibers to form the full heartbeat.

The first issue can be addressed by likening the slow influx of ions to a general diffusion process. The relation for the mass m of an ionic substance moving into the cells of a fiber is then expressible in dimensionless terms as

$$\frac{m}{\Delta C d^3} = f\left(\frac{\omega d^2}{D}\right) \tag{1.8}$$

where $f(\ )$ denotes a general function, D denotes a constant (in units of area per time), and ΔC denotes the initial difference between concentrations outside and inside the cell (in units of mass per volume). The left side of this equation, with concentration difference ΔC assumed scale-invariant, is proportional to the mass influx per unit cell volume, and this may be expected to be independent of mammal size. With the constant D also scale-invariant, as expected, it can be seen that the product of heart rate and square of cell dimension must likewise be constant under change of scale:

$$\omega d^2 \propto M^0 \tag{1.9}$$

Using the definition of cardiac cell dimension of relation (1.7), the follow relation thus results

$$\omega \propto M^{-2/3} N_c^{2/3} \tag{1.10}$$

For the second matter, it is assumed that the propagation speed of the voltage pulse through cardiac fiber is, like nerve fiber, expressible as a power-law relation with fiber diameter; that is, as d^b, where b denotes a constant. From experimental studies with small isolated nerve fibers (generally considered analogous to heart fibers), a value of b can be expected to be between 0.57 [13] and 0.78 [14]. A value of b equal to $\frac{2}{3}$ was used by the author in earlier work [1] and will be assumed here. Now, the period between heartbeats (reciprocal of the heart rate) must be proportional to the ratio of heart length traveled by the voltage pulse to the propagation speed. Assuming that overall heart dimensions scale with mammal mass to the one-third power (like ventricular dimensions noted earlier), the following relation can be obtained:

$$\omega \propto M^{-1/9} N_c^{-2/9} \tag{1.11}$$

Relations (1.10) and (1.11) provide the scaling laws for the heart rate and capillary number, and the second of relations (1.5) and (1.6) then provide the scaling laws for the radius and length of capillary vessels. The results are expressible in the form

$$\omega \propto M^{-1/4} \tag{1.12}$$

$$R_c \propto M^{1/12}, \quad L_c \propto M^{5/24}, \quad N_c \propto M^{5/8} \tag{1.13}$$

It is worthwhile to note that this solution for the scaling laws of the capillary vessels is independent of the assumption that inertial resistance dominates in the macroscopic arterial system and depends on the less stringent assumption that viscous effects dominate in the microscopic vessels, irrespective of the conditions applying in the macroscopic system.

With the above solution available, the first and third of relations (1.5) and (1.6) then provide the remaining scaling laws for the radius and length of the macroscale arterial and venous vessels. The solutions are expressible as

$$R_a \propto M^{3/8}, \quad L_a \propto M^{1/4}, \quad N_a \propto M^0 \tag{1.14}$$

and

$$R_v \propto M^{7/24}, \quad L_v \propto M^{5/12}, \quad N_v \propto M^0 \tag{1.15}$$

where it is also noted that the number of arterial and venous connecting vessels N_a and N_v are invariant with scale change.

1.7. OBSERVATIONS ON THE SCALING LAWS

Heart Rate

The reciprocal one-fourth scaling law for heart rate of relation (1.12) is intimately connected to the scaling laws for the vascular system, and its validity is therefore essential to the validity of the scaling laws themselves. The law is in fact consistent with the generally accepted empirical relation for resting mammals that has existed for many years [11,12,15,16]. Typical data are indicated in Figure 1.5. Predictions are also shown from the scaling law when expressed with average coefficient as

$$\omega = 230M^{-1/4} \tag{1.16}$$

The agreement between theory and measurement can be seen to be very good over the entire range from mouse to elephant. When applied to the human having typical body mass of 70 kg, the equation predicts a heart rate of 80 beats/min, which is about 14% greater than the value of 70 beats/min that usually applies for resting and relaxed conditions. For predictions for such a state, the coefficient should therefore be reduced from 230 to 200.

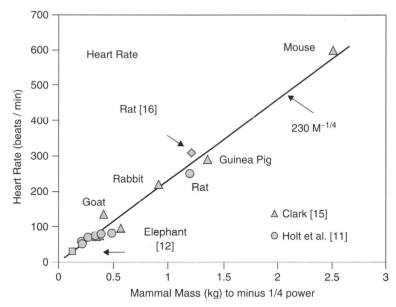

Figure 1.5.   Measurements (symbols) confirming the scaling law for resting heart rate, with data from typical mammals identified.

It is interesting to note that the physical explanation for increased or decreased heart rate of mammals relative to the human is provided by relation (1.9), which requires that heart rate vary inversely with the square of cardiac cell dimensions. Thus, for example, the diameter of the cardiac cells of the mouse must (according to this description) be approximately one-third smaller than that of the human in order to provide the observed increase in the resting heart rate by a factor of 9.

Ventricular Outflow

As a further preliminary examination of the vascular scaling theory, the related scaling laws associated with ventricular outflow will be developed and compared with measurements. These relations will be needed in the following work where the applicability of the theory is examined for mammals larger and smaller than the human (in the manner of results already presented in Table 1.2 for the human). For this purpose, it is convenient to return to the basic relation (1.4) and replace the dependent dimensionless stroke volume on the left side with the dimensionless ratio of flow Q to the product of ventricular volume V and heart rate ω, and also include the dimensionless time ωt on the right side. Similarity requires that this variable and all the original variables in the relation to remain fixed under change of scale. Ventricular volume is proportional to mammal mass under scale change, as noted earlier, so that flow in this revised relation at any fixed time ωt is predicted to vary directly as the product of mammal mass and heart rate.

A corresponding treatment indicates that flowrate Q_r must vary directly with the product of mammal mass and the square of heart rate at any fixed time ωt. Thus, the scaling relations for ventricular flow and flowrate at any time t in the process may thus be written as

$$Q \propto M^{3/4}, \quad Q_r \propto M^{1/2}, \quad t \propto M^{1/4} \tag{1.17}$$

With these relations, the entire time history of ventricular outflow of one mammal can be predicted from that of another. An illustration of their applicability is shown in Figure 1.6, where the outflow history for the human, as indicated earlier in Figure 1.2, has been scaled to the horse and compared with measurements reported by Noordergraaf et al. [17]. Here, a typical body mass of 70 kg was assumed for the human and an effective mass of 450 kg for the horse. No specific value was given for the latter in the cited reference, and the effective value was determined using the known condition that the ratio of areas under the two flow history graphs is equal to the ratio of stroke volumes and hence is equal to the corresponding ratio of mammal masses. The agreement shown in Figure 1.6 can be seen to be remarkably good considering the difference in scale between the two.

Range of Applicability

The general applicability of the scaling laws for the macroscale arterial vessels of the vascular system depends on the continued dominance of inertial resistance

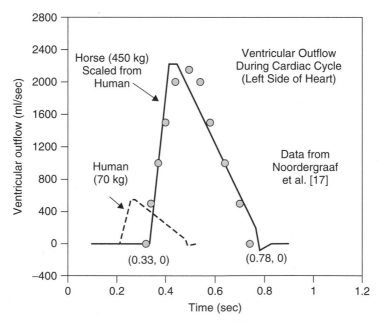

Figure 1.6. Ventricular outflow of horse as scaled from the human and as reported (circles) by Noordergraaf et al. [17].

to blood flow in these vessels as attention is shifted to mammals larger and smaller than the human. This matter can be investigated by projecting vessel characteristics of the human (Table 1.1) to the horse and rat using the previously developed vascular scaling laws and then calculating the flow resistances, as done earlier for the results given in Table 1.2, with the help now of the scaling relations (1.17).

Calculations of the vessel resistances for the horse (of 450 kg body mass) are listed in Table 1.3 for scaled values of flow acceleration and one-half maximum flow (27,900 mL/s^2, 1110 mL/s at 0.374 s). When compared with those given in Table 1.2, it can be seen that a scale change from the human to the horse leaves unchanged the inertial resistances in the arteries and the viscous resistances in the capillary networks and veins. This is as expected from the theory. The viscous resistances in the arteries do change some but are still negligible overall compared with the inertial resistances and are, in fact, somewhat less than those in the human because of the increase in scale. Calculated blood pressures accordingly remain unchanged from those determined for the human. The scaling relations derived under the assumptions of dominant inertial resistances in the arteries can thus generally be expected to apply at least to mammals of the size of the human and larger.

Similar calculations are also shown in Table 1.3 for the rat (0.3 kg body mass), using scaled values of flow acceleration and one-half maximum flow (720 mL/s^2, 4.6 mL/s at 0.060 s). The inertial resistance in the arteries and the viscous resistances in the capillary networks and veins are found to remain unchanged, as in the case of horses and humans. However, the total calculated viscous resistance in the arteries is found to be about 23% of the total inertial resistance and is therefore no longer negligible. The calculated diastolic blood pressure remains the same as for the human and the horse because this depends only on the inertial resistance in the arteries, which continues to be scale-independent. The calculated systolic blood pressure (for maximum flow) does change, though,

TABLE 1.3. Estimated Flow Resistances (dyn/cm^2) for Horse and Rat at One-Half Maximum Flow

Vessel	Horse (450 kg)		Rat (0.3 kg)	
	Inertial	Viscous	Inertial	Viscous
Aorta	91,200	170	91,200	6,580
Large arteries	15,300	380	15,300	14,900
Small arteries	380	90	380	3,340
Arterioles	4	19,100	0.8	19,100
Capillaries	0.4	6,790	0.7	6,790
Venues	0.5	600	1.0	600
Small veins	—	220	—	220
Large veins	—	130	—	130
Venae cavae	—	110	—	110

from 122 to 158 mmHg, and this is a direct result of the appreciable viscous resistance calculated for the arteries of the rat. These calculations suggest that relations (1.14) for scaling the macroscale arterial vessels, and the associated prediction of identical blood pressures, could not apply for smaller mammals such as the rat.

The latter observation is, however, inconsistent with the original blood pressure measurements of small mammals by Greg et al. [18] and Woodbury and Hamilton [19], which showed values for the mouse and dog to be the same as those for the human. More recently, Marque et al. [16] have reported measurements in connection with other work that confirm these earlier results specifically for the rat. The indication is therefore that viscous resistances in the arteries are, in fact, much less than calculated values from equation (1.3). In contrast, the calculations in Table 1.3, as well as those in Table 1.2, indicate that equation (1.3) does indeed apply to the capillary networks.

Evidence for the legitimacy of both of these indications can be found in the theory of starting motion of viscous fluids under constant driving pressure, as developed by Szymanski [20]. According to this theory, the initiated flow will first resemble that occurring in the absence of viscous effects (Figure 1.7a) and then proceed to become the fully developed Hagen–Poiseuille flow (Figure 1.7b), on which equation (1.3) is based (with the constant driving pressure then equal to the viscous resistance for the resulting flow). For fully developed flow in a vessel of radius R after time τ since initiation, the theory requires the value of the ratio $\rho R^2/\mu\tau$ to be equal to or less than unity, with ρ and μ denoting blood density and viscosity coefficient, respectively, as earlier.

If the driving pressure continually increases during the period τ (as in ventricle outflow during the period of interest here), smaller time intervals must be

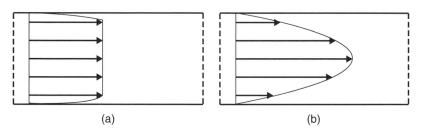

(a)   (b)

Rat (0.3 kg) with $\tau = 0.013$ s

Vessel	Radius (cm)	$\rho R^2/\mu\tau$	Condition
Aorta	0.14	53	Underdeveloped
Large artery	0.04	4	Underdeveloped
Small artery	0.01	0.3	Underdeveloped
Capillary	0.0003	0.0004	Fully developed

Figure 1.7. Velocity distributions illustrating flow development in blood vessels from starting condition [underdeveloped, early flow (a)] to fully developed viscous flow [later flow (b)] and illustration of its measure with the dimensionless number indicated.

considered for which the condition of constant driving pressure is effectively satisfied. Thus, taking the smaller increments as $\tau/100$, the criterion for fully developed flow in each interval is expressible as $\rho R^2/\mu\tau \leq 0.01$. Application of this requirement for the rat is included in the flow illustrations in Figure 1.7, with the time τ measured from the beginning of the heart cycle and equal to that at which maximum flow occurs.

It can be seen from the results in Figure 1.7 that the values of the flow development ratio for the arterial vessels of the rat are not small in the required sense for fully developed flow, in contrast with the capillary vessel, where this condition is satisfied to an extent far exceeding minimum requirements. The conclusion is therefore that viscous flow is not fully developed in the arterial vessels and that equation (1.3) cannot be expected to apply to flow resistances in these vessels, but that this is not the case for the vessels of the capillary networks.

The matter of apparent viscous resistance in the arterial vessels of the rat and other small mammals is thus clarified; calculations with equation (1.3) greatly overestimate the actual viscous resistance in the arteries so that, as with larger mammals, inertial resistance dominates in the arterial vessels and viscous resistance dominates in the capillary networks and the venous vessels. The vascular scaling relations developed under this condition are thus applicable to smaller mammals such as the rat as well as to larger ones such as the horse. Blood pressures in these circumstances are also predicted to be the same for both small and large mammals.

Within the capillary networks, the scaling laws of relations (1.13) can be expected to apply to the number and dimensions of the capillaries for all mammals. These relations depend only on the assumptions leading to relations (1.10) and (1.11) and the second of relations (1.5) and (1.6). In fact, they may also be established using the requirement that capillary blood volume is proportional to mammal mass, together with the relation for scale-independent drop in blood pressure across the capillary networks and the scaling relation for oxygen transfer to surrounding tissue [3]. The scaling relations (1.13) will also apply to the microscopic arterioles and venules that connect to the capillaries, as assumed here, provided only that their numbers scale directly with the capillary numbers.

The scaling laws of relations (1.15) for macroscale venous vessels can similarly be expected to apply to the upper and lower vena cava and to the large veins of all mammals. They may also apply to the small veins, as assumed here, provided their number is scale-independent like that of the larger veins.

1.8. EXAMINATION OF SCALING LAWS FOR VESSEL DIMENSIONS

The scaling laws for vessel dimensions are compared below with measurements reported by others for arterial, capillary, and venous vessels. In each case considered, the scaling relation has been cast in equation form, with its coefficient determined from a best-fit (least-square) analysis of the data involved.

Arterial Vessels

Holt et al. [8] measured the aortic radius (in the absence of any significant vessel distension from mean blood pressure) over the range from mouse to cow. Similar autopsy measurements of Clark [15] of the aortic radius are also available. The first of relations (1.14) requires the aortic radius to vary with mammal mass to the power $\frac{3}{8}$. Figure 1.8 illustrates the excellent agreement existing between the measurements (ascending aorta) and theoretical predictions when the scaling relation is expressed in the form indicated in the figure. Similar agreement exists with the earlier data of Clark.

Holt et al. [8] also measured the length of the aorta (heart to bifurcation) for the same mammals as used for the aortic radius. These data are shown in Figure 1.9 together with predictions from the second of relations (1.14) in the form of the equation indicated.

The theoretical scaling predictions for the aortic length can be seen to agree very well with the measurements from mammals ranging from the rabbit to the cow. There is, however, some overestimate of the measured values from mouse and rat. For these mammals, it may simply be that other conditions enter to prevent closer agreement with the theoretical projections.

Capillary Vessels

Measurements of capillary vessels are limited for the systemic side of the circulation, but the data available are consistent with the present theory [1,3]. Fortunately, for the pulmonary side of the circulation there are estimates (based

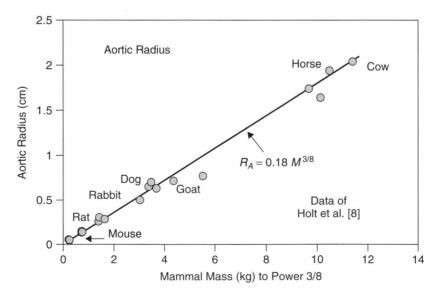

Figure 1.8.   Comparison of data with $\frac{3}{8}$th scaling law for aortic radius.

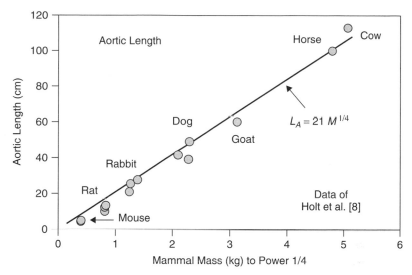

Figure 1.9. Comparison of data with 1/4-th scaling relation for aortic length.

on tissue samplings) of the net volume and surface area of the capillaries present in the oxygen transfer surfaces of the lung of mammals [21]. These data have been examined for individual mammals and the capillary radius and net capillary length determined from simple geometry. The results have been considered earlier [1,2]. Typical values for the capillary radius are shown in Figure 1.10 together with predictions from the first of relations (1.13) in the form of the $\frac{1}{12}$th power law indicated.

It can be seen that considerable scatter exists in the data, so that nothing definitive can be said about the predictions other than that they follow the trend of the data and provide a good representation of their average variation. The data do confirm the theoretical indication of a dependence of capillary radius on mammal size, and this alone provides an endorsement of the theoretical description. It also offers a striking illustration of the level of detail present in the vascular system of all mammals.

Similar data are shown in Figure 1.11 for the net length of the pulmonary capillaries, defined as the product of the capillary length and the number present. From the second and third of relations (1.13), the scaling relation for this net length involves mammal mass to the power $\frac{5}{6}$. Predictions from the indicated equation having this form are also shown in the figure. Here the scatter is minimal and the data and predictions can be seen to agree very well with one another.

Venous Vessels

Considering next the venous vessels, the measurements of Holt et al. [8] may again be used. Figure 1.12 shows these data for the radius of the inferior vena

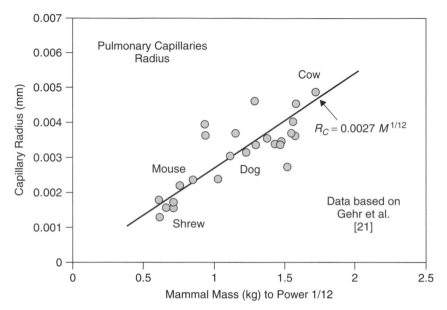

Figure 1.10.   Data from pulmonary side of circulation for capillary radius compared with $\frac{1}{12}$th relation.

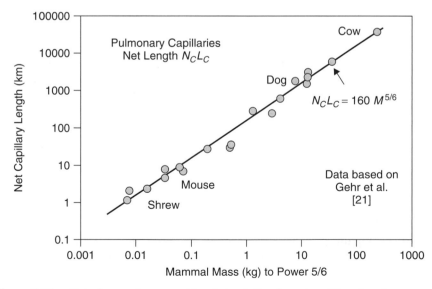

Figure 1.11.   Data from pulmonary side of circulation for net capillary length compared with $\frac{5}{6}$th relation.

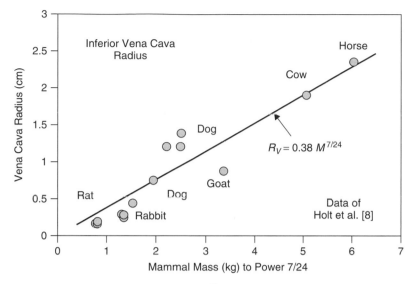

Figure 1.12. Comparison of data with $\frac{7}{24}$th scaling law for radius of vena cava.

cava. Predictions are also shown from the first of relations (1.15) when expressed in the form indicated. Some variability can be seen to exist in the measurements, and this renders the comparisons less definitive than might otherwise have been the case. Nevertheless, the theoretical predictions do provide a good average representation of the data.

Measurements of the length of the vena cava for various mammals are shown in Figure 1.13. In analyzing the data, the measurement for the horse appeared to be an anomaly and was neglected in determining the best-fit value for the coefficient of the scaling law. The remaining measurements can be seen to agree well with the predictions from the theoretical scaling relation.

1.9. APPLICATIONS OF SCALING THEORY

Indirect applications of the scaling laws for the vascular system have already been considered for heart rate, ventricular outflow, and blood pressures. More direct applications are described below concerning cardiac output and oxygen delivery, capillary density, circulation time of the blood, and kidney form and function. A final illustration involves the scaling of the time history of therapeutic drug concentration in the blood from the mouse to the human.

Cardiac Output and Oxygen Delivery

As is well known, a major role of the vascular system is to direct blood from the heart to the systemic capillaries for oxygen transfer to the cells. The transport

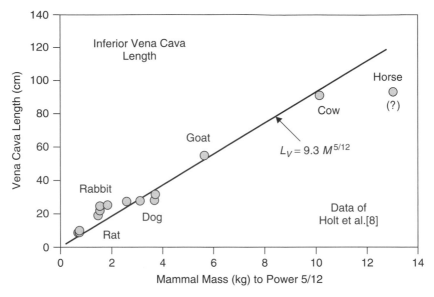

Figure 1.13.   Comparison of data with $\frac{5}{12}$th scaling law for length of vena cava.

activity is conveniently characterized by the cardiac output, which denotes the flow of blood into the system when averaged over a heart cycle. Cardiac output is thus equal to the product of stroke volume and heart rate and scales as mammal mass to the power $\frac{3}{4}$, consistent with the measurements shown in Figures 1.4 and 1.5.

For the resting mammal, mixed venous blood is approximately 75% saturated with oxygen (with maximum of 20 mL per 100 mL of blood), so that about 5 mL of oxygen is delivered to the cells for every 100 mL of blood from the heart. Oxygen consumption rate (or metabolic rate) is thus equal to 5% of the cardiac output and accordingly scales also as mammal mass to the power $\frac{3}{4}$. This scaling relation has been known for many years to be a result of direct measurements of oxygen utilization of mammals.

The associated rate of transfer of oxygen from the capillaries to surround tissue involves a basic diffusion process with driving force equal to the difference in oxygen partial pressures ΔP_O inside and outside the capillaries. The transfer rate is also proportional to the net surface area of the capillaries $N_C \times (2\pi R_C L_C)$ and inversely proportional to their wall thickness H_C. Thus, oxygen transfer rate V_{O_2} is expressible as

$$V_{O_2} \propto \Delta P_O \, \frac{N_C R_C L_C}{H_C} \tag{1.18}$$

Assuming that the partial pressures inside and outside are proportional under scale change and that the wall thickness and radius are similarly proportional, the following simplified relation results

$$V_{O_2} \propto P_O N_C L_C \propto M^{3/4} \tag{1.19}$$

where P_O denotes oxygen pressure in the blood and the second proportionality denotes the required scaling dependence of oxygen consumption rate noted above. The product $N_C L_C$ scales as mammal mass to the power $\frac{5}{6}$ so that the oxygen pressure in the blood must scale as mammal mass to the power $-\frac{1}{12}$ if the relation is to give the required $\frac{3}{4}$th scaling with body mass. This has, in fact, been shown to be the case by the author [1], based on detailed analysis of measurements of Schmidt-Nielsen and Larimer [22] for a saturation level of 75% or so.

Capillary Density

The number of capillaries per unit cross-sectional area of tissue is referred to as *capillary density*. It generally increases with decreasing mammal size, at least in muscle tissue, where the parallel arrangement of capillary vessels makes systematic investigation possible. Because of this arrangement, a simple scaling relation for capillary density of muscle can be established. In particular, the characteristic number of capillaries N_C per unit of cross-sectional area perpendicular to the capillary lengths must be proportional to the product of the volume density of the capillaries (number per unit of associated muscle volume) and the characteristic capillary length. With volume density proportional to muscle mass density and with muscle mass proportional to mammal mass, as is known to be the case, capillary density γ is thus expressible as

$$\gamma \propto \frac{N_C}{M} \times L_C \qquad \text{or} \qquad \gamma \propto M^{-1/6} \tag{1.20}$$

where the scaling relations (1.13) have been used in writing the second expression.

The variation of capillary density with mammal size has been studied in detail [23], and data for the masseter (jaw) muscle of mammals are shown in Figure 1.14. Also shown are predictions from the scaling relation (1.20) when cast in the indicated equation form.

Although some variability exists in the data, the scaling predictions can be seen to provide a good representation of the average increase associated with decreasing mammal size. Interestingly, the scaling relation (1.20) can also be established by assuming that capillary spacing is proportional to capillary radius. This, in turn, indicates geometric similarity under scale change in the array of capillaries and spacings in the cross-sectional areas of the muscle.

Circulation Time

As might be anticipated, the average time required for complete circulation of a small volume of blood around the vascular system is dependent on mammal size.

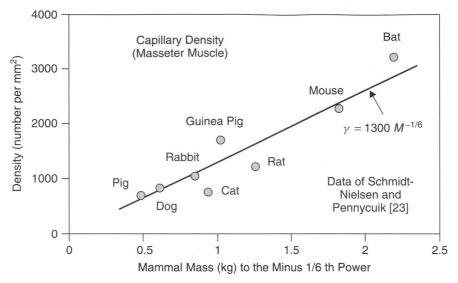

Figure 1.14.   Comparison of measurements with theory for capillary density.

This matter is readily discussed with the help of the present theory. Referring in particular to the idealized description illustrated in Figure 1.3, the circulation time for the systemic system involves the time for travel through the arterial connecting vessel, the capillary network, and the venous connecting vessel. The time of travel through each of these vessels is proportional to the length of the vessel L divided by the average velocity of the blood through it.

Considering, for example, the capillary network, this velocity is equal to the cardiac output Q_b divided by the total cross-sectional area of the network so that it is proportional to the ratio $Q_b/N_C R_C^2$. On substituting the scaling relations for the capillary vessels and the previously discussed $\frac{3}{4}$th relation for cardiac output, the velocity of the blood in the capillaries is found to be proportional to mammal mass to the power $-\frac{1}{24}$. Capillary length scales as mammal mass to the power $\frac{5}{24}$, so the travel time is thus found to be proportional to mammal mass to the power $\frac{1}{4}$. The same can be found true for the connecting vessels. Thus, the entire travel time for an element of blood through the systemic system must vary in this manner. This is also the case for the pulmonary system so that, assuming the time through the heart varies similarly, the circulation time T_B is predicted to obey the following scaling relation

$$T_B \propto M^{1/4} \tag{1.21}$$

Prosser and Brown [24] have collected measured values of circulation time for the rabbit (8 s), the dog (16 s), and the human (23 s). These may be examined in terms of the indicated scaling relation using the human ($M = 70$ kg) as reference. Assuming typical body masses for the rabbit and the dog of 2 and 20 kg, respectively, this equation provides a scaled circulation time of 9 s for the rabbit and 17 s for the dog. These findings are in good agreement with the indicated measurements of 8 and 16 s, respectively.

Vascular Form and Function of the Kidney

The kidney is the organ of the body responsible for removal of waste fluid from the blood. The vascular organization of the kidney is of special interest because it provides the means for both filtering fluid from the blood and reabsorbing the valuable portion for further use. This process is possible because of a series connection of capillary networks in the kidney, one that removes fluid from the blood and the other, that allows the useful parts to be returned to it.

The basic unit of the kidney is the *nephron*, which consists of a capillary network, referred to as the *glomerulus*, from which fluid is filtered, and a second capillary network, referred to as the *peritubular capillaries*, in which some of the fluid and valuable solutes are reabsorbed. A nephron unit is illustrated in Figure 1.15. The two kidneys of mammals contain many thousands of these units, each operating independently to produce urine, which is stored in the bladder for periodic discharge. The operation of the units is as follows. Blood flows into the glomerulus, and fluid is filtered through small pores in the capillary walls. The fluid is collected in a capsule and drained through a series of tubules to the pelvis of the kidney, where it then empties into the bladder. During this drainage,

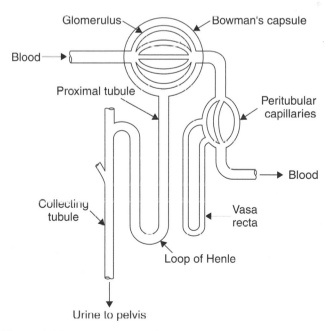

Figure 1.15.   Nephron or basic capillary unit in the kidney [1].

much of the fluid and valuable solutes are reabsorbed into the blood through the peritubular capillary vessels surrounding the tubules.

Interest here is in both form and function of the kidney for different mammals because both are connected to the scaling laws for the capillary networks. Form will involve the basic makeup of the nephron and the number present in the kidney of a mammal. Function will involve the rate of transfer of fluid from and to the capillaries and their difference, which equals the rate of urine production. The first will provide an independent confirmation of the scaling law for capillary number, and the second will indicate the scaling law for the thickness of the capillary walls. These issues have been discussed earlier [1] and will be summarized here.

With respect to form, it may be assumed tentatively that the basic construction pattern of the nephron is the same for all mammals and, in particular, that the number of capillaries in a nephron is the same for all. The product of this number and the total number of nephrons in a kidney will thus equal the number of capillaries involved in the kidney function. This number can be expected to be proportional under change of scale to the total number of capillaries in the kidney, with this number proportional, in turn, to the characteristic number of capillaries N_C for the entire body, as given by the third of relations (1.13). Thus, if N_N denotes the total number of nephrons in a kidney, it follows that this number should be proportional under change of scale to mammal mass to the power $\frac{5}{8}$:

$$N_N \propto N_C \propto M^{5/8} \tag{1.22}$$

Interestingly, Adolph [25] applied best-fit methods of analysis to data reported earlier by Kunkel [26] and found a power 0.62, which is essentially $\frac{5}{8}$ (0.625). Writing the exponent as $\frac{5}{8}$ and expressing the number of nephrons in units of 1000, the scaling equation may be written as

$$N_N = 94M^{5/8} \tag{1.23}$$

Predictions from this equation are compared with the original countings of Kunkel in Figure 1.16, where the data can be seen to follow closely the predictions of relation (1.23). Thus, as to form, the scaling law for capillary number determines the variation in number of nephrons with mammal size; or, alternatively, the scaling law for the number of nephrons provides confirmation of the scaling law for the number of capillaries.

With respect to function, the matter of interest is the rate of removal of waste fluid from the blood. The capillaries of the kidneys, like those elsewhere in the body, have numerous pores in their walls through which fluid can pass into or out of the circulating blood. The basic equation for this process resembles a diffusion process, except that the driving force is the net pressure ΔP in the capillaries arising from the blood pressure, the tissue pressure, and the osmotic pressure of the plasma proteins. In simplest terms, the equation for flow Q_f into or out of

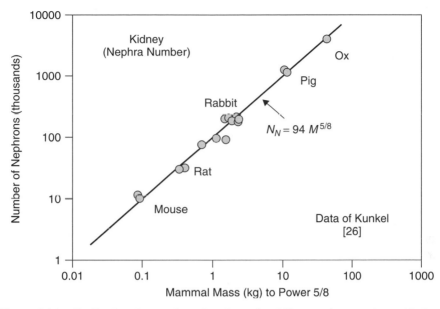

Figure 1.16. Scaling law for number of nephrons in a kidney and comparison with data.

a capillary network may be expressed like equation (1.18) for oxygen transfer, that is, as

$$Q_f \propto \Delta P \frac{R_C N_C L_C}{H_C} \tag{1.24}$$

If the net pressure is assumed to be scale-invariant and the capillary wall thickness is assumed to vary as the radius under scale change (as earlier in the case of oxygen transfer), the following relation must apply:

$$Q_f \propto N_C L_C \propto M^{5/6} \tag{1.25}$$

In the glomerular capillaries, the net pressure is outward, and water and solutes thus pass through theses capillaries and into the surrounding capsule. In contrast, in the peritubular capillaries, the net pressure is inward so that some of the glomerular flow is directed back to the blood through these capillaries. In both cases, the theoretical scaling law is that of relation (1.25). The difference in these rates is the rate of urine output Q_U whose scaling is thus also governed by the same law. Predictions from this law in equation form are shown in Figure 1.17 and compared with measurements summarized by Adolph [27]. The agreement can be seen to be very good.

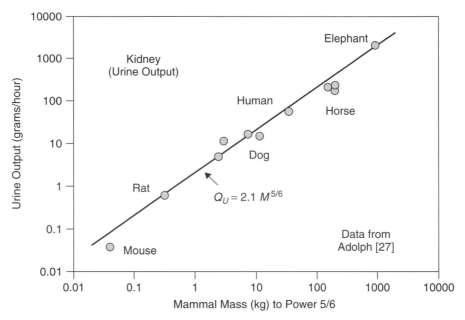

Figure 1.17. Comparison of measurements of urine output of mammals with the scaling law of relation (1.25) in best-fit equation form.

Application to Drug Therapy

The development of the scaling relation for the time history of therapeutic drug concentrations in small mammals and humans provides a practical application of the scaling laws considered here. This matter will be discussed briefly with attention restricted to the chemotherapy drug *methotrexate*, which is a well-known (nonmetabolized) drug used in the treatment of certain types of cancer. More than 37 years ago, Dedrick et al. [28] showed that data from various mammals could be consolidated reasonably well into a broad correlation by plotting the ratio of drug concentration in the blood to initial dose as a function of time since injection, when the latter was divided by mammal mass raised to the power $\frac{1}{4}$. From the previous discussion, it can now be seen that the times used in this description were expressed relative to the circulation time. Observed decreases in drug concentration in the blood with time can thus be attributed mainly to decreases associated with each cycle of blood circulation.

In considering this subject in terms of the present work, it may be anticipated that some refinement could be gained by including the capillary geometry and scaling into the correlation. This matter has been considered earlier by the writer [4]. For purposes of discussion and analysis, the drug is assumed to be injected on the systemic venous side in a relatively short period of time that is negligible in comparison with times of interest. It is also assumed that the injected drug in the blood follows the processes of filtration, absorption and diffusion that apply generally to the transfer of capillary fluid to and from the tissues and within the kidneys.

No information is available on the amount of the drug that is removed from the blood and then returned to it during a cycle of circulation. For scaling purposes, a simplified process may be assumed where the entire drug in the blood is removed and some of it returned during this period. In this case, the drug concentration at the injection site after each cycle will equal the amount returned to the blood. This assumption, if not strictly correct, would lead to a calculated concentration at the site that is less than that for the actual process. However, the same percentage difference would be expected for all mammals, so that correct scaling would still be possible.

The concentration of drug (in units of mass per volume of blood) after the first complete cycle of blood circulation in the process simplified above can now be considered. It has been shown earlier, in connection with scaling of kidney function, that the flow of fluid and dissolved substances associated with the filtering and absorption process can be considered proportional to the net capillary length $N_C L_C$ for scaling purposes. The same is also true for exchanges by diffusion. The net volume of drug reabsorbed into the blood over the time T_B for a complete cycle of circulation can be considered proportional to the product $N_C L_C T_B$. The mass of drug ΔM_D reabsorbed is proportional to this product when multiplied by the initial drug concentration M_{D0}/V_B. On dividing ΔM_D and $N_C L_C T_B$ by the blood volume, the expression for $\Delta M_D/V_B$ can thus be written as

$$\frac{\Delta M_D}{V_B} \propto \frac{M_{D0}}{V_B} \frac{N_C L_C T_B}{V_B} \quad \text{or} \quad C \propto D_0 \frac{N_C L_C T_B}{V_B} \qquad (1.26)$$

where $C\ (= \Delta M_D/V_B)$ denotes the concentration of the drug after the first cycle of circulation and $D_0 (= M_{D0}/V_B)$ denotes the initial concentration of the drug.

With additional cycles of blood circulation, a gradual reduction and redistribution of the drug in the blood will occur, as a result of transfer processes in the capillaries and net loss in the kidney, and this will further reduce the concentration at the injection site. This process depends on the number of cycles of circulation and can thus be described by a factor $f(t/T_B)$, where $f(\ )$ denotes an unspecified function. The concentration of drug in the blood is then described for scaling purposes by the following proportional relation:

$$\frac{C}{D_0} \propto \frac{N_C L_C T_B}{V_B} f\left(\frac{t}{T_B}\right) \qquad (1.27)$$

Now, if the ratio t/T_B is fixed, the ratio on the left side of this relation will be proportional to the first ratio on the right. This provides the scaling law for the relative concentration C/D_0 as a function of time. The product $N_C L_C$ varies with mammal mass to the power $\frac{5}{6}$, the total blood volume V_B varies directly with mammal mass, and the time for circulation T_B varies as mammal mass to the power $\frac{1}{4}$. The desired scaling relations may be written, for example, for the human relative to a smaller (or larger) mammal as

$$\left(\frac{C}{D_0}\right)_H = \left(\frac{M_H}{M_M}\right)^{1/12} \left(\frac{C}{D_0}\right)_M \quad \text{and} \quad t_H = \left(\frac{M_H}{M_M}\right)^{1/4} t_M \quad (1.28)$$

where the subscripts H and M denotes values for the human and mammal, respectively.

Figure 1.18 illustrates application of this scaling law in projecting measurements from the mouse (mass of 0.022 kg) to the human (mass of 70 kg) for the plasma concentration of methotrexate in the blood as a function of time. Here, concentration C is expressed in micrograms per milliliter of blood plasma and initial dose is expressed in terms of milligrams per kilogram of body weight, with 3 mg/kg used for the mouse and 10 mg/kg for the human. The basic measurements for the mouse, as used in developing the results of Figure 1.18, are due to Dedrick et al. [28], and the data for the human are due to Henderson et al. [29]. The solid curve shown in the figure is a simple "best fit" power-law expression for measured and scaled values and is included for comparison purposes.

The agreement of the scaled data from the mouse with that of the human is indeed very good. The factor $(M_H/M_M)^{1/12}$ in the first of the scaling relations (1.28) represents the effect of capillary process and is equal to 1.96. Without this factor, the predictions from the mouse would thus be reduced by a factor of ~ 2.

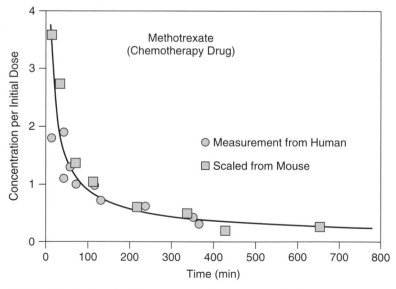

Figure 1.18. Graph showing drug concentration (μg/mL of blood plasma) per unit of initial dose (mg/kg of body weight) as a function of time for the human and as scaled from the mouse [4].

Overall, the factor can be seen to improve the predictions over what they would be otherwise.

1.10. EFFECTS OF STRENUOUS EXERCISE

The modeling of the vascular system discussed here is based on the assumption of resting or near-resting conditions. For the vascular system itself, the length and radius of the vessels of mammals do not change with exercise and there can be only one set of scaling equations for vessel dimensions. These are the relations developed and confirmed here. In contrast, the scaling relation for the number of capillary vessels is subject to change since it is well known from the original work of Krogh [30] that reserve capillaries exist in the locomotive musculature, which open and allow increased oxygen delivery during strenuous exercise.

For modest exercise, the same basic scaling relations discussed here for resting physiological functions can be expected to apply, with only the coefficients in the scaling equations changed to accommodate the physical changes involved. However, for the extreme case of strenuous exercise, this is not the case and associated empirical equations describing the scaling of heart rate, cardiac output, and oxygen consumption rate are known to be different from the scaling laws for the resting state [31–33]. No detailed modeling theory is yet available for the case of strenuous exercise, but the subject is of obvious interest in understanding the physiological adaptations required to handle this extreme condition [34].

REFERENCES

1. Dawson TH: *Engineering Design of the Cardiovascular System of Mammals*, Prentice-Hall, Englewood Cliffs, NJ, 1991.

2. Dawson TH: Similitude in the cardiovascular system of mammals, *J Exp Biol* **204**:395–407 (2001).

3. Dawson TH: Scaling laws for capillary vessels of mammals at rest and in exercise, *Proc Roy Soc Lond B* **270**:755–763 (2003).

4. Dawson TH: Modeling of vascular networks, *J Exp Biol* **208**:1687–1694 (2005).

5. Lambert R, Teissier G: Theorie de la similitude biologique (Theory of biological similitude), *Ann Physiol* **3**:212–246 (1927).

6. Kenner T: Flow and pressure in the arteries, in Fung YC, Perrone N, Anliker M, eds, *Biomechanics—Its Foundations and Objectives*, Prentice-Hall, Englewood Cliffs, NJ, 1972, pp 381–434.

7. Green HD: Circulation: Physical principles, in Glasser O, ed, *Medical Physics*, Yearbook Publishers, Chicago, 1944, Vol 1, pp 208–232.

8. Holt JP, Rhode EA, Holt WW, Kines H: Geometric similarity of aorta, venae cavae, and certain of their branches in mammals, *Am J Physiol* **241**:100–104 (1981).

9. Selkurt EE, Bullard RW: The heart as a pump: Mechanical correlates of cardiac activity, in Selkurt EE, ed, *Physiology*, Boston; Little Brown, 1971, pp 275–295.

10. Noordergraaf A: *Circulatory System Dynamics*, Academic Press, New York, 1978.
11. Holt JP, Rhode EA, Kines H: Ventricular volumes and body weight in mammals, *Am J Physiol* **215**:704–715 (1968).
12. Brody S: *Bioenergetics and Growth*, Reinhold, New York, 1945.
13. Burrows TMO, Campbell IA, Howe EJ, Young, JZ: Conduction velocity and diameter of nerve fibers of cephalopods, *J Physiol* **179**:39–40 (1965).
14. Pearson KG, Stein RB, Malhorta SK: Properties of action potentials from insect motor nerves, *J Exp Biol* **53**:299–316 (1970).
15. Clark AJ: *Comparative Physiology of the Heart*, Cambridge Univ Press, Cambridge, UK, 1927.
16. Marque V, Essen HV, Struijker-Boudier HAJ, Atkinson J, Lartoud-Idjouadiene I: Determination of aortic elastic modulus by pulse wave velocity and wall tracking in a rat model of aortic stiffness, *J Vasc Res* **38**:546–550 (2001).
17. Noordergraaf A, Li JKJ, Campbell KB: Mammalian hemodynamics: A new similarity principle, *J Theor Biol* **79**:485–489 (1979).
18. Gregg DE, Eckstein RW, Fineberg MH: Pressure pulses and blood pressure values in unanesthetized dogs, *Am J Physiol* **118**:399–410 (1937).
19. Woodbury RA, Hamilton WF: Blood pressure studies in small animals, *Am J Physiol* **119**:663–674 (1937).
20. Szymanski F: Quelques solutions exactes des equations de l'hydrodynamiquede fluide visqueux dans le cas d'un tube cylindrique (Some exact solutions to equations on hydrodynamics of viscous fluid in the case of a cylindrical tube), *J Math Pures Appl* **11**(9):67–107 (1932).
21. Gehr P, Mwangi DK, Ammann A, Malooig GMD, Taylor CR, Weibel ER: Design of the mammalian respiratory system. V. Scaling morphometric pulmonary diffusing capacity to body mass: Wild and domestic mammals, *Resp Physiol* **44**:61–86 (1981).
22. Schmidt-Nielsen K, Larimer JL: Oxygendissociation curves of mammalian blood in relation to body size, *Am J Physiol* **195**(2):424–428 (1958).
23. Schmidt-Nielsen K, Pennycuik P: Capillary density in mammals in relation to body size and oxygen consumption, *Am J Physiol* **200**(4):746–750 (1961).
24. Prosser CL, Brown FA, Jr: *Comparative Animal Physiology*, Saunders, Philadelphia, 1961.
25. Adolph EF: Quantitative relations in the physiological constitution of mammals, *Science* **109**:579–585 (1949).
26. Kunkel PA Jr: The number and size of the glomeruli in the kidney of several mammals, *Bull Johns Hopkins Hosp* **47**:285–291 (1930).
27. Adolph EF: *Physiological Regulation*, The Jaques Cattell Press, Lancaster, PA, 1943.
28. Dedrick RL, Bischoff KB, Zaharko DS: 1970. Interspecies correlation of plasma concentration history of methotrexate, *Cancer Chemotherapy Report*, US Natl Inst Health, Bethesda, MD, 1970, Vol 54, pp 95–101.
29. Henderson, ES, Adamson RH, Oliverio VT: The metabolic fate of tritiated methotrexate: Absorption and excretion in man, *Cancer Res* **25**:1018–1024 (1965).

30. Krogh A: A contribution to the physiology of capillaries, Nobel Lecture, Stockholm; also in *Nobel Lectures, Physiology or Medicine 1901–1921*, Elsevier, Amsterdam, 1967.

31. Bishop CM: Heart mass and the maximum cardiac output of birds and mammals: Implications for estimating the maximum aerobic power input of flying mammals, *Phil Trans Roy Soc Lond B* **352**:447–456 (1997).

32. Bishop CM: The maximum oxygen consumption and aerobic scope of birds and mammals: Getting to the heart of the matter, *Proc Roy Soc Lond B* **266**:2275–2281 (1999).

33. Weibel EH, Bacigalupe LD, Schmitt B, Hoppeler H: Allometric scaling of maximal metabolic rate in mammals: Muscle aerobic capacity as determinant factor, *Resp Physiol Neurobiol* **140**:115–132 (2004).

34. Weibel EH, Hoppeler H: Exercise-induced maximal metabolic rate scales with muscle aerobic capacity, *J Exp Biol* **208**:1635–1644 (2005).

CHAPTER 2

Wall Shear Stress in the Arterial System In Vivo: Assessment, Results, and Comparison with Theory

ROBERT S. RENEMAN

Department of Physiology, Cardiovascular Research Institute Maastricht, Maastricht University, The Netherlands

THEO ARTS and ARNOLD P. G. HOEKS

Department of Biophysics, Cardiovascular Research Institute Maastricht, Maastricht University, The Netherlands

Abstract. In this chapter we discuss theoretical aspects of wall shear stress (WSS) and its assessment in the arterial system in vivo, with emphasis on the results obtained. The limitations of the methods in use are discussed as well. Comparisons are made between the WSS values derived from in vivo measurements and those derived theoretically. Based on theory, WSS, an important determinant of endothelial function and gene expression, is considered to be constant along the arterial tree and similar in a particular artery across species. In vivo measurements, however, avoiding theoretical assumptions, show that these considerations are far from valid. In humans mean WSS is on the average higher in the carotid artery (1.1–1.3 Pa) than in the brachial (0.4–0.5 Pa) and femoral (0.3–0.5 Pa) arteries. Mean WSS also varies within artery bifurcations. In animals mean WSS is not constant along the arterial tree. In arterioles mean WSS varies on average between 1.8 and 4.7 Pa. Across species mean WSS in a particular artery decreases linearly with body mass, in the descending aorta from 8.8 Pa in mica to 0.5 Pa in humans. The observation that mean WSS is far from constant along the arterial tree indicates that Murray's cube law on flow-diameter relations cannot be applied to the whole arterial system. These findings also imply that in in vitro investigations no average shears stress value can be taken to study cellular adhesion and the effects on endothelial cells derived from different vascular areas or from the same artery in different species.

Vascular Hemodynamics: Bioengineering and Clinical Perspectives, Edited by Peter J. Yim
Copyright © 2008 John Wiley & Sons, Inc.

2.1. INTRODUCTION

During left ventricular ejection the forces generated by the heart expel blood into the arterial system, resulting in the exertion of hemodynamic forces on the artery wall. The endothelial cells, lining the artery wall on the luminal side, are subjected to a pressure pulse, specifically, the difference between diastolic and systolic blood pressure, and a tangential stress exerted by the flowing blood. The pressure pulse induces distension of the artery wall, resulting in mainly radial and circumferential wall strain, namely, the systolic increase in diameter and cross-sectional area relative to the end-diastolic level, respectively. The radial strain induces compression of the artery wall and, hence, a reduction of intima–media thickness (IMT) during the systolic phase of the cardiac cycle [1]. The tangential stress is known as *wall shear stress* (WSS). It can be estimated as the product of *wall shear rate* (WSR) and local blood viscosity, where WSR is defined as the radial derivative of blood flow velocity at the wall.

It has been well established that, in addition to biochemical mediators, these biomechanical forces are important determinants of endothelial cell function. For example, WSS regulates arterial diameter by modifying the production of vasoactive mediators by endothelial cells [2–5], while WSS and radial and circumferential strain are determinants of endothelial gene expression [6,7]. Endothelial genes upregulated by shear stress include transcription factors, growth factors, adhesion molecules, and enzymes; they can be transiently or more permanently upregulated [8]. Shear stress downregulates endothelin-1 [9] and thrombomodulin [10]. It is of interest to note that the type [11–13] and the level [14] of shear stress applied to endothelial cells determine whether genes are up- or downregulated. These findings indicate that endothelial cells can discriminate between subtle variations in loading conditions.

Atherosclerotic lesions preferentially originate in areas of disturbed flow associated with low shear stress [15–17]. It has been shown that genes are differently expressed in areas of undisturbed and in areas of disturbed flow [18,19] and that shear stresses ranging from 1.0 [20] to 1.5 Pa [20,21] induce atheroprotective endothelial gene expression profiles, while a shear stress of 0.4 Pa stimulates the expression of an atherogenic phenotype [21]. In an in vivo study, Cheng and colleagues [22] showed the development of atherosclerotic lesions in areas with lower shear stress is associated with the expression of proatherogenic inflammatory mediators. The plaques formed in these areas are more vulnerable, showing intraplaque hemorrhage, than those in the areas with disturbed flow. Despite the increasing evidence that fluid dynamical forces play a role in endothelial gene expression in relation to atherogenesis, further investigations are needed to rate these findings at their true values.

Biomechanical forces also affect endothelial cell structure. Endothelial cells tend to align with WSS: the higher the WSS is, the more elongated the cells will be [23–25]. These changes are associated with redistribution and rearrangement of intracellular stress fibers [24] and with their number [26]. The shape change may also depend on the type of shear stress applied [23]. By means of atomic force microscopy [24] combined with computational fluid mechanics [27], it could be demonstrated that the shear stress-induced reorganization of endothelial cells results in flattening of these cells, thereby reducing the shear stress difference along endothelial cells; this difference will be smaller, the higher the WSS is.

Especially in vivo, it is difficult to distinguish between pressure- and shear stress-induced changes in endothelial cell function, because changes in radial and circumferential strain and changes in WSS are inextricably connected and even may interact [4]. Therefore, except for the WSS-induced changes in arterial diameter, the studies on the effect of cyclic strain or shear stress on endothelial cell function and gene expression as well as on their structure are performed mostly in vitro. In these experiments the level of shear stress applied is generally calculated based on theory, assuming WSS to be constant along the arterial tree, as predicted by theory, and to be about the same in a particular artery across species. Thus, the endothelial cells are exposed to average calculated shear stress values, regardless of the area or the species from which they are derived. To rate the results obtained in the in vitro studies at its true value, it is important to be informed of the level of WSS in vivo along the arterial tree and in particular arteries across species.

The first assessments of WSS in vivo were performed in arterioles, either directly by means of pressure, length, and diameter measurements [28], or indirectly by deriving WSR [29] from velocity profiles, that is, the velocity distribution over the cross-sectional area of the vessel, using fluorescently labeled platelets [30] as velocity tracers and estimating WSS from the product of shear rate and plasma viscosity [31]. More recently fluorescently labeled nanometer particles [32,33], with a better spatial resolution are in use as velocity tracers. It was not until the 1990s that ultrasound [34,35] and magnetic resonance imaging (MRI) [36,37] techniques became available to noninvasively assess time-dependent velocity profiles in human central and peripheral arteries directly, enabling the determination of WSR in these vessels. In large arteries whole-blood viscosity is used to convert WSR to WSS. In human coronary arteries WSS has been estimated from flow velocity measurements and angiography [38] or three-dimensional (3D) arterial reconstruction from arterial images and computational fluid dynamics [39]. These developments have improved our insights into the level of WSS in arteries and its distribution along the arterial tree as well as into the differences across species. Especially in large arteries, however, the measurement of WSS remains an approximation, due mainly to the limited spatial resolution of the systems in use to determine time-dependent velocity profiles noninvasively.

In this chapter we will discuss theoretical aspects of WSS and its assessment in the arterial system in vivo, with emphasis on the results obtained. The limitations of the methods in use are discussed as well. Comparisons are made between the WSS values derived from in vivo measurements and those derived theoretically. Some biological aspects and the consequences of the WSS values obtained in vivo for in vitro experiments are considered.

2.2. THEORETICAL ASPECTS

In theoretical considerations and in in vitro and in vivo experiments on the interaction between shear stress (τ) and endothelial cell function, this tangential force is usually calculated from the measured flow q, the lumen radius r, and the viscosity of the medium or of the blood η on the basis of Poiseuille's law, according to

$$\tau = \frac{4\eta q}{\pi r^3} \tag{2.1}$$

In clinical studies shear stress is often calculated from whole-blood viscosity and shear rate (γ) as estimated from the measured blood flow velocity and internal diameter of the artery, assuming Poiseuille flow according to [40]

$$\gamma = \frac{8v_m}{d} \tag{2.2}$$

where v_m is the mean flow velocity of the blood and d the end-diastolic internal arterial diameter. Alternatively, only centerline flow velocity is determined. When peak flow velocity v_{max} is used to calculate γ, and assuming a parabolic velocity profile, the numerator in this equation becomes $4v_{max}$. Equation (2.2) has also been applied in animal experiments.

The shear stress values calculated in this way might hold in vitro, provided that the conditions meet Poiseuille's law. This law certainly does not hold in arteries in vivo, where we are dealing with non-Newtonian fluid, distensible vessels, unsteady flow, and, as a result of the branching arterial tree, the effect of too short entrance lengths. This prevents, among other things, the velocity profiles from developing to a full parabola.

The shear stress value for arteries as obtained by applying Poiseuille's law is estimated to be 1.5 Pa (15 dyn/cm^2) $\pm$ 50% [41]. On the basis of the principle of minimal work according to Murray's law [42], which states that the cube of the radius of a parent vessel is equal to the sum of the cubes of the radii of the daughter vessels, it is assumed that mean WSS is constant along the arterial tree [43,44]. Because the latter is certainly not true [45], as will also be shown in this chapter, the validity of the "cube law" for the whole arterial tree has been challenged [46]. Zamir and colleagues [46] showed that in the major branches of the aortic arch the relation between flow and diameter is governed by a "square law." They indicated, however, that the cube law may hold for more downstream vessels, implying that the exponent in the power law varies along the arterial tree. In line with this idea are the earlier observations that the exponent was found to be 2.55 in coronary arteries [47] and 3.01 in arterioles [48]. A varying exponent in the power law along the arterial tree is supported by the finding that mean blood flow velocity is not constant along the arterial tree either, either in animals (Table 2.1) [49,50] or in humans (Table 2.2) [35,51–55], which should have been the case if the square law held for the whole arterial system [46]. In the same artery, however, mean blood flow velocity is similar across species. From the allometric scaling data of Dawson [56], an average mean blood flow velocity in the ascending aorta of ~30 cm/s can be estimated for all species. This value is not too far from the values of 23 cm/s as measured in mice [49,50], and of 25 cm/s as estimated from data in anesthetized humans (Tables 2.1 and 2.2) [51].

Because shear stress critically depends on the radius of the artery [equation (2.1)], adaptation of the arterial diameter to changes in blood flow to maintain this tangential force within limits has been considered from early on [57–60]. To date, this adaptation mechanism to maintain mean WSS within limits has been well established, not only with changing flow requirements [4,5,61] but also with changes in blood viscosity [59,62,63].

In arteries the velocity profile will not develop to a full parabola as a consequence of unsteady blood flow and short entrance lengths due to branching of the arterial tree. In arterioles (diameter $<\sim100$ μm), where flow is practically steady, the velocity profile will not develop to a full parabola, either, owing to the dominating viscous forces in the center of these vessels and branching. In both arteries and arterioles the velocity profiles are flattened parabolas. Therefore, shear rate, that is, the velocity gradient relative to the arterial radius (dv/dr), is low in the center of the vessel and high toward the artery wall. The viscosity is high in the center of the vessel where red blood cells tend to stream. Towards the artery wall, where mainly blood platelets are traveling, partly in a thin layer of plasma, viscosity is low. The platelets are dispersed from the center of the vessel due to collision with the larger red blood cells [64,65]. The velocity profiles are not only flattened but often also skewed as a result of curvature effects (Figure 2.1c). As a consequence, WSR can be different near opposite walls (Figure 2.1d).

Blood flow velocity, and, hence, WSS, is high in systole and low in diastole. Because diastole comprises approximately two-thirds of the cardiac cycle, the level of WSS during diastole dominates calculated mean WSS. The increase in WSS during systole is limited because of the increase in arterial diameter,

TABLE 2.1. Peak and Mean Blood Flow Velocity (cm/s)^a in Ascending and Abdominal Aorta and Common Carotid Artery in Mice

	Peak Velocity	Mean Velocity	Reference
Ascending aorta	90 ± 11	23 ± 4	49
	86 ± 9	23 ± 3	50
Abdominal aorta	40 ± 11	13 ± 3	50
Common carotid artery			
Right	34 ± 7	10 ± 3	50
Left	31 ± 7	10 ± 3	50

^{a}Mean velocity is the temporal mean of centerline velocity. Mean values $\pm$ SD (standard deviation) are presented.

TABLE 2.2. Peak and Mean Blood Flow Velocity (cm/s)[a] in Ascending Aorta, Pulmonary Artery, Common Carotid Artery, and Brachial Artery in Young and Old Males

	Peak Velocity	Mean Velocity	Reference(s)
Ascending aorta[b]	Not determined	25	51
Pulmonary artery[b]	Not determined	22	51
Common carotid artery[c]			
Young	$87 \pm 26 - 105 \pm 21$	$30 \pm 4 - 32 \pm 5$	35,52,53
Old	$57 \pm 13 - 67 \pm 10$	$20 \pm 6 - 30 \pm 7$	35,53
Brachial artery[c]			
Young	$59 \pm 15 - 68 \pm 16$	$7.5 \pm 2.0 - 7.7 \pm 2.7$	54,55
Old	49 ± 12	8.3 ± 6.4	55

[a]Mean velocity is the temporal mean of centerline velocity. The mean values $\pm$ SD found in the various studies are presented. Ranges are given in the event that data from more than one study are available.
[b]Determined in anesthetized patients during surgery [51].
[c]Determined in presumed healthy volunteers.

especially in elastic arteries [66]; this reduces WSR by ~30% as compared with rigid arteries [67, 68] .

At branch points the laminar flow field is disturbed. This has been well established in model studies [69,70], in numerical analyses [71,72], and in in vitro [73] and in vivo [74] investigations. In bifurcations, regions with predominantly axial and unidirectional flow are observed on the side of the flow divider, while opposite to this divider flow separation occurs and areas of recirculation and flow reversal develop; flow remains laminar. WSS is high near the flow divider and low, and even negative (i.e., reversed through zero) opposite to this divider [75,76]. Both at and opposite to the flow divider the flow pattern is oscillatory in nature.

In arterioles plasma viscosity can be used to calculate WSS, because WSR can be measured close to the wall. In large arteries, however, shear rate is assessed at 250–300 μm from the wall because of the limited resolution of the ultrasound and MRI systems employed. Therefore, in these vessels the values obtained have to be considered as least estimates, because shear rate increases toward the wall. Whole-blood viscosity is used in the calculation of WSS in large arteries. In this calculation the influence of plasma viscosity can be ignored, because in arteries the plasma layer is only 3–7 μm thick [77], which is negligibly small relative to the size of the sample volumes of the ultrasound and MRI systems. Despite the underestimation of WSR, the WSS values as estimated at a distance from the artery wall will not be too different from those at the wall, because shear stress can be considered as a continuum from the center of the vessel to the wall. Although assessed in venules, extrapolation of the data on shear stress and shear rate as a function of vessel radius of Long and colleagues [32] indicates that shear stress determined at 250–300 μm from the wall, which converts to a relative radial position of 0.9 for an artery of 6 mm in diameter, will underestimate shear stress at the wall by about 10%.

2.3. DETERMINATION OF WALL SHEAR STRESS IN VIVO

In arterioles WSS can be determined in vivo directly or calculated from WSR, as derived from measured velocity profiles, and plasma viscosity. In large arteries, WSS is generally calculated from WSR, as derived from noninvasively recorded velocity profiles, and whole-blood viscosity. In the following sections we will discuss consecutively the different approaches in arterioles and in arteries.

In Arterioles

Direct Assessment. In cat mesenteric arterioles WSS was determined by means of micropressure measurements upstream and downstream, and length and diameter measurements [28]. The measurement of micropressure, however, needs a lot of skill and can be realized in only a limited number of experienced centers.

Assessment of Velocity Profiles. In arterioles optical techniques are employed, using fluorescent particles as velocity tracers. To assess velocity profiles, pairs of flashes of light are given and a short preset time interval between the two flashes provides in one video field two images of the same tracer displaced over a certain distance for the given time interval. The time interval between the two flashes is selected so that the concomitant images of the tracer show no or only negligible overlap. To construct velocity profiles, the centroids of the images of the tracers are identified and the displacement of the tracer in the preset time interval, yielding its velocity, and its relative radial position in the vessel are measured. By triggering the sequence of light flashes by the R wave of the ECG and using a preset delay, velocity profiles can be determined in systole and diastole. Originally, fluorescently labeled blood platelets were used as velocity tracers [30]. With blood platelets no data points could be obtained closer to the wall than 0.5 μm because of their physical size [78] and their orientation [79]. In more recent years nanometer particles have been used to assess the flow velocity distribution, basically using similar processing techniques [32,33]. Because of their smaller size (0.4–0.5 μm in diameter), flow velocities can be determined as close to the wall as ~0.2 μm. Originally displacement of the tracers and their position were determined by hand, a time-consuming procedure, but more recently a computerized two-dimensional correlation technique has been developed to assess displacement and position of the tracers [33].

Description of the Velocity Profile and Determination of WSR. The experimentally determined velocity profiles can be adequately described with the following equation, modified after Roevros [80]

$$v(r) = v_{\max}\left(1 - \left|a\frac{r}{R} + b\right|^{K}\right), \ a > 0 \tag{2.3}$$

where $v(r)$ is the flow velocity at the radial position r, the vertical lines denote absolute values, $v_{\max}$ is the maximal center stream flow velocity in the vessel, R is the radius of the vessel, a is a scale factor allowing a nonzero intercept of the fit with the vessel wall, b is a parameter correcting for a shift of the top of the profile away from the vessel center (note that a and b are interrelated), and K describes the degree of flattening of the profile. For a fully developed parabolic velocity profile $K = 2$; the flatter the velocity profile is, the higher K will be.

The velocity profiles as assessed with labeled blood platelets as tracers and described in this way are flattened parabolas in both systole and diastole [30,31], with K factors varying between 2.3 and 4. The ratio of the maximum and the mean velocity of the profile, which is 2 in case of a parabolic profile, was found to range from 1.39 to 1.54, which also indicates flattening of the profile. Because of asymmetry of the velocity profiles, differences in WSR at opposite walls may have to be appreciated [29]. In arterioles the velocity profile of fluorescently labeled red blood cells is similar to that of blood platelets, but most of the red blood cells are traveling at streamlines with higher velocities (see section on theoretical aspects), that is, more toward the center of the vessel [30,31].

By describing the velocity profiles as recorded by the best fit through the measuring points with the use of equation (2.3), and a linear extrapolation from the point closest to the wall where velocity can be measured (transition point) to zero flow at the wall, a least estimate of WSR can be determined by means of the following equation [29]

$$\mathrm{WSR} = \frac{2v(x)}{D(1 - |x|)} \tag{2.4}$$

where $v(x)$ is the velocity at x, which is the relative radial position of the transition point, and D is the vessel diameter. This equation holds for x close to 1.

The WSR values expected in the case of a parabolic velocity distribution (WSR_P), but with the same volume flow in the arteriole can be derived with the following equation:

$$\mathrm{WSR}_P = \frac{4v_{\max}}{D} = \frac{8v_{\mathrm{mean}}}{D} \tag{2.5}$$

The extent to which the WSR values as derived from the actual velocity profiles in vivo are higher than those calculated on the basis of a parabolic velocity distribution for the same volume flow is given by the following relation:

$$\frac{\mathrm{WSR}}{\mathrm{WSR}_P} = \frac{0.25v(x)}{(1 - |x|)v_{\mathrm{mean}}} \tag{2.6}$$

In Large Arteries

Recording of Velocity Profiles by Means of Ultrasound. Initially the velocity distribution in large arteries was assessed by means of multigate pulsed Doppler systems [74,81]. With these systems interesting information could be obtained about velocity patterns and artery wall dynamics in, for example, the carotid artery bifurcation [74]. Although this Doppler technique has been improved substantially, notably the inherent determination of the Doppler observation angle and the circumvention of Doppler highpass filtering [82], it has several important limitations, including a limited spatial resolution. In the 1990s ultrasound techniques became available to more accurately determine velocity profiles in large arteries [34,35].

To accurately determine velocity profiles in vivo, precise measurement of low blood flow velocities close to the vessel wall is required. This can be achieved only when the high-amplitude low-frequency signals reflected by the artery wall are adequately suppressed without loosing the low blood flow velocity information near the wall. This can be accomplished by considering the time-dependent aspects of the reflections and using a bandstop filter that adapts its rejection range to the mean frequency of the reflections from the artery wall [83]. In this adaptive filtering technique these reflections are suppressed by shifting the temporal frequency distribution toward zero frequency, with the shift given by the estimated mean frequency of the reflected signal. Subsequently, the reflections, then centered around zero frequency, are selectively suppressed by a highpass filter with a low cutoff frequency.

For the assessment of WSR a conventional 2D imager (Mark 9 HDI, ATL, Bothell, Washington, USA) with a C9-5 curved array is combined with dedicated signal processing to measure the blood flow velocity distribution along a selected line of observation across the center of the artery. After localization of the region of interest, the system is switched to a single line of observation (motion mode; M-mode) with short emission bursts (2 periods) to retain spatial resolution and a high pulse repetition frequency to facilitate blood flow velocity detection. The radiofrequency (RF) signals are captured at a sample rate of 20 MHz and stored on a computer for offline analysis. After automatic identification of the wall–lumen interfaces, cursors, representing sample volumes, are positioned on the reflections from the anterior and posterior walls [84]. The time-dependent blood flow velocity distribution is obtained with the use of a modeled cross-correlation function applied to the RF data between the cursors after elimination of the wall signals with the adaptive highpass filter. Calculation of mean blood flow velocity for all RF segments provides a time-dependent velocity profile (Figures 2.1a and 2.1c). The length of the RF segments is selected according to the actual bandwidth of the RF signals (2.5 MHz) and corresponds to 300 μm in depth; the segments are spaced at 150-μm intervals (50% overlap). For further details regarding this ultrasound technique the reader is referred to previous publications of our group [34,35,83].

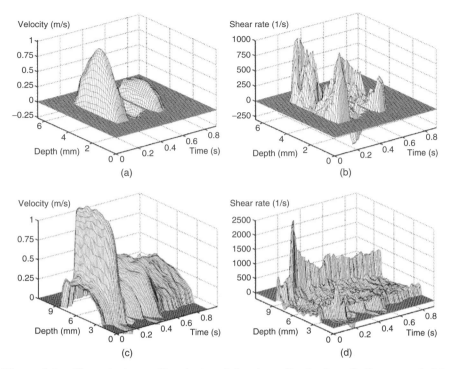

Figure 2.1. The velocity profiles (a,c) and the shear distributions (b,d) as recorded in the brachial (a,b) and the common carotid (c,d) artery of a presumed healthy volunteer. (After Reneman et al. [45], with permission.)

Recording of Velocity Profiles by Means of MRI.

MRI also allows the non-invasive recording of velocity profiles in humans [36,37,85]. In this technique, flow velocity distribution in a cross-section of an artery can be visualized as a function of time by placing the artery of interest in a strong static magnetic field ($\sim 1-2$ T) and modulating the static field with high-frequency magnetic pulses. In this way a small fraction of the hydrogen atoms (protons) is brought into resonance (~ 150 MHz). After the addition of a gradient field to the static magnetic field, the phase shift of the resonating atoms becomes position-dependent. If there is no flow-related motion, a linear gradient in phase shift is generated. However, if an atom travels along the direction of the magnetic gradient, the phase shift of the position where the atom was excited is brought to a new position in the image. Thus, proportionally with blood flow velocity, an additional phase shift is generated. The related deviation in phase shift can be detected by means of the velocity encoded phase contrast method. In this method two images are acquired: a reference scan and a velocity-encoded sensitized scan. The phase shift between both images is denoted as the phase contrast image. A velocity map is obtained by multiplication of the observed phase shift with a calibration factor, defined as the aliasing velocity (AVL) divided by 180°.

In MRI flow velocity mapping, the settings have to be optimized for a given experimental condition, because the sensitivity to blood flow velocity increases with decreasing AVL. If blood flow velocity exceeds AVL, the phase shift exceeds the interval of ±180° and it will be falsely interpreted as a phase shift within this interval. This artifact, known as *aliasing*, requires that AVL be at least as high as the maximum blood flow velocity to be measured. In finding the optimum value for AVL, one should realize that AVL cannot be elevated too much, because of the tradeoff with a reduced signal-to-noise ratio in the phase assessment, resulting in enhancement of noise in the velocity signal.

The spatial resolution of MRI in the assessment of blood flow velocity is determined by the pixel size in the imaging plane and by slice thickness in the direction perpendicular to the imaging plane. In humans a convenient pixel size is 0.3–1.0 mm. For reliable blood flow velocity measurements, the information of 4 pixels has to be collected, limiting the true spatial resolution of velocity assessment to about 1–2 mm. Slice thickness is generally around 4–8 mm. Diminution of slice thickness would enhance the resolution in depth, but at the cost of signal power. Misalignment of the artery with the perpendicular direction of the image further deteriorates spatial resolution. Fortunately, the latter effect is of limited importance in most applications.

The temporal resolution of blood flow velocity mapping is determined by three factors: (1) the number of cardiac beats for averaging, (2) the measurement interval, and (3) the acquisition duration within the cardiac cycle. Averaging over several heartbeats requires good periodicity of the flow velocity signal, which may be improved by breath holding during the MRI measurement. By averaging over 2–16 heartbeats, flow velocity profiles during the cardiac cycle can be obtained with a repetition time of 25 ms [37]. In complicated flow fields as in turbulence, such as, near valves or stenoses, the periodicity of the flow velocity signal becomes a problem, hampering reliable multiple-beat averaging. The latter is also difficult during such interventions as reactive hyperemia, when the flow velocity signal becomes noisy because of unsteadiness. For further details regarding flow velocity imaging in arteries by means of MRI, the reader is referred to a review by Gatehouse and colleagues [86].

Following the approach as described above, in the common carotid artery flow velocity maps over the cross section of an artery can be obtained with a spatial resolution generally of 1–2 mm and a temporal resolution of 25 ms, while averaging over 10 heartbeats [37,87]. Taking special precautions, spatial resolutions, similar to those in ultrasound systems (i.e., ~300 μm), can be obtained [88]. Since the flow velocity map provides simultaneously flow velocities at various distances from the artery wall, the velocity profile and, hence, shear rate can be accurately determined in the field of observation.

Description of the Velocity Profile and Derivation of WSR. Using similar approaches as in arterioles, it could be demonstrated that the velocity profile is also substantially flattened in the common carotid artery (Figure 2.1c) with a K factor of 4 in systole [54]. Also in the femoral artery the velocity profile is flattened in systole [85]. In the brachial artery, however, in systole the velocity profile was found to be close to parabolic [85] (Figure 2.1a) with a K factor of 2.1 [54]. This difference can likely be explained by the greater relative distension of the common carotid artery [54,68] and a relatively longer entrance length in the brachial artery. The smaller diameter of the brachial artery, relative to the resolution of the ultrasound system, may also contribute to the more parabolic profile measured in this vessel.

In the ultrasound systems presently in use, the shear rate distribution in an artery is derived from the radial derivative of the velocity profile at each site and each time instant (Figures 2.1b and 2.1d). Because blood flow velocities cannot be determined at the wall, the maximum value of the radial derivative of the velocity profile is considered as the estimate of instantaneous WSR [34,35]. From the shear distribution mean WSR, the time-averaged shear rate over one cardiac cycle, peak WSR, the value at peak systole, and the maximal cyclic change in WSR within a cardiac cycle can be determined.

In MRI, generally a quadratic curve is fitted through the velocity data points as a function of the distance to the wall in a certain distance range (e.g., 0.3–1.3 mm), and the slope at the site where the extrapolated curve crosses zero is considered to represent a measure of WSR [37,85].

When WSR values in a particular artery are of interest, the values as recorded near the anterior and the posterior wall are usually averaged to minimize the influence of skewness of the velocity profile and of secondary flows. In studies on the relation between WSR and artery wall structure, the shear rate values as assessed locally are used.

Accuracy and Limitations. When assessed with ultrasound, in the common carotid artery the intrasubject intersession variability on different days varies between 13 and 15% for peak WSR and between 10 and 12% for mean WSR (coefficient of variation), while the intersubject variability varies between 16% and 19% for peak WSR and between 11% and 17% for mean WSR [52]. In the femoral artery [89] and the brachial artery [55], these values are somewhat higher. Therefore, measurements over $\sim$16 cardiac cycles are considered to obtain reliable values of peak and mean WSR, that is, a methodological variation about 4 times lower than the biological one.

As a consequence of the limited spatial resolution, the WSR values obtained with ultrasound and MRI are underestimations. Moreover, with these techniques WSR can be determined reliably only in relatively straight arteries.

Calculation of WSS. In arterioles plasma viscosity is used to calculate WSS. Plasma viscosity can be accurately determined in vitro by means of commercially available glass capillary viscometry systems.

In large arteries whole-blood viscosity is used to calculate WSS. Whole-blood viscosity (WBV) can be determined by using the approximation proposed by

TABLE 2.3. Units of Parameters Described in This Chapter

Description	Units
Velocity	
Microcirculation	mm/s
Large arteries	cm/s
WSR	s^{-1}
WSS	Pa[a]
Viscosity	mPa·s[b]
Distension (Δd)	mm
Wall strain ($\Delta d/d$)	Dimensionless
Distensibility	MPa^{-1}
Compliance	mm^2/MPa
Intima–media thickness (IMT)	mm

[a] 1 Pa $= 10$ dyn/cm^2.
[b] 1 mPa·s $= 0.01$ dyn·s/cm^2.

Source: After Reneman et al. [45], with permission.

Weaver et al. [90].

$$\log(\text{WBV}) = \log(\eta_0) + (0.03 - 0.0076\log(\gamma))\text{Ht} \qquad (2.7)$$

where η_0 is plasma viscosity, γ is WSR, and Ht is hematocrit.

Under the shear rate conditions found in vivo (i.e., $100\ s^{-1} < \gamma < 1000\ s^{-1}$ in large arteries), the effect of changes in plasma viscosity on whole-blood viscosity, as calculated by means of equation (2.7), is negligible [54], leaving shear rate and hematocrit as the relevant parameters. Alternatively, whole-blood viscosity can be determined in vitro by means of a cone plate viscometer. A limitation of this method is that viscosity cannot be determined at appropriate and sufficiently high shear rates in all subjects studied [91], resulting in too high estimates of whole-blood viscosity.

The units of the parameters, as described in this chapter and commonly used, are presented in Table 2.3 .

2.4. WALL SHEAR RATE DATA OBTAINED IN VIVO

In Humans

Mean and peak WSR are higher in elastic than in muscular conduit arteries. In the common carotid artery, mean and peak WSR varies in the different study populations between 310 and 414 s^{-1} and between 900 and 1,338 s^{-1}, respectively [45]. In the brachial artery mean and peak WSR was found to be on the average 95 and 770 s^{-1}, respectively [45]. These data derived from velocity profiles recorded by means of ultrasound compare favorably with those derived from velocity profiles recorded by means of MRI [88]. In the superficial femoral artery mean and peak WSR was found to be on the average 130 and 736 s^{-1}, respectively [88]. The lower WSR in the brachial than in the common carotid artery implies that whole-blood viscosity is higher [equation (2.7)] in the former artery, which is indeed the case, ranging from 4.8 to 5.0 mPa·s in the brachial artery and from 2.9 to 3.2 mPa·s in the common carotid artery [45].

In Animals

In mesenteric arterioles of the rabbit, mean WSR was found to be on the average 1,700 s^{-1}, ranging from 472 to 4,712 s^{-1} [29,31]. This substantial spread in WSR in these arterioles can be explained by the variations in blood flow velocity, peak flow velocity varying between 1.3 and 14.4 mm/s, and the absence of any regulatory property of these arterioles: their diameters do not change in response to changes in blood flow velocity [92]. To the best of our knowledge, no data are available on WSR in large arteries in experimental animals.

2.5. WALL SHEAR STRESS DATA OBTAINED IN VIVO

In Humans

An important observation made in human arteries is that mean WSS is far from constant along the arterial tree [45] as predicted by theory. In the common carotid artery of presumed healthy volunteers, Reneman et al. [45] reported mean WSS to be within the limits of the theoretically predicted value of 1.5 Pa±50%, varying on the average between 1.1 and 1.4 Pa in the different study populations (Table 2.4) [52–55]. In muscular conduit arteries of presumed healthy volunteers, however, mean WSS is substantially lower, reaching average values in the common femoral artery, the superficial femoral artery, and the brachial artery varying between 0.3 and 0.4 Pa, around 0.5 Pa and between 0.4 and 0.5 Pa, respectively, in the different populations studied (Table 2.4) [45]. The WSS values presented are based on the average of the shear rate values recorded near the anterior and posterior walls. Although large arteries adapt their diameters to changes in blood flow velocity, maintaining mean WSS within limits, interindividual variations in this parameter have to be appreciated [45].

The lower mean WSS in these conduit arteries at rest can be explained by the high peripheral resistance in these vessels, reducing mean volume flow and inducing reflections. In the femoral artery, adaptation of the peripheral resistance during vasodilatation results in mean WSS values close to those in the common carotid artery [93]. This indicates that mean WSS is regulated locally and strongly depends on the characteristics of the peripheral circulation. In case of matching of the characteristic and input impedances, as in the brain circulation, reflections are practically absent, while they are dominant in the arm and leg circulations where these impedances are not well matched at rest.

In normal coronary arteries mean shear stress, as derived from intracoronary velocity measurements and coronary angiography, using a modification of equation (2.1), was found to average 0.68 Pa (range 0.33–1.24 Pa) [38]. These values, however, may be underestimations.

Peak WSS is not significantly different between elastic and muscular arteries and varies between 2.5 and 4.3 Pa in the common carotid artery, between 3.4 and 4.0 Pa in the femoral arteries, and between 2.7 and 3.9 Pa in the brachial artery in the different populations studied (Table 2.4) [45].

In humans, mean WSS also varies within artery bifurcations. In the femoral artery bifurcation mean WSS was found to be significantly lower in the common than in the superficial femoral artery; the former artery seeing reflections from both the superficial and the deep femoral artery, resulting in a longer-lasting negative flow during diastole in the common femoral artery [93]. Peak and maximal

TABLE 2.4. Peak and Mean Wall Shear Stress (Pa)^a in Common Carotid, Common Femoral, Superficial Femoral, and Brachial Arteries in Presumed Healthy Young and Old Males and Females as Determined by Ultrasound

	Peak WSS	Mean WSS	Reference(s)
Common carotid artery			
Males			
Young	$3.4 \pm 0.8 - 4.3 \pm 1.3$	$1.2 \pm 0.2 - 1.4 \pm 0.2$	52,53,54
Old	2.6 ± 0.3	1.2 ± 0.2	
Females			
Young	$2.9 \pm 0.5 - 3.3 \pm 0.7$	$1.1 \pm 0.2 - 1.2 \pm 0.2$	52,53
Old	2.5 ± 0.4	1.1 ± 0.2	53
Common femoral artery			
Males			
Young	4.0 ± 1.3	0.4 ± 0.3	93
Old	3.8 ± 1.2	0.3 ± 0.1	93
Superficial femoral artery			
Males			
Young	3.4 ± 0.6	0.5 ± 0.1	93
Old	4.0 ± 0.1	0.5 ± 0.2	93
Brachial artery			
Males			
Young	$3.3 \pm 0.7 - 3.9 \pm 0.8$	$0.5 \pm 0.1 - 0.5 \pm 0.2$	54,55
Old	3.3 ± 0.5	0.5 ± 0.3	55
Females			
Young	2.7 ± 0.6	0.4 ± 0.2	55
Old	2.9 ± 1.2	0.5 ± 0.2	55

^{a}The mean values $\pm$ SD found in the various studies are presented. Ranges are given in the event that data from more than one study are available.

cyclic WSS are not significantly different between the common and superficial femoral arteries [93]. Similarly, in the common carotid artery mean WSR, and, hence mean WSS, was found to be lower near the bifurcation than ∼3 cm more proximally, probably because at the latter site the influence of reflections from the external carotid artery has greatly disappeared [94]. It is of interest to note that in both the femoral [89] and the carotid artery bifurcation [94] IMT at the posterior wall is greater in the areas with lower WSS. Also, in normal coronary arteries, wall thickness and shear stress correlate negatively [39].

No significant differences in mean WSS could be detected between men and women, either in the common carotid artery [53] or in the brachial artery [55]. Only peak WSS in the common carotid artery was found to be higher in males than in females [53].

In Animals

Most of the shear stress data obtained in anaesthetized animals are calculated from blood flow, as recorded electromagnetically or by means of ultrasound, diameter, and blood viscosity, using equation (2.1). These shear stress data are likely to be underestimations and do not necessarily represent the shear stress value near the artery wall. Despite these limitations and the substantial spread in the data, for example, varying in the common carotid artery between 1.6 and 4.6 Pa in dogs and between 1.2 and 8.4 Pa in mice, the data collected by Cheng and colleagues [95] show that mean shear stress is not constant along the arterial tree in animals, either. The error made in estimating the internal diameter of the artery is likely responsible for this spread in the data.

Across species mean shear stress decreases with an increase in estimated internal artery diameter. In their allometric scaling study, Greve and colleagues [96] showed that across species, including mice, rats, dogs, and humans, mean WSS in the infrarenal aorta decreases linearly with body mass on a log/log scale. In this part of the aorta mean WSS was estimated to be about 0.5 Pa in men, about 7 Pa in rat and about 8.8 Pa in mice. Thus, the lesson to be learned is that in a particular artery mean shear stress will be higher, the smaller the animal is. In the common carotid artery mean shear stress varies on the average from about 1.2 Pa in humans to on the average about 7.0 Pa in mice [95].

In mesenteric rabbit arterioles the average WSS as calculated from measured shear rate and a plasma viscosity of 1.07 mPa·s, a value commonly found in rabbits, was found to be 1.82 Pa with a range of 0.51–5.0 Pa [31]. These values are significantly lower than the values of 4.71 ± 2.34 Pa [mean ± standard deviation (SD)] as found by direct measurement in arterioles of the cat mesentery [28]. In the latter study, however, the reduced velocity, defined as mean flow velocity divided by vessel diameter, was significantly higher than those found in the rabbit mesentery (on the average 208 vs. 87 s^{-1}). Considering the nonregulatory properties of mesenteric arteries [92], differences in reduced velocity may explain the differences in WSS values as found in these studies.

2.6. COMPARISON BETWEEN THEORY AND DATA OBTAINED IN VIVO

According to theory, mean WSS in arteries should be 1.5 Pa ± 50% and constant along the arterial tree. As shown, however, in vivo at rest mean WSS varies substantially along the human arterial tree and is comparable to the theoretically predicted value only in the human common carotid artery; it is substantially lower in the femoral and brachial arteries (Table 2.4) [45]. In animals shear stress also varies along the arterial tree and is substantially higher than the theoretically predicted value in all arteries studied [95]. The smaller the animal is, the higher WSS will be in a particular artery [96].

Using equation (2.6), it was found that in arterioles WSR is on the average 2.1 times lower (range 1.5–3.9 times) when derived from a parabolic than from an actually measured velocity profile [29]. This underestimation of WSR, and, hence, of WSS, is even more pronounced when nanometer particles [32], allowing flow velocity assessments closer to the wall, rather than platelets [30] are used as velocity tracers.

As in arterioles, in large arteries the WSR and WSS values calculated on the basis of a parabolic velocity profile are substantially lower than those derived from the actually measured profiles. In the common carotid artery mean WSR is underestimated by a factor of 2–3 [35,54] and mean WSS by a factor of 2 [54], when assuming a parabolic velocity profile. In the brachial artery the underestimation of mean WSR and mean WSS is less pronounced [54], likely due to the more parabolic shape of the velocity profile in this artery (Figure 2.1a). The underestimation, when assuming a parabolic velocity profile, is also illustrated by the low mean and peak shear rate values (260 and 640 s^{-1}, respectively) as obtained by Gnasso and colleagues [91] in the common carotid artery and the low peak shear stress values as found by Silber and colleagues [85] in the brachial and femoral arteries (averaging 1.2 and 1.3 Pa, respectively). Erroneously, "correct" WSS values can be obtained when assuming a parabolic velocity profile |91|. When underestimating WSR and using these excessively low values to assess whole-blood viscosity, excessively high viscosity values will be found [see equation (2.7)], resulting in calculated WSS values close to the values derived from the in vivo recorded velocity profiles.

In line with theory are the in vivo findings that mean WSS is regulated via diameter adaptation; the arterial diameter adapts to forced changes in volume flow, thereby restoring mean WSS toward its baseline value. This adaptation occurs not only in large arteries [59,97], but also in arterioles [61]. Diameter adaptation to maintain mean WSS within limits also holds for changes in blood viscosity [62,63]. In the latter adaptation the reciprocal change in WSR also plays a role. Also in embryogenesis, mean shear rate, and, hence, mean shear stress, is rather constant along the arterial tree in the developing arterial system down to a diameter of ~40 μm [98], indicating that during development arterial segments adapt their lumen size to the flow to be carried.

Mean WSS is maintained at its basic level not only when hemodynamics change acutely, but also when hemodynamic changes occur more chronically as in aging. Only in the elastic common carotid artery mean WSS decreases slightly with increasing age, reaching values still within the range of optimal values as predicted by theory [53]. Mean WSS does not change with age in conduit arteries, as the brachial [55] and the common and superficial femoral arteries [93]. The decrease in mean WSS in the common carotid artery with increasing age may be explained by the increase in arterial diameter to reduce the loss of arterial compliance, namely, the absolute change in arterial cross-sectional area for a given increase in pulse pressure, at older age [66,99], a good example of interaction between two parameters to be regulated.

2.7. CONCLUSIONS

The lessons learned from the in vivo measurements are that mean WSS is neither constant along the arterial tree in a particular species (Table 2.4), nor the same in a particular artery across species. In humans, the values found in vivo may deviate substantially from the theoretically predicted value of 1.5 Pa ± 50% [41] 1984). Only in the human common carotid artery is the mean WSS within the limits of the value predicted by theory [45]. In the human femoral and brachial arteries mean WSS is substantially lower, varying on the average between 0.3 and 0.5 Pa and between 0.4 and 0.5 Pa, respectively, in the populations studied [45]. The lower mean WSS in the latter arteries can be explained by the high peripheral resistance in these arteries, reducing volume flow and causing reflections, thereby reducing mean WSS. This observation and the finding that during vasodilatation mean WSS is similar in these conductive arteries and in the common carotid artery indicate that the level of mean WSS is regulated locally [93]. The low mean WSS in the femoral and brachial arteries at rest is logical from a physiological perspective; it allows for an increase in mean WSS during exercise without reaching high levels that could be damaging to endothelial cells. Within artery bifurcations differences in mean WSS have to be appreciated, too—differences that do have structural consequences [89,94]. Despite the substantial spread in the data and the possible underestimations, it can be concluded that also in species such as dog, rat, and mouse, WSS is not constant along the arterial tree, either [95]. Across species WSS in a particular artery is substantially different and will be higher, the smaller the animal is [96]. For example, in the common carotid artery WSS is about 1.5 Pa in humans and around 7 Pa in mice. The arteriolar WSS values presented, about 2.0–5.0 Pa on the average, are determined in nonregulating mesenteric arterioles and are not necessarily representative of the values in regulating arterioles as in skeletal muscle. In line with theory are the in vivo observations that WSS is a regulated parameter.

Using nanometer particles, shear rate can be determined close to the wall in arterioles, but in large arteries WSR is determined at a distance from the wall and, hence, the values obtained in arteries are least estimates because shear rate increases toward the wall. Despite this underestimation, WSS as estimated at a distance from the wall will not differ much from the value at the wall, because shear stress can be considered as a continuum from the center of the vessel to the wall. The underestimation of shear stress at the wall will be approximately 10%. Calculation of WSR on the basis of a parabolic velocity profile leads to an additional underestimation (by a factor of ~2), because the in vivo recorded velocity profiles are generally flattened parabolas, in both arterioles and large arteries. Such an underestimation does affect not only calculated WSS, but also calculated or determined whole-blood viscosity, which strongly depends on shear rate.

The finding that WSS is not constant along the arterial tree implies that the "cube law" for flow–diameter relations [42] does not hold for the whole arterial tree, and indeed in the major branches of the aortic arch, the relation between flow and diameter was found to be governed by a "square law" [46]. A square law cannot be applied to the whole arterial tree, either, because mean blood flow velocity also varies along this tree. At the present state of the art, it may be concluded that the power-law exponent varies along the arterial tree, possibly from 2 in larger arteries to 3 in smaller ones.

WSS is an important determinant of endothelial cell function [2–5] and gene expression [6,7,9,10] by these cells as well as of their structure [23–26]. Most of the studies on the interaction between shear stress and endothelial cell gene expression and structure have been performed in vitro, exposing these cells to a general shear stress value, often derived from theory. From the in vivo findings, it may be concluded that no general value of shear stress can be taken for endothelial cells derived from different vascular areas or from the same artery in different species; the cells have to be studied under the shear stress conditions to which they are exposed in real life. This is especially important, because genes are expressed differently, depending on the level [14] and the type [11–13] of shear stress that they are exposed to.

The transduction of biomechanical forces into biomolecular responses is called mechanotransduction, This intriguing mechanism has been subject of investigation in previous decades [6,100–104]. In mechanotransduction the mechanical forces acting on the luminal side of the endothelial cells, thereby deforming these cells, are transmitted through the cytoskeleton to other sites in the cell [105]. These forces are especially sensed at the basal adhesion points, where the endothelial cell is attached to the extracellular matrix, cell junctions, and the nuclear membrane, leading to redistribution of forces throughout endothelial cells [100] and to acute and more delayed processes in these cells [6,100]. In the cellular membrane, that may respond to the induced deformation directly, shear stress activates, among others, stretch-sensitive ion channels, phospholipids, and integrins [6,100]. The biomechanical forces transferred to the nuclei can be sensed by the shear stress-sensitive sequences in the promoter of a variety of genes [7,101]. There are indications that the glycocalyx, a mesh of sulfated proteoglycans, glycoproteins, and associated glycosamineglycans of a few hundred nanometers to a micrometer in thickness covering the endothelial cells [106–108], senses the fluid dynamic forces that the cells are exposed to [104,108–110]. It has been proposed that the core proteins in the glycocalyx are especially suited to act as a transducer of fluid shearing stresses [111] and that the glycocalyx transfers the fluid dynamic forces into tensile stress [107]. These findings indicate that the glycocalyx may act as the first step in the process of mechanotransduction.

It should be realized that the ultrasound and MRI techniques presently available to noninvasively assess WSR, and, hence, WSS, in vivo do have their limitations. Not only is the spatial resolution of the systems limited, but at the present state of the art WSR can reliably be determined only in relatively straight arteries. This is a serious limitation, because information about the level of WSS and its direction in artery bifurcations, especially opposite to the flow divider, is of utmost importance when studying the role of WSS in atherogenesis. In our institute we are working on a different approach to the assessment of velocity profiles, using multiple lines of observation (multiple M-line technique), which may allow assessment of the shear rate distribution in the carotid artery bulb.

REFERENCES

1. Meinders JM, Kornet L, Hoeks AP: Assessment of spatial inhomogeneities in intima media thickness along an arterial segment using its dynamic behavior, *Am J Physiol Heart Circ Physiol* **285**:H384–H391 (2003).
2. Furchgott RF: Role of endothelium in responses of vascular smooth muscle, *Circ Res* **53**:557–573 (1983).
3. Pohl U, Holtz J, Busse R, Bassenge E: Crucial role of endothelium in the vasodilator response to increased flow in vivo, *Hypertension* **8**:37–44 (1986).
4. Busse R, Fleming I: Pulsatile stretch and shear stress; physical stimuli determining the production of endothelium-derived relaxing factors, *J Vasc Res* **35**:73–84 (1998).
5. Koller A, Huang A: Development of nitric oxide and prostaglandin mediation of shear stress-induced arteriolar dilation with aging and hypertension, *Hypertension* **34**:1073–1079 (1999).
6. Davies PF, Tripathi SC: Mechanical stress mechanisms and the cell. An endothelial paradigm. *Circ Res* **72**:239–245 (1993).
7. Gimbrone MA, Topper JN: Biology of the vessel wall, in *Molecular Basis of Cardiovascular Disease*, Chien KR, eds, Saunders, Philadelphia, 1999, pp 331–348.
8. Topper JN, Gimbrone MA: Blood flow and vascular gene expression: Fluid shear stress as a modulator of endothelial phenotype, *Mol Med Today* **5**:40–46 (1999).
9. Malek AM, Greene AL, Izumo S: Regulation of endothelin 1 gene by fluid shear stress is transcriptionally mediated and independent of protein kinase C and cAMP, *Proc Natl Acad Sci USA* **90**:5999–6003 (1993).
10. Malek AM, Izumo S: Molecular aspects of signal transduction of shear stress in the endothelial cell, *J Hypertens* **12**:989–999 (1994).
11. Ando J, Tsuboi H, Korenaga R, Takada Y, Toyama-Sorimachi N, Miyasaka M, Kamiya A: Shear stress inhibits adhesion of cultured mouse endothelial cells to lymphocytes by downregulating VCAM-1 expression, *Am J Physiol* **267**:C679–C687 (1994).
12. Chappell DC, Varner SE, Nerem RM, Medford RM, Alexander RW: Oscillatory shear stress stimulates adhesion molecule expression in cultured human endothelium, *Circ Res* **82**:532–539 (1998).

13. De Keulenaer GW, Chappell DC, Ishizaka N, Nerem RM, Alexander RW, Griendling KK: Oscillatory and steady laminar shear stress differentially affect human endothelial redox state: Role of a superoxide-producing NADH oxidase, *Circ Res* **82**:1094–1101 (1998).

14. Walpola PL, Gotlieb AI, Cybulsky MI, Langille BL: Expression of ICAM-1 and VCAM-1 and monocyte adherence in arteries exposed to altered shear stress, *Arterioscler Thromb Vasc Biol* **15**:2–10 (1995).

15. Zarins CK, Giddens DP, Bharadvaj BK, Sottiura VS, Mabon RF, Glagov S: Carotid bifurcation atherosclerosis. Quantitative correlation of plaque localization with flow velocity profiles and wall shear stress, *Circ Res* **53**:502–514 (1983).

16. Ku DN, Giddens DP, Phillips DJ, Strandness DE: Hemodynamics in the normal human carotid bifurcation: In vitro and in vivo studies, *Ultrasound Med Biol* **11**:13–26 (1985).

17. Friedman MH, Deters OJ, Bargeron CB, Hutchins GM, Mark FF: Shear-dependent thickening of the human arterial intima, *Atherosclerosis* **60**:161 171 (1986).

18. Davies PF, Shi C, Depaola N, Helmke BP, Polacek DC: Hemodynamics and the focal origin of atherosclerosis: A spatial approach to endothelial structure, gene expression, and function, *Ann NY Acad Sci* **947**:7–16; discussion 16–17 (2001).

19. Passerini AG, Polacek DC, Shi C, Francesco NM, Manduchi E, Grant GR, Pritchard WF, Powell S, Chang GY, Stoeckert CJ Jr, Davies PF: Coexisting proinflammatory and antioxidative endothelial transcription profiles in a disturbed flow region of the adult porcine aorta, *Proc Natl Acad Sci USA* **101**:2482–2487 (2004).

20. Topper JN, Cai J, Falb D, Gimbrone MA Jr: Identification of vascular endothelial genes differentially responsive to fluid mechanical stimuli: Cyclooxygenase-2, manganese superoxide dismutase, and endothelial cell nitric oxide synthase are selectively up-regulated by steady laminar shear stress, *Proc Natl Acad Sci USA* **93**:10417–10422 (1996).

21. Malek AM, Alper SL, Izumo S: Hemodynamic shear stress and its role in atherosclerosis, *JAMA* **282**:2035–2042 (1999).

22. Cheng C, Tempel D, van Haperen R, van der Baan A, Grosveld F, Daemen MJ, Krams R, de Crom R: Atherosclerotic lesion size and vulnerability are determined by patterns of fluid shear stress, *Circulation* **113**:2744–2753 (2006).

23. Helmlinger G, Geiger RV, Schreck S, Nerem RM: Effects of pulsatile flow on cultured vascular endothelial cell morphology, *J Biomech Eng* **113**:123–131 (1991).

24. Barbee KA, Davies PF, Lal R: Shear stress-induced reorganization of the surface topography of living endothelial cells imaged by atomic force microscopy, *Circ Res* **74**:163–171 (1994).

25. Sato M, Ohshima N: Flow-induced changes in shape and cytoskeletal structure of vascular endothelial cells, *Biorheology* **31**:143–153 (1994).

26. Walpola PL, Gotlieb AI, Langille BL: Monocyte adhesion and changes in endothelial cell number, morphology, and F-actin distribution elicited by low shear stress in vivo, *Am J Pathol* **142**:1392–1400 (1993).

27. Barbee KA, Mundel T, Lal R, Davies PF: Subcellular distribution of shear stress at the surface of flow-aligned and nonaligned endothelial monolayers, *Am J Physiol* **268**:H1765–H1772 (1995).

28. Lipowsky HH, Kovalcheck S, Zweifach BW: The distribution of blood rheological parameters in the microvasculature of cat mesentery, *Circ Res* **43**:738–749 (1978).

29. Tangelder GJ, Slaaf DW, Arts T, Reneman RS: Wall shear rate in arterioles in vivo: Least estimates from platelet velocity profiles, *Am J Physiol* **254**:H1059–H1064 (1988).

30. Tangelder GJ, Slaaf DW, Muijtjens AM, Arts T, Egbrink MG, Reneman RS: Velocity profiles of blood platelets and red blood cells flowing in arterioles of the rabbit mesentery, *Circ Res* **59**:505–514 (1986).

31. Reneman RS, Woldhuis B, Egbrink MGA, Slaaf DW, Tangelder GJ: Concentration and velocity profiles of blood cells in the microcirculation, in Hwang NHC et al. eds, *Advances in Cardiovascular Engineering,* Plenum Press, New York, 1992, pp 25–40.

32. Long DS, Smith ML, Pries AR, Ley K, Damiano ER: Microviscometry reveals reduced blood viscosity and altered shear rate and shear stress profiles in microvessels after hemodilution, *Proc Natl Acad Sci USA* **101**:10060–10065 (2004).

33. Vennemann P, Kiger KT, Lindken R, Groenendijk BC, Stekelenburg-de Vos S, ten Hagen TL, Ursem NT, Poelmann RE, Westerweel J, Hierck BP: In vivo micro particle image velocimetry measurements of blood-plasma in the embryonic avian heart, *J Biomech* **39**:1191–1200 (2006).

34. Brands PJ, Hoeks APG, Hofstra L, Reneman RS: A noninvasive method to estimate wall shear rate using ultrasound, *Ultrasound Med Biol* **21**:171–185 (1995).

35. Hoeks APG, Samijo SK, Brands PJ, Reneman RS: Assessment of wall shear rate in humans: An ultrasound study, *J Vasc Invest* **1**:108–117 (1995).

36. Oyre S, Pedersen EM, Ringgaard S, Boesiger P, Paaske WP: In vivo wall shear stress measured by magnetic resonance velocity mapping in the normal human abdominal aorta, *Eur J Vasc Endovasc Surg* **13**:263–271 (1997).

37. Oyre S, Ringgaard S, Kozerke S, Paaske WP, Erlandsen M, Boesiger P, Pedersen EM: Accurate noninvasive quantitation of blood flow, cross-sectional lumen vessel area and wall shear stress by three-dimensional paraboloid modeling of magnetic resonance imaging velocity data, *J Am Coll Cardiol* **32**:128–134 (1998).

38. Doriot PA, Dorsaz PA, Dorsaz L, De Benedetti E, Chatelain P, Delafontaine P: In vivo measurements of wall shear stress in human coronary arteries, *Coron Artery Dis* **11**:495–502 (2000).

39. Wentzel JJ, Janssen E, Vos J, Schuurbiers JC, Krams R, Serruys PW, de Feyter PJ, Slager CJ: Extension of increased atherosclerotic wall thickness into high shear stress regions is associated with loss of compensatory remodeling, *Circulation* **108**:17–23 (2003).

40. Hoeks APG, Reneman RS: Flow patterns and arterial wall dynamics, in *Cerebrovascular Ultrasound,* Hennerici MG, Meairs, SP, eds, Cambridge Univ Press, Cambridge, UK, 2001, pp 77–87.

41. Kamiya A, Bukhari R, Togawa T: Adaptive regulation of wall shear stress optimizing vascular tree function, *Bull Math Biol* **46**:127–137 (1984).

42. Murray CD: The physiological principle of minimum work: I. The vascular system and the cost of blood volume, *Proc Natl Acad Sci USA* **12**:207–214 (1926).

43. LaBarbera M: Principles of design of fluid transport systems in zoology, *Science* **249**:992–1000 (1990).

44. Kassab GS, Fung YC: The pattern of coronary arteriolar bifurcations and the uniform shear hypothesis, *Ann Biomed Eng* **23**:13–20 (1995).

45. Reneman RS, Arts T, Hoeks AP: Wall shear stress—an important determinant of endothelial cell function and structure—in the arterial system in vivo, discrepancies with theory. *J Vasc Res* **43**:251–269 (2006).

46. Zamir M, Sinclair P, Wonnacott TH: Relation between diameter and flow in major branches of the arch of the aorta, *J Biomech* **25**:1303–1310 (1992).

47. Arts T, Kruger RT, van Gerven W, Lambregts JA, Reneman RS: Propagation velocity and reflection of pressure waves in the canine coronary artery, *Am J Physiol* **237**:H469–H474 (1979).

48. Mayrovitz HN, Roy J: Microvascular blood flow: Evidence indicating a cubic dependence on arteriolar diameter, *Am J Physiol* **245**:H1031–H1038 (1983).

49. Hartley CJ, Michael LH, Entman ML: Noninvasive measurement of ascending aortic blood velocity in mice, *Am J Physiol* **268**:H499–H505 (1995).

50. Li YH, Reddy AK, Taffet GE, Michael LH, Entman ML, Hartley CJ: Doppler evaluation of peripheral vascular adaptations to transverse aortic banding in mice, *Ultrasound Med Biol* **29**:1281–1289 (2003).

51. Reneman RS, Schneider H, Wieberdink J, Brouwer FAS: Elektro-magnetische stroomsterktemeting van het bloed (Electromagnetic flow measurements of the blood). *Ned T Geneesk* **114**:1090–1101 (1970).

52. Samijo SK, Willigers JM, Brands PJ, Barkhuysen R, Reneman RS, Kitslaar PJEHM, Hoeks APG: Reproducibility of shear rate and shear stress assessment by means of ultrasound in the common carotid artery of young human males and females, *Ultrasound Med Biol* **23**:583–590 (1997).

53. Samijo SK, Willigers JM, Barkhuysen R, Kitslaar PJEHM, Reneman RS, Hoeks APG: Wall shear stress in the common carotid artery as function of age and gender, *Cardiovasc Res* **39**:515–522 (1998).

54. Dammers R, Stifft F, Tordoir JH, Hameleers JM, Hoeks AP, Kitslaar PJ: Shear stress depends on vascular territory: Comparison between common carotid and brachial artery, *J Appl Physiol* **94**:485–489 (2003).

55. Dammers R, Tordoir JHM, Hameleers JMM, Kitslaar PJEHM, Hoeks APG: Brachial artery shear stress is independent of gender or age and does not modify vessel wall mechanical properties, *Ultrasound Med Biol* **28**:1015–1022 (2002).

56. Dawson TH. *Engineering Design of the Cardiovascular System*, Prentice-Hall, Englewood Cliffs, NJ, 1991.

57. Rodbard S: Vascular caliber, *Cardiology* **60**:4–49 (1975).

58. Zamir M: Shear forces and blood vessel radii in the cardiovascular system, *J Gen Physiol* **69**:449–461 (1977).

59. Kamiya A, Togawa T: Adaptive regulation of wall shear stress to flow change in the canine carotid artery, *Am J Physiol* **239**:H14–H21 (1980).

60. Sherman TF: On connecting large vessels to small. The meaning of Murray's law, *J Gen Physiol* **78**:431–453 (1981).

61. Koller A, Kaley G: Shear stress dependent regulation of vascular resistance in health and disease: Role of endothelium, *Endothelium* **4**:247–272 (1996).

62. Melkumyants AM, Balashov SA: Effect of blood viscocity on arterial flow induced dilator response, *Cardiovasc Res* **24**:165–168 (1990).

63. Melkumyants AM, Balashov SA, Khayutin VM: Control of arterial lumen by shear stress on endothelium, *News Physiol Sciences* **10**:204–210 (1995).

64. Eckstein EC: Rheophoresis—a broader concept of platelet dispersivity, *Biorheology* **19**:717–724 (1982).

65. Tangelder GJ, Teirlinck HC, Slaaf DW, Reneman RS: Distribution of blood platelets flowing in arterioles, *Am J Physiol* **248**:H318–H323 (1985).

66. Reneman RS, Meinders JM, Hoeks AP: Non-invasive ultrasound in arterial wall dynamics in humans: What have we learned and what remains to be solved, *Eur Heart J* **26**:960–966 (2005).

67. Duncan DD, Bargeron CB, Borchardt SE, Deters OJ, Gearhart SA, Mark FF, Friedman MH: The effect of compliance on wall shear in casts of a human aortic bifurcation, *J Biomed Eng* **112**:183–188 (1990).

68. Perktold K, Thurner E, Kenner T: Flow and stress characteristics in rigid walled and compliant carotid artery bifurcation models, *Med Biol Eng Comput* **32**:19–26 (1994).

69. Bharadvaj BK, Mabon RF, Giddens DP: Steady flow in a model of the human carotid bifurcation. Part I—flow visualization, *J Biomech* **15**:349–362 (1982).

70. Bharadvaj BK, Mabon RF, Giddens DP: Steady flow in a model of the human carotid bifurcation. Part II—laser-Doppler anemometer measurements, *J Biomech* **15**:363–378 (1982).

71. Rindt CC, Steenhoven AA: Unsteady flow in a rigid 3-D model of the carotid artery bifurcation, *J Biomech Eng* **118**:90–96 (1996).

72. Rindt CCM, Van Steenhoven AA, Janssen JD, Reneman RS, Segal A: A numerical analysis of steady flow in a three-dimensional model of the carotid artery bifurcation, *J Biomech* **23**:461–473 (1990).

73. Motomiya M, Karino T: Flow patterns in the human carotid artery bifurcation, *Stroke* **15**:50–56 (1984).

74. Reneman RS, Van Merode T, Hick P, Hoeks APG: Flow velocity patterns in and distensibility of the carotid artery bulb in subjects of various ages, *Circulation* **71**:500–509 (1985).

75. Van de Vosse FN, Van Steenhoven AA, Janssen JD, Reneman RS: A two-dimensional numerical analysis of unsteady flow in the carotid artery bifurcation. A comparison with three-dimensional in-vitro measurements and the influence of minor stenoses, *Biorheology* **27**:163–189 (1990).

76. Reneman RS, Hoeks APG, Van de Vosse F, Ku D: Three-dimensional blood flow in bifurcations: Computational and experimental analyses and clinical applications, *Cerebrovasc Disc* **3**:185–192 (1993).

77. Wazer JR: Viscosity and flow measurements, in *A Laboratory Handbook of Rheology*, Interscience, New York, 1963.

78. Frojmovic MM, Panjwani R: Geometry of normal mammalian platelets by quantitative microscopic studies, *Biophys J* **16**:1071–1089 (1976).

79. Teirlinck HC, Tangelder GJ, Slaaf DW, Muijtjens AM, Arts T, Reneman RS: Orientation and diameter distribution of rabbit blood platelets flowing in small arterioles, *Biorheology* **21**:317–331 (1984).

80. Roevros JMJG: Analogue processing of C.W.-Doppler flowmeter signals to determine average frequency shift momentaneously without the use of a wave analyzer, in Reneman RS, ed, *Cardiovascular Applications of Ultrasound*, North-Holland, Amsterdam, 1974, pp 43–54.

81. Reneman RS, Van Merode T, Hick P, Hoeks APG: Cardiovascular applications of multi-gate pulsed Doppler systems, *Ultrasound Med Biol* **12**:357–370 (1986).

82. Tortoli P, Morganti T, Bambi G, Palombo C, Ramnarine KV: Noninvasive simultaneous assessment of wall shear rate and wall distension in carotid arteries, *Ultrasound Med Biol* **32**:1661–1670 (2006).

83. Brands PJ, Hoeks APG, Reneman RS: The effect of echo suppression on the mean velocity estimation range of the rf cross-correlation model estimator, *Ultrasound Med Biol* **21**:945–959 (1995).

84. Meinders JM, Brands PJ, Willigers JM, Kornet L, Hoeks AP: Assessment of the spatial homogeneity of artery dimension parameters with high frame rate 2-D B-mode, *Ultrasound Med Biol* **27**:785–794 (2001).

85. Silber HA, Ouyang P, Bluemke DA, Gupta SN, Foo TK, Lima JA: Why is flow-mediated dilation dependent on arterial size? Assessment of the shear stimulus using phase-contrast magnetic resonance imaging, *Am J Physiol Heart Circ Physiol* **288**:H822–H828 (2005).

86. Gatehouse PD, Keegan J, Crowe LA, Masood S, Mohiaddin RH, Kreitner KF, Firmin DN: Applications of phase-contrast flow and velocity imaging in cardiovascular MRI, *Eur Radiol* **15**:2172–2184 (2005).

87. Nayak KS, Hargreaves BA, Hu BS, Nishimura DG, Pauly JM, Meyer CH: Spiral balanced steady-state free precession cardiac imaging, *Magn Reson Med* **53**:1468–1473 (2005).

88. Wu SP, Ringgaard S, Oyre S, Hansen MS, Rasmus S, Pedersen EM: Wall shear rates differ between the normal carotid, femoral, and brachial arteries: An in vivo MRI study, *J Magn Reson Imag* **19**:188–193 (2004).

89. Kornet L, Hoeks APG, Lambregts J, Reneman RS: In the femoral artery bifurcation differences in mean wall shear stress within subjects are associated with different intima-media thicknesses, *Arterioscler Thromb Vasc Biol* **19**:2933–2939 (1999).

90. Weaver JPA, Evans A, Walder DN: The effect of increased fibrinogen content on the viscosity of blood, *Clin Sci* **36**:1–10 (1969).

91. Gnasso A, Carallo C, Irace C, Spagnuolo V, De Novara G, Mattiolo PL, Pujia A: Association between intima-media thickness and wall shear stress in common carotid artery in healthy male subjects, *Circulation* **94**:3257–3262 (1996).

92. Broeders MA, Tangelder GJ, Slaaf DW, Reneman RS, Egbrink MG: Endogenous nitric oxide protects against thromboembolism in venules but not in arterioles, *Arterioscler Thromb Vasc Biol*; **18**:139–145 (1998).

93. Kornet L, Hoeks AP, Lambregts J, Reneman RS: Mean wall shear stress in the femoral arterial bifurcation is low and independent of age at rest, *J Vasc Res* **37**:112–122 (2000).

94. Kornet L, Lambregts JAC, Hoeks APG, Reneman RS: Differences in near-wall shear rate in the carotid artery within subjects are associated with different intima-media thicknesses, *Arterioscl Thromb Vasc Biol* **18**:1877–1884 (1998).

95. Cheng C, Helderman F, Segers D, Hierck B, Poelman R, van Tol A, Tempel D, Duncker JD, Robbers-Visser D, Ursem N, van Haperen R, Wentzel J, Gijsen F, van der Steen A, de Crom R, Krams R: Large variations in absolute wall shear stress levels within one and between species, *Atherosclerosis* **195**:225–235 (2007).

96. Greve JM, Les AS, Tang BT, Draney Blomme MT, Wilson NM, Dalman RL, Pelc NJ, Taylor CA: Allometric scaling of wall shear stress from mice to humans: quantification using cine phase-contrast MRI and computational fluid dynamics, *Am J Physiol Heart Circ Physiol* **291**:H1700–H1708 (2006).

97. Zarins CK, Zatina MA, Giddens DP, Ku DN, Glagov S: Shear stress regulation of artery lumen diameter in experimental atherogenesis, *J Vasc Surg* **5**:413–420 (1987).

98. le Noble F, Fleury V, Pries A, Corvol P, Eichmann A, Reneman RS: Control of arterial branching morphogenesis in embryogenesis: Go with the flow, *Cardiovasc Res* **65**:619–628 (2005).

99. Reneman RS, Van Merode T, Hick P, Muytjens AMM, Hoeks APG: Age-related changes in carotid artery wall properties in man, *Ultrasound Med Biol* **12**:465–471 (1986).

100. Davies PF: Flow-mediated endothelial mechanotransduction, *Physiol Rev* **75**:519–560 (1995).

101. Resnick N, Gimbrone MAJ: Hemodynamic forces are complex regulators of endothelial gene expression, *Faseb J* **9**:874–882 (1995).

102. Chien S: Molecular and mechanical bases of focal lipid accumulation in arterial wall, *Prog Biophys Mol Biol* **83**:131–151 (2003).

103. Li YS, Haga JH, Chien S: Molecular basis of the effects of shear stress on vascular endothelial cells, *J Biomech* **38**:1949–1971 (2005).

104. Moon JJ, Matsumoto M, Patel S, Lee L, Guan JL, Li S: Role of cell surface heparan sulfate proteoglycans in endothelial cell migration and mechanotransduction, *J Cell Physiol* **203**:166–176 (2005).

105. Helmke BP, Davies PF: The cytoskeleton under external fluid mechanical forces: Hemodynamic forces acting on the endothelium, *Ann Biomed Eng* **30**:284–296 (2002).

106. Vink H, Duling BR: Identification of distinct luminal domains for macromolecules, erythrocytes, and leukocytes within mammalian capillaries, *Circ Res* **79**:581–589 (1996).

107. Smith ML, Long DS, Damiano ER, Ley K: Near-wall micro-PIV reveals a hydrodynamically relevant endothelial surface layer in venules in vivo, *Biophys J* **85**:637–645 (2003).

108. Gouverneur M, Spaan JA, Pannekoek H, Fontijn RD, Vink H: Fluid shear stress stimulates incorporation of hyaluronan into endothelial cell glycocalyx, *Am J Physiol Heart Circ Physiol* **290**:H458–H462 (2006).

109. Florian JA, Kosky JR, Ainslie K, Pang Z, Dull RO, Tarbell JM: Heparan sulfate proteoglycan is a mechanosensor on endothelial cells, *Circ Res* **93**:e136–e142 (2003).

110. Tarbell JM, Pahakis MY: Mechanotransduction and the glycocalyx, *J Intern Med* **259**:339–350 (2006).

111. Weinbaum S, Zhang X, Han Y, Vink H, Cowin SC: Mechanotransduction and flow across the endothelial glycocalyx, *Proc Natl Acad Sci USA* **100**:7988–7995 (2003).

CHAPTER 3

Relating Cerebral Aneurysm Hemodynamics and Clinical Events

JUAN R. CEBRAL

Center for Computational Fluid Dynamics, George Mason University, Fairfax, Virginia

CHRISTOPHER M. PUTMAN

Interventional Neuroradiology, Inova Fairfax Hospital, Falls Church, Virginia

Abstract. This chapter summarizes more recent investigations of the role of hemodynamics in the process of cerebral aneurysm progression and rupture. These studies are based on patient-specific computational fluid dynamics models constructed from medical images and used to relate aneurysmal hemodynamics and clinical information indicative of aneurysm evolution or rupture. After a brief introduction of the image based methodology for computational modeling of cerebral aneurysms, the chapter describes studies relating hemodynamic characteristics such as the concentration of the inflow jet, the size of the flow impingement region, and the stability and complexity of the intraaneurysmal flow pattern to aneurysmal rupture. Subsequently, studies of the role of hemodynamics in the processes of aneurysmal wall weakening are described, particularly the relationship between the distribution of wall shear stress and regions of nonuniform aneurysm pulsation observed with dynamic imaging techniques and the formation of secondary lobulations or blebs. All these studies suggest that hemodynamics, and in particular abnormal wall shear stress values, plays an important role in the initiation, progression and rupture of intracranial aneurysms.

3.1. INTRODUCTION

Cerebral aneurysms are pathological dilatations of the arterial wall frequently located near arterial bifurcations in the circle of Willis [1–3]. The most serious consequence is their rupture and intracranial hemorrhage, with an associated high mortality–morbidity rate [4–7]. Intracranial aneurysms are particularly difficult to treat, and seldom produce symptoms before they rupture [8]. Improvements of neuroradiological techniques have resulted in more frequent detection of aneurysms before they have bled. Bleeding from an aneurysm most commonly causes subarachnoid hemorrhage. Because the prognosis from aneurismal bleeding is still poor, preventive surgery is increasingly considered as a therapeutic option. But every treatment carries a risk, which sometimes matches or exceeds the yearly risk of aneurysm rupture. Therefore, the best patient care would be to treat only those patients who are likely to rupture [9–11]. Currently, clinicians rely on size for estimation of the risk of an aneurysm to rupture, but this predictor is relatively poor. Physicians need better predictors of the risk of future bleeding so that they can minimize unnecessary and potentially dangerous surgeries. Identifying useful predictors requires a better understanding of the process of aneurysm formation, progression, and rupture. These processes are not well understood. Previous studies [1,12–21] have identified the major factors involved in these processes: (1) hemodynamics, (2) wall biomechanics, (3) mechanobiology, and (4) perianeurysmal environment.

The flow dynamics of cerebral aneurysms have been studied in numerous experimental models and clinical studies to investigate the role of hemodynamics in their initiation, growth, and rupture [14,22–29]. Although this work has characterized the complexity of intraaneurysmal hemodynamics, the studies have focused largely on idealized aneurysm geometries or surgically created aneurysms in animals. Each of these approaches has significant limitations because they do not allow the connection of the clinical outcomes to the hemodynamic factors. Animal models can have quite realistic anatomies and hemodynamics but do not progress and rupture as do intracranial aneurysms.

Computational models of blood flows offer the attractive possibility for overcoming the limitations seen in previous experiments. The ability to study any vessel geometry and isolate the hemodynamics from other factors when combined with medical imaging techniques allows for the construction of patient-specific geometry [30–34]. Therefore, the models and their hemodynamic factors can be connected to the clinical outcomes for use in clinical studies. In this chapter we will concentrate only on computational models and their use in investigating connections between hemodynamic variables and clinical events indicative of aneurysm progression or rupture.

3.2. IMAGE-BASED COMPUTATIONAL HEMODYNAMICS MODELING

The modeling process of patient-specific hemodynamics from medical images can be divided into two major stages: (1) anatomic modeling and (2) blood flow modeling. Each of these stages can be further subdivided into more basic steps: (1a) image processing, (1b) geometric modeling, (1c) grid generation, (2a) flow simulation, (2b) postprocessing, and (2c) visualization. The set of sequential modeling stages is called a *computational modeling pipeline* or *chain*. Several alternative approaches exist for each stage of the modeling chain, and different investigators have used different combinations of computational tools to assemble their pipelines. In what follows a brief description of the pipeline used by the authors is provided [35].

Vascular Modeling

The anatomic images are first smoothed to reduce noise by alternative application of blurring and sharpening operators that tend to smooth the image without shrinking or enlarging vascular structures [33,35]. A seeded region growing algorithm is then used to segment the vessels, and an initial surface model is obtained by isosurface extraction [36]. Both the intensity level for the region growing segmentation and the isosurface extraction are selected by trial and error. This reconstructed triangulation is then used as the initialization of a geometrically deformable model [37]. The nodes of the triangulation are allowed to deform under the action of internal smoothing forces and external forces computed from the image intensity gradients. This algorithm tends to place the surface nodes on the edges of vascular structures, thus achieving subvoxel accuracy and making the anatomical model less dependent on the selected intensity threshold. In some cases, because of limited image resolution, small vessels are not properly modeled by this procedure and are independently reconstructed. For this purpose, a tubular deformable model along the vessel axis of each such artery is constructed [38]. The triangulation of the small vessel is subsequently fused to the final model using an adaptive voxelization technique [39].

Once all the components have been merged into a single watertight vascular model, this model is smoothed using the nonshrinking algorithm developed by Taubin [40] in order to eliminate high-frequency noise from the triangulation. The surface model is then optimized using edge collapses and diagonal swaps in order to increase the quality of the triangular elements [36]. Very small or highly distorted triangles (i.e., aspect ratio larger than a given threshold, e.g., 10) are deleted by collapsing the edges shared by such elements. Diagonal swaps aim at minimizing the maximum internal angle of the triangular elements. This is done by swapping the diagonal of quadrilaterals formed by two adjacent triangles if such a swap yields smaller maximum angles. Terminal vessel branches are then truncated perpendicularly to the vessel axis [36].

The reconstructed anatomic models are used to generate high quality volumetric grids composed of tetrahedral elements suitable for finite-element calculations of blood flow dynamics. This is done utilizing an advancing front method to create a new surface triangulation using the reconstructed model as a support surface or definition of the computational domain [36,41]. Newly created points are placed on the original surface by linear interpolation. Surface features automatically detected on the original reconstructed model are preserved in the final grid [42]. Starting from the new surface triangulation, the advancing front algorithm then marches into the volume of the computational domain generating tetrahedral elements [43]. The element size distribution is prescribed using source functions and adaptive background grids [44].

Hemodynamics Modeling

Blood is mathematically modeled as a continuous incompressible fluid. The governing equations are the unsteady 3D Navier–Stokes equations, which can be written as

$$\rho \left(\frac{\partial \mathbf{u}}{\partial t} + \mathbf{u} \cdot \nabla \mathbf{u} \right) = -\nabla p + \nabla \cdot \tau + \mathbf{F} \tag{3.1}$$

$$\nabla \cdot \mathbf{u} = 0 \tag{3.2}$$

where $\mathbf{u}$ is the velocity field, ρ is the density, p is the pressure, τ is the deviatoric stress tensor, and $\mathbf{F}$ represents any externally applied body forces such as gravity. For Newtonian fluids the deviatoric stress tensor can be written as

$$\tau_{ij} = 2\mu\varepsilon_{ij} \tag{3.3}$$

where μ is the viscosity, and the strain rate tensor is defined as

$$\varepsilon_{ij} = \frac{1}{2} \left(\frac{\partial u_i}{\partial x_j} + \frac{\partial u_j}{\partial x_i} \right) \tag{3.4}$$

Typical values for blood are $\rho = 1.0$ g/cm^3 and $\mu = 0.04$ dyn·s/cm. The non-Newtonian model of Casson [45] has been used to approximate the rheologic behavior of blood. In this case, the relationship between the shear stress and strain rate is given by:

$$\sqrt{\tau} = \sqrt{\tau_0} + \sqrt{\mu_0 \dot{\gamma}} \tag{3.5}$$

where τ_0 is the yield stress and μ_0 the asymptotic Newtonian viscosity. Typical values used for these constants that fit empirical data for blood are $\tau_0 = 0.04$ dyn/cm^2 and $\mu = 0.04$ dyn·s/cm. The values of these constants depend on the hematocrit, which is the volume fraction of red blood cells. The strain rate is computed from the second invariant of the strain rate tensor [46], which for incompressible fluids takes the form

$$\dot{\gamma} = 2\sqrt{\varepsilon_{ij}\varepsilon_{ij}} \tag{3.6}$$

The apparent viscosity can be written as

$$\mu = \left(\sqrt{\tau_0/\dot{\gamma}} + \sqrt{\mu_0} \right)^2 \tag{3.7}$$

Since the apparent viscosity grows indefinitely as the strain rate is reduced, alternative expressions have been used for numerical simulations. One such formula is [47]

$$\mu = \left(\sqrt{\tau_0 \, (1 - e^{-m\dot{\gamma}})/\dot{\gamma}} + \sqrt{\mu_0} \right)^2 \tag{3.8}$$

with values of $m > 100$ reported to produce satisfactory results [48].

The governing equations are numerically solved using an implicit finite-element formulation based on unstructured grids [35,49]. This approach allows arbitrary timestep sizes. Typically 100–200 timesteps are taken per cardiac cycle and the simulations run for at least two cardiac cycles.

Physiologic inflow conditions can be derived from phase contrast magnetic resonance measurements of blood flowrates obtained in the major cerebral vessels [50,51]. Each flow rate curve is decomposed into Fourier modes

$$Q(t) = \sum_{n=0}^{N} Q_n e^{in\omega t} \tag{3.9}$$

where N is the number of modes and ω is the angular frequency obtained from the period of the cardiac cycle. The velocity profile corresponding to this flowrate curve can be computed from the Womersley solution [52]. The Womersley profile is the analytic solution for a fully developed sinusoidally varying flow of an incompressible Newtonian fluid in a rigid circular pipe. The velocity profile is then obtained as a superposition of Womersley solutions corresponding to each Fourier mode [53]:

$$\mu(r,t) = \frac{2Q_0}{\pi a^2}\left[1 - \left(\frac{r}{a}\right)^2\right] + \sum_{n=1}^{N} \frac{2Q_n}{\pi a^2}\left[\frac{1 - \dfrac{J_0\,(\beta_n r/a)}{J_0\,(\beta_n)}}{1 - \dfrac{2J_1\,(\beta_n)}{\beta_n J_0\,(\beta_n)}}\right] e^{in\omega t} \tag{3.10}$$

where

$$\beta_n = i^{3/2}\alpha_n = i^{3/2}\sqrt{\frac{n\omega}{\nu}} \tag{3.11}$$

with α_n the Womersley number (a dimensionless parameter characterizing the frequency of the pulsatile flow) and ν the kinematic viscosity. In order to impose pulsatile flow boundary conditions, this velocity profile is mapped to the inflow boundary.

In vivo, the flow division among different arterial branches is determined by the impedance of the distal arterial tree. Currently there are no means of measuring this impedance in vivo, so an approximation of this is needed for computational models. Different authors have used different approaches for prescribing outflow boundary conditions, depending on the availability of flow measurements in the different branches of the models. The different options are (1) impose traction free boundary conditions in all the model outlets with the implicit assumption that all vascular trees have the same impedance [31,33]; (2) impose flow divisions determined by the area ratio of the outflow vessels, which implies that the distal impedance is proportional to the area [27,54]; (3) prescribe flow impedances computed from arterial tree models generated for each outflow boundary [50,55,56], (4) couple the 3D simulations to 1D models of the systemic circulation [57]; and (5) impose flowrates measured in all the model outlets [41,58].

At the vessel wall, the no-slip boundary condition implies that the fluid velocity must be equal to the velocity of the arterial wall. If the vessel walls are assumed rigid, this implies a zero velocity at the wall. Vessel wall compliance is an important effect that may alter the local hemodynamics. Vessel wall compliance can be incorporated into the models in two basic ways: (1) directly impose the motion of the vessel wall measured using dynamic imaging techniques such as 4D-CTA or high-frame-rate biplane angiography [59,60], and (2) perform coupled fluid–solid interaction simulations [41,58,61–63]. The former option is very attractive as more recent advances in dynamic imaging modalities are making this possibility a reality. The latter option has several difficulties, such as a proper model for the solid or biomechanical modeling of the vessel wall, estimations of the distribution of the wall elasticity and thickness, estimation of the intraarterial pressure waveform required for proper boundary condition specification, and larger CPU requirements. However, this approach can yield detailed biomechanical information useful for studying the interplay of hemodynamics and wall mechanobiology.

3.3. CEREBRAL ANEURYSM HEMODYNAMICS AND RUPTURE

Central to any hypothesis of the pathogenesis of growth and rupture of aneurysms is the interaction between the hemodynamic forces with the vessel wall biology and the resulting impact on the mechanics of the wall. Ultimately, any rupture is the consequence of the inability of the wall to contain the force of the flowing blood. Yet hemodynamic studies have not found evidence of excessive elevations of peak pressure within cerebral aneurysms to explain the wall failure on a purely mechanical basis. Consequently, there must be an alteration of the aneurysmal wall that results in its mechanical weakening over time. Histological studies have found a decreased number or degeneration of endothelial cells, degeneration of the internal elastic lamina, and thinning of the medial layer [22,23]. Because the internal elastic lamina and vascular extracellular matrix are considered the main contributors to the structural integrity of the vessel, investigators have examined a variety of enzymes related to their remodeling and potential degeneration. Circulating levels of serum gelatinase or elastase are increased in patients with cerebral aneurysms [24]. Increased matrix metalloproteinase have been found in aneurysm walls [25]. Finally, a genetic locus for cerebral aneurysms has been found to lie within or close to the elastin gene locus on chromosome 7 in Japanese patients [26]. These enzymes are largely responsible for intracellular matrix degradation as part of the process of wall remodeling, and therefore increased activity could cause weakening of the wall. Thinning of the medial layer in the aneurysm wall seen histologically largely explained by a decreased number of smooth muscle cells [22,23,27]. In both experimental [27] and clinical studies [27,28] the decrease of smooth muscle cells has been attributed to apoptosis of smooth muscle cells. Consequently, it is widely believed that smooth muscle cell apoptosis and elastin/collagen fiber reconstitution mechanisms are central to the process of wall weakening.

The interplay of genetics and biomechanical stimuli generated by blood flow seems to be the critical element in the pathogenesis of cerebral aneurysms. Animal studies have pointed to endothelial degeneration and cell loss as the initiating event of aneurysm wall remodeling [29]. Endothelial gene expression is related to WSS. Studies demonstrate that prolonged laminar WSS regulates the expression to only a small percentage (1–5%) of endothelial genes, and this transcriptional profile produces an endothelial phenotype that is quiescent, as it is protected from apoptosis, inflammation, and oxidative stress [30]. Therefore, triggering for genetic traits, potentially affecting arterial wall mechanical load tolerance, may be attributed to a hemodynamic condition.

The formation of cerebral aneurysms is believed to be related to an interaction between high flow hemodynamic forces and the arterial wall because of several clinical and experimental observations. Cerebral aneurysms are commonly associated with anatomic variations and pathological conditions such as hypoplasia or occlusion of a segment of the circle of Willis [21,31–34], or high flow arteriovenous malformations [35,36], which cause locally increased flow in the cerebral circulation, and at points of flow bifurcation, a site of flow separation and elevated WSS. Observations from animal models have shown that elevations of WSS to levels that can be found in these conditions can cause fragmentation of the internal elastic lamina of blood vessels [37] as well as alterations in endothelial phenotype or endothelial damage [22]. Additionally, increased flow and systemic hypertension are required for creating experimental cerebral aneurysms in rats and primates [38–42].

Despite this agreement in the mechanism of aneurysm initiation there is significant controversy regarding the mechanisms responsible for growth and ultimate rupture of a cerebral aneurysm. The controversy can be divided into two main schools of thought: high flow effects and low flow effects. In each theory, the hemodynamic environment within the aneurysm interacts with the cellular elements of the aneurysmal wall to result in a weakening of the wall. From histological observations, investigators have concluded that the mechanical properties of the aneurysmal wall are related mainly to collagen. Measurements of the strength of the aneurysm walls from cadaveric and surgical specimens have shown that the yield stress of tissue in the fundi of aneurysms was mildly in excess of the calculated systolic stresses in contrast to normal arterial wall, which were higher by a factor of 10–20 [43]. Furthermore, this analysis showed that the stress tolerated by aneurysm walls for a prolonged period was in the range of the stress that is imposed in vivo by the mean blood pressure. So, aneurysm growth could be understood as a passive yield to blood pressure and reactive healing and thickening of the wall with increasing aneurysm diameter. The distinguishing feature between the two schools of thought is in the mechanisms responsible for wall weakening.

The high-flow theory focuses on the effects of elevation of WSS. Elevation of maximal WSS can cause endothelial injury and thus initiate wall remodelling and potential degeneration [44]. A vascular endothelium malfunction or/and an abnormal shear stress field can cause an overexpression of endothelium-dependent nitric oxide (NO) production, which leads to a lower, nonphysiological local arterial tone via processes connected with scarcity and apoptosis of wall-embedded smooth muscle cells and wall remodeling [28,45–47]. This would result in a disturbance of the equilibrium between the blood pressure forces and the internal wall stress forces, in favor of the first, and would subsequently dilate the arterial wall locally. The resulting abnormal blood shear stress field is the driving factor for further growth of the aneurysmal geometry. This geometric growth stretches the collagen and elastin fibers of the medial and adventitial layers and gives rise to internal stresses that are contributing to the arterial stiffness. Eventually, the biomechanical system equilibrates at a state where the internal wall stresses and the transmural pressure are equal while, the local hemodynamics can no longer alter the arterial properties. At this point, the elastin and the collagen fibers are constantly under a nonphysiological large mechanical load and eventually undergo remodeling.

The low-flow theory points to low flows within aneurysms as causing localized stagnation of blood flow against the wall in the dome. Blood stagnation is known to cause a dysfunction of flow-induced NO, which is usually released by mechanical stimulation from increased shear stress. This dysfunction results in the aggregation of red blood cells, as well as accumulation and adhesion of both platelets and leukocytes along the intimal surface [48–51]. This process may cause intimal damage, leading to infiltration of white blood cells and fibrin inside the aneurysm wall, all of which have been seen in pathological examinations of aneurysm walls [52,53]. The inflammation would lead to localized degeneration of the aneurysm wall, resulting in a lower pressure threshold at which physiological tensile forces could be supported. The aneurysm wall would progressively thin and may result finally in a tearing of the tissue.

Current opinion is divided on which mechanism takes precedence in causing an aneurysm to rupture. Proponents of the low-shear-stress theories rely on several clinical observations and CFD data they consider to be incompatible with the high shear stress mechanisms. First, prior CFD modeling has shown that focal elevations in WSS are largely confined to the downstream lip of an aneurysm yet clinically the dome is the most common site of rupture [54] and WSS in the dome is low. Thus, they reason, shear stress can be related to aneurysm growth only if one assumes that the active matrix of aneurysm growth is located at the orifice. Yet, angiographically documented cases of aneurysm growth show in general progression of the dome but only rarely changes in the neck region [55]. Second, the strongest known predictor of aneurysm's rate of rupture is size with larger sizes corresponding to elevated rates of rupture. Flow velocities in aneurysms depend on the volume, with velocity inversely proportional to the square of the maximum diameter of the fundus [56–60]. Also, a direct relationship exists between the area of the orifice and the intraaneurysmal flow velocities [61]. These observations have led to a clinical measure called the *aspect ratio* (depth of aneurysm divided by neck width). An aspect ratio greater than 1.6 has been found in some studies to be correlated to risk of rupture [62]. Finally, CFD analysis and experimental in vitro measurements of WSS have shown that the magnitude of the WSS of the aneurysm region is significantly lower than that of the vessel region and WSS inversely correlated with the aspect ratio [63]. Naturally, their conclusion is that high shear stress cannot be the cause of aneurysm rupture.

Despite these admittedly compelling arguments, the low-shear-stress theory may not be the correct explanation for aneurysm rupture. First, low WSS at the bifurcations of the carotid arteries are causally connected with proliferative degenerative alterations (i.e., atheromas). Although atheromas are found in a minority of cerebral aneurysms, presence of an atheroma is not a common finding in histological examinations of ruptured aneurysms. Why would we anticipate the biological response to be different intra-aneurysmally? Second, much of the previous CFD work was performed using idealized lateral wall aneurysm models that are not representative of the wide range of geometries found in patients.

Since there is a significant controversy, a pilot clinical study of cerebral aneurysm hemodynamics was conducted in order to explore possible relationships between hemodynamic characteristics and aneurysm rupture [64]. In this study, a total of 62 patient-specific models of cerebral aneurysms were constructed from 3D rotational angiography images, and computational fluid dynamics simulations were performed under pulsatile flow conditions. The aneurysms were classified into different categories depending on the complexity and stability of the flow pattern, the location and size of the flow impingement region, and the size of the inflow jet. A large variety of flow patterns was observed. Interesting trends in the distribution of ruptured and unruptured aneurysms among these categories were found. It was found that 72% of ruptured aneurysms had complex or unstable flow patterns, 80% had small impingement regions, and 76% had small jet sizes. Conversely, unruptured aneurysms accounted for 73%, 82%, and 75% of aneurysms with simple stable flow patterns, large impingement regions, and large jet sizes, respectively. Although the sample size was not very large, it was possible to establish one statistically significant correlation; namely, aneurysms with small impingement sizes were 6.3 times more likely to have experienced rupture than those with large impingement sizes ($p = .01$). Figure 3.1 presents examples of two aneurysms with small impaction zones (top row) and two aneurysms with large impaction zones (bottom row). Our findings support the high-flow theory as the mechanism responsible for aneurysm rupture because of the link with impaction zones an area of elevated WSS. However, our findings also differ from previous works on idealized aneurysms because the large majority of aneurysms in our study had focalized regions of elevated WSS within the body or dome. This led to further studies to understand why idealized models yielded differing results.

Until recently computational studies have been performed only on idealized aneurysm geometries or approximations of a specific patient geometry [29,65,66]. These experiments have greatly influenced thinking about the

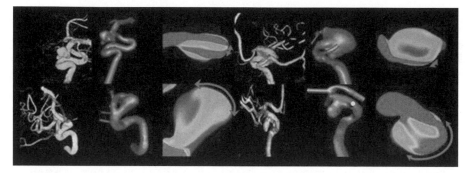

Figure 3.1. Examples of cerebral aneurysms with small (top row) and large (bottom row) flow impaction regions. (See insert for color representation).

mechanisms of aneurysm development as researchers have attempted to make generalized statements about aneurysmal hemodynamics from these simplified models. As computational methods and modeling have improved, more refined models have been constructed, leading to a transition from idealized geometries to "realistic" models based on typical patient anatomies. Most recently, studies have tried to replicate the exact anatomy of specific patients from medical images [30–35,62]. Implicit in computational modeling has been the study of the aneurysmal system in effect disconnected from the systemic circulation. A portion of the vascular tree including the aneurysm is reconstructed, and inflows and outflow are assigned on the basis of a variety of assumptions. Early "idealized" models used a short straight tube as the parent artery and therefore largely neglected the potential effects of parent artery geometry. More recently, "realistic" approximations of patient anatomies and patient-specific anatomic models have been used. When comparing the models used in these studies, there is a wide variation in the amount of parent artery used. Considering that cerebral arteries, like aneurysms, widely vary between patients, the effects of the segmentation of the parent artery upstream of an aneurysm could be significant on the intraaneurysmal hemodynamics. A more recent study showed that models that ignore secondary flows produced by the curvature and tortuosity of the parent arteries upstream of the aneurysm (those with idealized parent artery geometries) tend to result in flow impaction zones located at the distal neck of the aneurysm with an associated low-WSS distribution in the aneurysm [67]. In contrast, realistic models show a large number of aneurysms with flow impaction zone in the body or dome of the aneurysm and a region of elevated wall shear stress in the aneurysm [64]. An example is presented in Figure 3.2. The flow pattern in a model with a truncated parent artery (right) is parallel in the parent artery and impacts at the neck of the aneurysm, while in a realistic model (left) the secondary flows present in the parent artery cause the flow to impact on the body and dome of the aneurysm. This is an important observation because it can affect the way we think about the

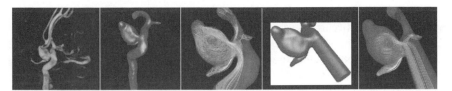

Figure 3.2. Effect of parent artery geometry on intraaneurysmal hemodynamics. (See insert for color representation).

mechanisms responsible for the initiation, evolution, and rupture of cerebral aneurysms.

3.4. HEMODYNAMICS AND RUPTURE OF ANTERIOR COMMUNICATING ARTERY ANEURYSMS

The anterior communicating artery (ACoA) is a recognized site of aneurysm predilection accounting for nearly a fourth of all cerebral aneurysms in several large studies [68–70]. The anterior communicating artery has a unique function in the body's vascular system as it serves as a collateral channel between the cerebral anterior circulations. The anterior communicating artery is the only cerebral artery that evolves from an arterial plexus in the deep intrahemispheric fissure, which may account for the high frequency of anomalies such as duplication, fenestration, and plexus formation at this location. Inequality of the proximal segment of the anterior cerebral artery (ACA) has been reported to occur in 7–46% of selected cases [71], adding to the complexity of the flow patterns in this region. Lifelong physiological factors and aging may further influence the geometry over time as a result of vascular remodeling and pathological responses. Considering the complexity and diversity to the geometry of the ACoA, it is not surprising that aneurysms of the ACoA are considered the most complex of the anterior circulation. The anterior communicating artery receives blood flow from the two A1 segments of the anterior cerebral arteries, so inequality in pressures transmitted from the internal carotid arteries (ICAs) determines the flow in the anterior communicating artery. Thus, in addition to the complex geometry of the sac and parent arteries, study of ACoA aneurysms is more difficult because of the interaction of two sources of inflow [72].

Unlike CTA and MR angiography, cerebral angiography visualizes only a single avenue of flow at a time because vessels are seen by the injection of a contrast agent into the flow stream of a single feeding vessel and images taken through the course of a single passage of contrast through the vasculature. For the majority of aneurysms, this poses no problems because most aneurysms arise from a vessel with only one source of inflow. However, a significant number of aneurysms arise from vessels of the circle of Willis with the potential of receiving blood flow from two sources. This is seen in the basilar artery, in the posterior communicating arteries, and, most commonly, in the anterior communicating arteries, which act as a collateral pathway between the internal carotid arteries via the anterior cerebral arteries. The inability to directly obtain a complete 3D model of aneurysms of this type has limited the ability to study these aneurysms using patient-specific CFD methods. On the other hand, the highest-resolution images of the cerebral vessels are from rotational angiographic images. For this reason, a new methodology was developed for constructing subject-specific models of cerebral aneurysms with multiple avenues of flow from multiple rotational angiography images using a combination of image coregistration and surface-merging techniques [73]. Briefly, rotational angiography images are obtained by contrast injection in each vessel that provides inflow to the aneurysm. Anatomic models are independently constructed of each of these vascular trees and fused together into a single model using an adaptive voxelization technique [39]. The anatomic model is then used to construct a finite element grid for CFD simulations of hemodynamics including all sources of inflow to the aneurysm. The methodology is schematically shown in Figure 3.3.

In order to extend our study of the relationship between hemodynamics and aneurysm rupture to aneurysms of the anterior communicating artery, a total of 26 patients with anterior communicating artery aneurysms and imaged with rotational angiography from our database were analyzed [74]. Of these patients, 11 had unilateral ACoA aneurysms; thus one of the A1 segments was missing, and 15 had bilateral ACoA aneurysms, that is, with both A1 segments present. Two three-dimensional rotational angiography (3DRA) images were acquired by

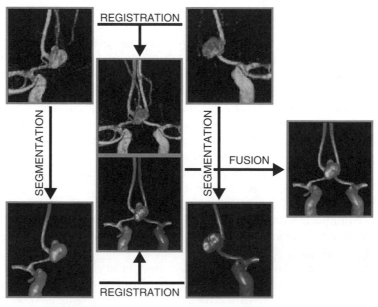

Figure 3.3. Construction of patient-specific models of anterior communicating artery aneurysms from bilateral 3D rotational angiography images.

injection in each internal carotid artery for the bilateral aneurysms. The patient's medical and radiological records were reviewed and evaluated for evidence of aneurysmal intracranial hemorrhage. In patients with multiple aneurysms, clinical and radiological information was considered and the most likely source of the hemorrhage was determined. The other coincident aneurysms were classified as unruptured. Corresponding CFD models were constructed using our image-based computational modeling pipeline [35]. Flow patterns were visualized using streamlines and classified into the four categories shown in the top row of Figure 3.4 by counting the number of streamlines from the parent vessel(s) entering the aneurysm and flowing into each of the daughter A2 segments of the ACAs. Examples each flow type are presented in the bottom row of Figure 3.4.

It was found that only 25% of the bilateral aneurysms accepted blood from both A1 segments [flow type (a)]. The remaining 75% of bilateral aneurysms together with the unilateral aneurysms (85% of the sample) accepted blood from a single A1 segment. According to the clinical information, the percentage of ruptured aneurysms was 70%: 73% in the unilateral group and 67% in the bilateral one. The number of ruptured and unruptured aneurysms in each flow category was counted. It was found that the number of ruptured aneurysms varied with the flow type. Most aneurysms in group (a) were unruptured (75%). Ruptured and unruptured aneurysms were equally distributed in group (b), while aneurysms in groups (c) and (d) had the highest rupture ratio: 87% and 67%, respectively. The maximum intra-aneurysmal wall shear stress magnitude at the systolic peak (MWSS) was computed for each aneurysm, and the average was

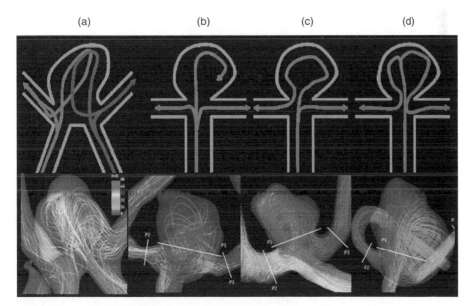

Figure 3.4. Classification of blood flow patterns in anterior communicating artery aneurysms. (See insert for color representation).

calculated for each group. It was found that all the unruptured aneurysms in group (a) had a low WSS (63 dyn/cm^2), while the only ruptured aneurysm in that flow type had a MWSS one order of magnitude higher. Aneurysms in group (b) showed a relatively small MWSS, which is slightly higher in ruptured aneurysms (78 dyn/cm^2) than in unruptured ones (60 dyn/cm^2). In contrast, aneurysms in groups (c) and (d), which have a higher rupture rate, have a larger MWSS. Specifically, the average MWSS for unruptured and ruptured aneurysms in group (c) were 225 and 306 dyn/cm^2, while those for group (d) were 150 and 163 dyn/cm^2, respectively. Although the current sample is not large enough to achieve statistical significance, an interesting trend in the distribution of ruptured and unruptured aneurysms among the proposed categories was observed. In each category, the maximum wall shear stress at the systolic peak is higher in the ruptured subgroup than in the unruptured one. Aneurysms where the two inflow jets collide and disperse inside the aneurysm showed the lowest rupture rate. The highest ratio of ruptured aneurysms was observed in categories (c) and (d), where a significant amount of flow from the parent vessel enters the aneurysm, suggesting that this subset of aneurysms may be at a higher rupture risk. The data also suggest that the number of ruptured aneurysms in each category increases with the maximum wall shear stress in the aneurysm at the systolic peak. Further studies with larger samples are necessary to confirm these trends statistically. If these trends are proved correctly, this simple classification system could be used to better assess the rupture risk of anterior communicating artery aneurysms.

3.5. HEMODYNAMICS AND WALL WEAKNESS

Previous studies found that unruptured aneurysms tended to have large flow impingement regions (more dispersed inflow jets) and simple stable flow patterns, while ruptured aneurysms tended to have small impaction zones (more concentrated inflow jets) and complex or unstable intraaneurysmal flow patterns [64]. This suggests that elevated wall shear stress caused by the impaction of a concentrated inflow jet may have a damaging effect on the arterial wall. A study of the relationship between wall shear stress and aneurysm formation in animal models showed that elevated wall shear stress gradients tend to damage the arterial wall promoting aneurysm formation [75]. Another study of the motion of the arterial wall of cerebral aneurysms based on dynamic digital subtraction angiography (DSA) showed that the bleb of an aneurysm had a larger deformation amplitude (by a factor of ~2) than the rest of the aneurysm sac [59]. In this study, the wall motion was quantified from high-frame-rate biplane angiography images obtained during an 8-s contrast injection. Nonrigid image registration algorithms, which establish correspondences between points in two different images, were used to track landmark points selected on the aneurysm and vessel walls [59,76]. An example is presented in Figure 3.5. The top row shows the propagation of landmark points between different frames of the dynamic image sequence. The left panel of the bottom row shows the regions selected to quantify the motion in

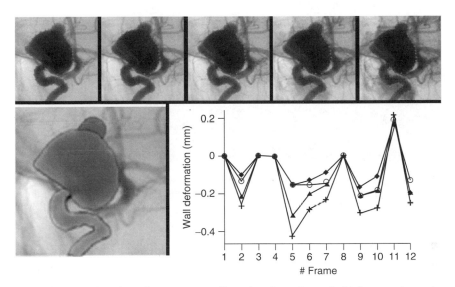

Figure 3.5. Estimation of aneurysm wall motion from dynamic biplane angiography.

the bleb, the aneurysm and the parent artery. The right panel of the bottom row shows the deformation amplitude of each region during the acquisition time. In these curves, the amplitude of the pulsation of the bleb is larger than that of the aneurysm and the parent artery. Similar observations were reported in a study of wall motion based on dynamic computed tomography angiography (CTA) [77]. These observations suggest that blebs deform at a larger rate because of a locally weaker aneurysm wall. Therefore, a focalized injury of the arterial wall is likely the reason for the formation of the bleb. So, what caused this focalized injury to the arterial wall? Our hypothesis is that mechanobiological processes modulated by elevated wall shear stress caused by the impaction of the inflow jet on the aneurysm wall are responsible for this local damage and thus for the formation of a bleb [78].

In order to investigate this hypothesis, a total of seven patients with intracranial aneurysms harboring well-defined blebs and imaged by 3DRA were selected from the database. A bleb was considered well defined if its neck was visually easily recognizable, in other words, if one could mentally remove the bleb and imagine the surface of the aneurysm without the bleb. The selected aneurysms varied in size, location, and morphology. Realistic vascular models were constructed for each patient from the corresponding 3DRA images using geometrically deformable models [37]. A second anatomic model was created for each patient by removing the bleb. This was achieved by applying a Laplacian smoothing to the bleb region of the original anatomic model. A Laplacian smoothing procedure tends to shrink the surface being smoothed [40]. Thus, fixing the boundaries of the bleb region (the neck of the bleb) and applying the Laplacian smoothing iteratively effectively smoothes out the bleb while preserving a smooth

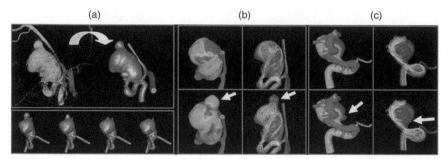

Figure 3.6.   (a) Construction of patient-specific models of cerebral aneurysms before and after bleb formation; (b) bleb formation at flow impaction zone; (c) bleb formation at outflow zone. (See insert for color representation).

surface at all times. The bleb regions were manually selected on the anatomic models. The procedure for removing the blebs is illustrated in Figure 3.6a. The top row of Figure 3.6a shows the original 3DRA image of an aneurysm located in the left internal carotid artery with a well-defined bleb in the superior part of the dome and the reconstructed anatomic model. The bottom row of Figure 3.6a shows the progressive smoothing out of this bleb. The final model without the bleb (rightmost model in the bottom row of Figure 3.6a) was considered to represent the stage of the aneurysm evolution just prior to formation of the bleb. In what follows, this model is denoted "pre–bleb formation," while the original model harboring the bleb is denoted "post–bleb formation." Volumetric grids, with the same resolutions and element size distributions, were generated for the pre–bleb formation models of each patient.

Two CFD simulations were carried out for each patient, corresponding to the pre– and post–bleb formation anatomic models. The intraaneurysmal flow patterns were visualized using instantaneous streamlines colored according to the flow velocity magnitude. Maps of wall shear stress magnitude were created to visualize the distribution of shear forces on the aneurysm wall. Inspection of these visualizations revealed that in the majority ($n = 6$) of these aneurysms the bleb formed in a region that was previously exposed to relatively elevated wall shear stress. An example of this type of aneurysm is presented in Figure 3.6b. The regions of highest wall shear stress in the aneurysms were associated with the impaction zone of the inflow jets. However, the sites where the blebs were formed did not necessarily coincide with the maximum of the wall shear stress or the center of the inflow jet impaction zones. The blebs were sometimes found in locations adjacent to the main flow impaction point. The magnitude of the wall shear stress in the regions of elevated WSS varied from patient to patient. However, in these six aneurysms, the blebs coincided with the region of maximal wall shear stress over the aneurysm. Once the blebs were formed, new flow recirculation regions were created inside the blebs and the blebs progressed to a state of lower wall shear stress. In general, the direction of flow recirculation inside the blebs was opposite to the direction of flow recirculation outside the blebs. In one patient, the bleb was found in a location previously subjected to low wall shear stress near the outflow zone of the aneurysm (Figure 3.6c). It was observed that in this case, the inflow jet maintained a fairly coherent and concentrated structure all the way to the outflow zone, while in the other six aneurysms the flow jet dispersed after the primary impaction against the aneurysm wall. As in the previous cases, once the bleb was formed, a new flow recirculation region was created inside the bleb, rotating in the opposite direction to the mean flow in the aneurysm.

In summary, we hypothesize that blebs form as a result of a locally weaken aneurysm wall, or in other words, that the region where blebs form is a marker of focal aneurysm wall injury. The results of this study seem to indicate that the localized injury of the vessel wall may be caused by elevated wall shear stress associated with the inflow jet. However, the final shape of the aneurysm is probably also influenced by the perianeurysmal environment, which can provide extra structural support in the form of contact with structures such as bone or dura matter. Further studies with a larger number of aneurysms and considering the perianeurysmal environment should be carried out to confirm this trend and to better understand the role of hemodynamic forces in the process of aneurysm growth and rupture.

3.6. CONCLUSIONS

Understanding the natural history of cerebral aneurysms is a challenging problem because the mechanisms responsible for their initiation, evolution, possible stabilization, or rupture are influenced by a variety of different factors such as genetics, hemodynamics, wall biomechanics, and perianeurysmal environment. Patient-specific computational models of the hemodynamics of intracranial aneurysms can provide information about the intraaneurysmal flow patterns and wall shear stress distributions. This patient-specific data can be combined with clinical information and observations to better understand the role of hemodynamics in the natural history of brain aneurysms. Connecting hemodynamic variables to clinical events requires population-based studies including large numbers of patient-specific computational models in order to obtain statistically significant results. This, in turn, requires high-throughput computational modeling pipelines that can be used to construct these models in a timely manner. With steady improvements in medical imaging systems, computer hardware and computational modeling software conducting such studies is becoming a reality.

ACKNOWLEDGMENTS

We would like to thank the American Heart Association and Philips Medical Systems for financial support. We would also like to express our gratitude to the work and effort of our collaborators: Marcelo Castro and Rainald Löhner of George Mason University in Fairfax, Virginia; Michael Sheridan and Richard Pergolizzi of Inova Fairfax Hospital in Virginia; and Alejandro Frangi, Alessandro Radaelli, Estanislao Oubel, Mathieu de Crane, and Laura Dempere-Marco of the Pompeu Fabra University in Barcelona, Spain.

REFERENCES

1. Stehbens WE: Intracranial aneurysms, in *Pathology of the Cerebral Blood Vessels*, 1972, pp 351–470.

2. Weir B: Unruptured intracranial aneurysms: A review, *J Neurosurg* **96**:3–42 (2002).

3. Foutrakis GN, Yonas H, Sclabassi RJ: Saccular aneurysm formation in curved and bifurcation arteries, *Am J Neuroradiol* **20**:1309–1317 (1999).

4. Tomasello F et al: Asymptomatic aneurysms. Literature meta-analysis and indications for treatment, *J Neurosurg Sci*, **42**(1):47–51 (1998).

5. Winn HR et al: Of asymptomatic incidental aneurysms: Review of 4568 arteriograms, *J Neurosurg* **96**(1):43–49 (2002).

6. Linn FH et al: Incidence of subarachnoid hemorrhage: Role of region, year, and rate of computed tomography: A meta-analysis, *Stroke* **27**(4):625–629 (1996).

7. Kaminogo M, Yonekura M, Shibata S: Incidence and outcome of multiple intracranial aneurysms in a defined population, *Stroke* **34**(1):16–21 (2003).

8. Kim C et al: In vivo study of flow pattern at human carotid bifurcation with regard to aneurysm development, *Acta Neurochir* (Wien) **115**(3–4):112–117 (1992).

9. Kassell NF et al: The International Cooperative Study on the Timing of Aneurysm Surgery. Part 1: Overall management results, *J Neurosurg* **73**(1):18–36 (1990).

10. Nishioka H et al: Cooperative study of intracranial aneurysms and subarachnoid hemorrhage: A long-term prognostic study. II. Ruptured intracranial aneurysms managed conservatively, *Arch Neurol* **41**(11):1142–1146 (1984).

11. White PM, Wardlaw JM: Unruptured intracranial aneurysms, *J Neuroradiol* **30**(5):336–350 (2003).

12. Kerber CW, Heilman CB: Flow in experimental berry aneurysms: Method and model, *Am J Neuroradiol*, **4**(3):374–377 (1983).

13. Kerber CW, Imbesi SG, Knox K: Flow dynamics in a lethal anterior communicating artery aneurysm, *Am J Neuroradiol* **20**(10):2000–2003 (1999).

14. Gobin YP, Counard JL, Flaud P: In vitro study of haemodynamics in a giant saccular aneurysm model: Influence of flow dynamics in the parent vessel and effects of coil embolization, *Neuroradiology* **36**(7):530–536 (1994).

15. Kyriacou SK, Humphrey JD: Influence of size, shape and properties on the mechanics of axisymmetric saccular aneurysms, *J Biomech* **29**(8):1015–1022 (1996).

16. Ortega HV: Computer simulation helps predict cerebral aneurysms, *J Med Eng Technol* **22**(4):179–181 (1998).

17. Buonocore MH: Visualizing blood flow patterns using streamlines, arrows, and particle paths, *Magn Reson Med* **40**(2):210–226 (1998).

18. Boecher-Schwarz HG et al: Ex vivo study of the physical effect of coils on pressure and flow dynamics in experimental aneurysms, *Am J Neuroradiol* **21**(8):1532–1536 (2000).

19. Groden C et al: Three-dimensional pulsatile flow simulation before and after endovascular coil embolization of a terminal cerebral aneurysm, *J Cereb Blood Flow Metab* **21**(12):1464–1471 (2001).

20. Metcalfe RW: The promise of computational fluid dynamics as a tool for delineating therapeutic options in the treatment of aneurysms, *Am J Neuroradiol* **24**(4):553–554 (2003).

21. Kayembe KNT, Sasahara M, Hazama F: Cerebral aneurysms and variations of the circle of Willis, *Stroke* **15**:846–850 (1984).

22. Nakatani H, Hashimoto N, Kang Y: Cerebral blood flow patterns at major vessel bifurcations and aneurysms in rats, *J Neurosurg* **74**:258–262 (1991).

23. Gonzalez CF, Choi YI, Ortega V: Intracranial aneurysms: Flow analysis of their origin and progression, *Am J Neuroradiol* **13**:181–188 (1992).

24. Burleson AC, Strother CM, Turitto VT: Computer modeling of intracranial saccular and lateral aneurysms for the study of their hemodynamics, *Neurosurgery* **37**:774–784 (1995).

25. Tenjin H, Asakura F, Nakahara Y: Evaluation of intraaneurysmal blood velocity by time-density curve analysis and digital subtraction angiography, *Am J Neuroradiol* **19**:1303–1307 (1998).

26. Ujiie H, Tachibana H, Hiramtsu O: Effects of size and shape (aspect ratio) on the hemodynamics of saccular aneurysms: A possible index for the surgical treatment of intracranial aneurysms, *Neurosurgery* **45**:119–130 (1999).

27. Tateshima S, Murayama Y, Villablanca JP: Intraaneurysmal flow dynamics study featuring an acrylic aneurysm model manufactured using computerized tomography angiogram as a mold, *J Neurosurg* **95**(6):1020–1027 (2001).

28. Satoh T, Onoda K, Tsuchimoto S: Visualization of intraaneurysmal flow patterns with transluminal flow images of 3D MR angiograms in conjunction with aneurysmal configurations, *Am J Neuroradiol* **24**:1436–1445 (2003).

29. Liou TM, Liou SN: A review of in vitro studies of hemodynamic characteristics in terminal and lateral aneurysm models, in *National Scientific Council ROC(B)*, 1999.

30. Butty VD et al: Residence times and basins of attraction for a realistic right internal carotid artery with two aneurysms, *Biorheology* **39**:387–393 (2002).

31. Steinman DA et al: Image-based computational simulation of flow dynamics in a giant intracranial aneurysm, *Am J Neuroradiol* **24**(4):559–566 (2003).

32. Jou LD et al: Computational approach to quantifying hemodynamic forces in giant cerebral aneurysms, *Am J Neuroradiol* **24**(9):1804–1810 (2003).

33. Cebral JR et al: Subject-specific modeling of intracranial aneurysms, in *SPIE (Society of Photo-Optical Instrumentation Engineers) Medical Imaging*, San Diego, CA, 2004.

34. Hassan T et al: Computational simulation of therapeutic parent artery occlusion to treat giant vertebrobasilar aneurysm, *Am J Neuroradiol*, **25**(1):63–68 (2004).

35. Cebral JR et al: Efficient pipeline for image-based patient-specific analysis of cerebral aneurysm hemodynamics: Technique and sensitivity, *IEEE Trans Med Imag* **24**(1):457–467 (2005).

36. Cebral JR, Löhner R: From medical images to anatomically accurate finite element grids, *Int J Num Meth Eng* **51**:985–1008 (2001).

37. Yim PJ et al: A Deformable isosurface and vascular applications, in *SPIE Medical Imaging*, San Diego, CA, 2002.

38. Yim PJ et al: Vessel surface reconstruction with a tubular deformable model, *IEEE Trans Med Imag*, **20**(12):1411–1421 (2001).

39. Cebral JR et al: Merging of intersecting triangulations for finite element modeling, *J Biomech* **34**:815–819 (2001).

40. Taubin G: A signal processing approach to fair surface design, *Comput Graph* 351–358 (1995).

41. Cebral JR et al: Blood flow modeling in carotid arteries using computational fluid dynamics and magnetic resonance imaging, *Acad Radiol* **9**:1286–1299 (2002).

42. Löhner R: Regridding surface triangulations, *J Comput Phys* **126**:1–10 (1996).

43. Löhner R: Automatic unstructured grid generators *Finite Elem Anal Design* **25**:111–134 (1997).

44. Löhner R: Extensions and improvements of the advancing front grid generation technique, *Comput Meth Appl Mech Eng* **5**:119–132 (1996).

45. Casson M: *Rheology of Dispersive Systems*, Pergamon Press, New York, 1959.

46. Perktold K, Peter R, Resch M: Pulsatile non-Newtonian blood flow simulation through a bifurcation with an aneurysm, *Biorheology* **26**(6):1011 (1989).

47. Papanastasiou TC: Flow of materials with yield, *J Rheol* **31**:385–404 (1987).

48. Neofitou P, Drikakis D: Non-Newtonian modeling effects on stenotic channel flows, in *ECCOMAS CFD*, Swansea, Wales, UK 2001.

49. Cebral JR, Löhner R: Efficient simulation of blood flow past complex endovascular devices using an adaptive embedding technique, *IEEE Trans Med Imag* **24**(4):468–477 (2005).

50. Cebral JR et al: Blood flow models of the circle of Willis from magnetic resonance data, *J Eng Math* **47**(3–4):369–386 (2003).

51. Cebral JR et al: Multi-modality image-based models of carotid artery hemodynamics, in *SPIE Medical Imaging*, San Diego, CA, 2004.

52. Womersley JR: Method for the calculation of velocity, rate of flow and viscous drag in arteries when the pressure gradient is known, *J Physiol* **127**:553–563 (1955).

53. Taylor CA, Hughes TJR, Zarins CK: Finite element modeling of blood flow in arteries, *Comput Meth Appl Mech Eng* **158**:155–196 (1998).

54. Tateshima S et al: Three-dimensional blood flow analysis in a wide-necked internal carotid artery-ophthalmic artery aneurysm, *J Neurosurg* **99**(3):526–533 (2003).

55. Vignon-Clementel IE et al: Outflow boundary conditions for three-dimensional finite element modeling of blood flow and pressure in arteries, *Comput Meth Appl Mech Eng* **195**:3776–3796 (2006).

56. Olufsen MS et al: Numerical simulation and experimental validation of blood flow in arteries with structured-tree outflow conditions, *Ann Biomed Eng* **28**:1281–1299 (2000).

57. Formaggia L et al: Multiscale modeling of the circulatory system: A preliminary analysis, *Comput Visual Sci* **2**:75–83 (1999).

58. Zhao SZ et al: Blood flow and vessel mechanics in a physiologically realistic model of a human carotid arterial bifurcation, *J Biomech* **33**:975–984 (2000).

59. Dempere-Marco L et al: Estimation of wall motion in intracranial aneurysms and its effects on hemodynamic patterns, *Lecture Notes Comput Sci* **4191**:438–445 (2006).

60. Dempere-Marco L et al: Wall motion and hemodynamics of intracranial aneurysms, in *World Congress on Biomechanics*, Munich, Germany, 2006.

61. Anayiotos AS et al: Shear stress in a compliant model of the human carotid bifurcation, *J Biomech Eng* **116**:98–106 (1994).

62. Shojima M et al: Magnitude and role of wall shear stress on cerebral aneurysm: Computational fluid dynamic study of 20 middle cerebral artery aneurysms, *Stroke* **35**(11):2500–2505 (2004).

63. Taylor CA, Draney MT: Experimental and computational methods in cardiovascular fluid mechanics, *Ann Rev Fluid Mech* **36**:197–231 (2004).

64. Cebral JR et al: Characterization of cerebral aneurysm for assessing risk of rupture using patient-specific computational hemodynamics models, *Am J Neuroradiol* **26**:2550–2559 (2005).

65. Steiger H et al: Haemodynamic stress in lateral saccular aneurysms: An experimental study, *Acta Neurchir* (Wein) **86**:98–105 (1987).

66. Liepsch DW et al: Hemodynamic stress in lateral saccular aneurysms, *Biorheology* **24**:689–710 (1987).

67. Castro MA, Putman CM, Cebral JR: Computational fluid dynamics modeling of intracranial aneurysms: Effects of parent artery segmentation on intra-aneurysmal hemodynamcis, *Am J Neuroradiol* **27**:1703–1709 (2006).

68. Horiuchi T, Tanaka T, Hongo K: Surgical treatment for aneurysmal subarachnoid hemorrhage in the 8th and 9th decade of life, *Neurosurgery* **56**(3):469–475 (2005).

69. Leipzip TJ, Morgan J, Horner TG: Analysis of intraoperative rupture in the surgical treatment of 1674 saccular aneurysms, *Neurosurgery* **56**(3):455–468 (2005).

70. Brilstra EH, Rinkel GJ, van der Graff Y: Treatment of intracranial aneurysms by embolization with coils: A systematic review, *Stroke* **30**(2):470–476 (1999).

71. Huber P: *Angiography*, Georg Thieme Verlag, Stuttgart, Germany, 1982, pp 79–93.

72. Castro MA, Putman CM, Cebral JR: Patient-specific computational fluid dynamics modeling of anterior communicating artery aneurysms: A study of the sensitivity of intra-aneurysmal flow patterns to flow conditions in the carotid arteries, *Am J Neuroradiol* **27**:2061–2068 (2006).

73. Castro MA, Putman CM, Cebral JR: Patient-specific computational modeling of cerebral aneurysms with multiple avenues of flow from 3D rotational angiography images, *Acad Radiol* **13**(7):811–821 (2006).

74. Castro MA, Putman CM, Cebral JR: Hemodynamic patterns of anterior communicating artery aneurysms: A possible association with rupture, in *SPIE Medical Imaging*, San Diego, CA, 2007.

75. Meng H et al: A model system for mapping vascular responses to complex hemodynamics at arterial bifurcations in vivo, *Neurosurgery* **59**(5):1094–1101 (2006).

76. Oubel E, et al: Analysis of intracranial aneurysm wall motion and its effects on hemodynamic patterns, in *SPIE Medical Imaging*, San Diego, CA, 2007.

77. Hayakawa M et al: CT angiography with electrocardiographically gated reconstruction for visualizing pulsation of intracranial aneurysms: Identification of aneurysmal protuberance presumably associated with wall thinning, *Am J Neuroradiol* **26**:1366–1369 (2005).

78. Cebral JR et al: Hemodynamics before and after bleb formation in cerebral aneurysms, in *SPIE Medical Imaging*, San Diego, CA, 2007.

CHAPTER 4

Prognostic Significance of Aortic Pulse-Wave Velocity

TINE WILLUM HANSEN

Department of Clinical Physiology, Hvidovre Hospital, University of Copenhagen, Hvidovre, Denmark

JØRGEN JEPPESEN

Department of Medicine, Glostrup University Hospital, Glostrup, Denmark

CHRISTIAN TORP-PEDERSEN

Department of Cardiology, Bispelbjerg University Hospital, Copenhagen, Denmark

Abstract. The measurement of aortic pulse-wave velocity (APWV) is generally accepted as the most simple and reproducible method to determine stiffness of the central arteries. There is growing evidence that increased APWV is a risk marker of cardiovascular events beyond traditional risk factors, including blood pressure. This chapter summarizes the exciting literature on the prognostic significance of APWV in studies of patients groups and studies of the general population. The results summarized clearly demonstrate that APWV is a promising risk marker and that APWV probably adds information on future cardiovascular events above traditional risk factors. However, interventions studies are required to determine whether a reduction in APWV is connected with a concomitant reduction in cardiovascular events, independently of the normalization of traditional risk factors.

4.1. INTRODUCTION

A pulse wave traveling through a tube has a traveling speed that depends on the stiffness of the tube, and as stiffness approaches complete rigidity, the speed of the pulse wave approaches that of the speed of light. This rigidity is also an expression of the compliance of the tube—and compliance is simply 1 divided by stiffness. The compliance of the circulation in relation to the pulse waves generated by the heart is determined in large part by the compliance of the

Vascular Hemodynamics: Bioengineering and Clinical Perspectives, Edited by Peter J. Yim
Copyright © 2008 John Wiley & Sons, Inc.

aorta, and therefore the pulse wave velocity of the arterial pulse wave through the aorta is a determinant of the compliance of the arterial bed of the body. Measurement of pulse-wave velocity of the aorta is simple and in practice is done by measuring the delay of the pulse between cutaneous pressure transducers placed on the carotid artery and the femoral artery. The problem inherent to this measurement is that the compliance/stiffness also depends on blood pressure with increasing stiffness and pulse-wave velocity as blood pressure increases. Because of its accessibility, APWV has been used frequently in surveys conducted to determine the prognostic importance of compliance of the vascular system, and because of the inherent relation to blood pressure it is important that such studies also take blood pressure into account when determining the prognostic importance of compliance. In the following we will summarize available studies of APWV for the ability to predict major cardiovascular events. We have subdivided the account into studies of patients groups and studies of the general population. A summary of these studies are provided in Tables 4.1 and 4.2 with focus on adjustment for blood pressure or not.

4.2. STUDIES CONDUCTED IN PATIENTS

There is accumulating evidence that APWV is a marker for risk of cardiovascular morbidity and mortality in patients with hypertension, renal disease, or diabetes, and in elderly hospitalized patients.

The first publication came in 1999 from Blacher et al. [1]. This study was conducted in 241 patients with end-stage renal disease. Subjects with clinical cardiovascular disease within the last 6 months were excluded. In this cohort, mean age was 51.5 ± 16.3 years, and 48% were on antihypertensive drug treatment. Information on all-causes and cardiovascular mortality was recorded, and during a mean follow-up of 6.0 ± 3.4 years, 73 deaths were documented, and 48 of these were cardiovascular. APWV was not studied as a continuous variable, but the cohort was divided into tertiles of APWV.

The odds ratio (95% confidence interval) adjusted for other significant risk factors [age, hemoglobin, and diastolic blood pressure (negative association)] was 5.4 (2.4–11.9) for subjects with PWV $\geq$ 12.0 m/s (upper tertile) when compared to subjects with PWV $\leq$ 9.4 m/s (lower tertile) for all-cause mortality and 5.9 (2.3–15.5) for cardiovascular mortality.

In 2003, the next paper from the same cohort was published [2], and here follow-up was extended to 6.5 ± 3.8 years and one more patient was included; 91 deaths were documented, 58 were cardiovascular. In that paper, the predictive value of APWV index was examined. A "control" population of 469 subjects without end-stage renal disease but comparable in terms of age, mean blood pressure, and gender was studied to obtain mean and range of APWV compared to the end-stage renal disease population. A theoretical APWV value was then calculated from multivariate analyses, including age, mean blood pressure, heart rate, and gender. APWV index was then computed as (measured APWV−theoretical APWV).

TABLE 4.1. Studies Conducted in Patients

First Authors (Year, Country) [Reference]	Number of Subjects	Mean Age (years)	Years of Follow-up	Outcome (Number of Events)[a]	Adjustments for Blood Pressure	Excluding Subjects with Previous CV Disease
Blacher (1999, France) [1]	241	51.5	6.0	All-cause (73) and CV mortality (48)	Yes	Yes
Blacher (2003, France) [2]	242	52	6.5	All-cause (91) and CV mortality (58)	No, but APWV was studied as index	Yes
Laurent (2001, France) [3]	1980	50	9.3	All-cause (107) and CV mortality (46)	No	No, but in a sensitivity analysis
Boutouyrie (2002, France) [4]	1045	51	5.7	Fatal and nonfatal CHD (53) and a combined CV endpoint (97)	Yes	Yes
Laurent (2003, France) [5]	1715	51	7.9	Fatal stroke (25)	Yes	Yes
Meaume (2001, France) [6]	141	87.1	2.5	All-cause (56) and CV mortality (27)	Yes	No
Cruickshank(2002, UK) [7]	571	60	10	All-cause mortality (219)	Yes	No

[a]CV, and CHD indicate cardiovascular and coronary heart disease, respectively.

TABLE 4.2. Studies Conducted in Subjects from the General Population

First Authors (Year, Country) [Reference]	Number of Subjects	Mean Age (years)	Years of Follow-up	Outcome (Number of Events)[a]	Adjustments for Blood Pressure	Excluding Subjects with Previous CV Disease
Shokawa (2005, Japan) [8]	492	63.7	10	All-cause (43) and CV mortality (14)	Yes	No
Sutton-Tyrrell (2005, USA) [9]	2488	73.7	4.6	All-cause (265) and CV mortality (111), fatal and nonfatal CHD (341), stroke (94), or CHF (181)	Yes	No
Mattace-Raso (2006, Netherlands) [10]	2835	71.7	4.1	Fatal or nonfatal CHD (101) or stroke (63)	Yes	Yes
Hansen (2006, Denmark) [11]	1678	54.8	9.4	CV mortality (62), fatal and nonfatal CHD (101), and a combined CV endpoint (154)	Yes	Yes

[a]CV, CHD and CHF indicate cardiovascular, coronary heart disease, and congestive heart failure respectively.

This index was shown to predict all-cause and cardiovascular mortality after adjustment for other significant risk factors (age, hemoglobin, and time on dialysis before inclusion). The adjusted hazard ratios associated with 1 m/s increase in APWV index were 1.14 (1.05–1.24) for all-causes mortality and 1.14 (1.03–1.26) for cardiovascular mortality. Additionally, it was shown that pulse pressure did not predict all-cause or cardiovascular mortality in adjusted analyses that included APWV index.

Another group that has contributed to the clarification of the predictive value of APWV includes Boutouyrie P, Laurent S, and colleagues from Paris. They have considered a cohort of outpatients with mild essential hypertension. The patients were recruited from the hypertension clinic of Hospital Broussais. In their first publication from 2001, they studied the risk of all-cause and cardio vascular mortality [3], in their 2002 publication they considered risk of fatal and nonfatal primary coronary events [4], and finally in 2003 they studied risk of fatal stroke [5].

In the 2001 paper [3], the cohort included 1980 patients, 182 of whom had a history of cardiovascular disease. Mean age was 50 ± 13 years, and mean follow-up was 9.3 ± 4.4 years. The endpoints considered were all-cause and cardiovascular mortality.

Multivariate adjustment included variables significant in univariate analyses, but APWV was not adjusted for any blood pressure component. Thus, APWV, pulse pressure, and systolic blood pressure were examined in three separate models. The adjusted odds ratios for APWV were 1.34 (1.04–1.74) for all-causes mortality and 1.51 (1.08–2.11) for cardiovascular mortality for each 5 m/s increase. Systolic blood pressure was predictive only of cardiovascular mortality with a hazard ratio of 1.15 (1.02–1.30) for each 10 mmHg increase of blood pressure, and pulse pressure was not predictive for any of the endpoints studied ($p \geq .06$). The outcome analyses after exclusion of the 182 subjects with a history of cardiovascular disease is reported in a sensitivity analyses, but only unadjusted results are described, here APWV was a significant ($p = .01$) predictor of cardiovascular mortality.

In the 2002 paper [4], the cohort included only 1045 patients; thus it was a subset of the previously published cohort (excluding 766 subjects without medical follow-up and 169 subjects with previous cardiovascular disease). Mean age was 51 years, and mean follow-up was reduced to 5.7 years. The paper examined the risk of fatal and nonfatal coronary events ($n = 53$) and also a combined cardiovascular endpoint ($n = 97$) consisting of fatal and nonfatal coronary events, strokes, abdominal aortic aneurysm, peripheral arterial disease, hypertension-related nephroangiosclerosis, and heart failure.

In multivariate analyses, APWV was adjusted for traditional cardiovascular risk factors in addition to either mean arterial pressure and pulse pressure, or systolic and diastolic blood pressure. Models were also formulated where APWV exclusively was adjusted for the Framingham Risk Score. In all of these models, APWV remained a significant predictor for coronary events ($p < .04$), but lost significance for the combined endpoint when adjusted for classical risk factors and blood pressure components ($p = .06$). While adjusting for the Framingham Risk Score, APWV was a predictor for the combined cardiovascular endpoint ($p = .04$). Similar results were obtained when APWV was analyzed in tertiles. However, when only subjects belonging to the first and second tertile of FRS (low-risk group) was analyzed, APWV was a significant predictor of all of the endpoints no matter what adjustment applied. In contrast, pulse pressure and systolic blood pressure lost significance in multivariate analyses including APWV.

In the last paper from 2003 [5], the cohort included 1715 patients, excluding 265 subjects with previous cardiovascular disease. Mean age was 51 ± 13 years, and mean follow-up was 7.9 years. Information on fatal stroke ($n = 25$) was recorded. In analyses adjusted for traditional cardiovascular risk factors in addition to either mean arterial pressure and pulse pressure or systolic and diastolic blood pressure, APWV remained a significant risk factor (relative risk per 4 m/s increase was 1.39 (1.08–1.72); $p = .02$). Pulse pressure was, on the other hand, not a significant predictor of fatal stroke in adjusted models.

In another study from 2001 [6], Meaume et al. followed 141 elderly subjects aged 70–100 years (mean 87.1 ± 6.6 years). The subjects were patients hospitalized in three geriatrics departments in a Paris suburb and 42% had a history of cardiovascular disease.

After 2.5 years of follow-up, information on all-cause and cardiovascular mortality was acquired. In total, 56 deaths were recorded, and 27 of the deaths were classified as cardiovascular.

Logistics regression was applied, and the odds ratio for 1 m/s increase in APWV was 1.19 (1.03–1.37) for cardiovascular mortality in a model also including systolic blood pressure, mean arterial pressure, and other significant risk factors. Notably, systolic blood pressure and pulse pressure were not significant predictors of cardiovascular mortality in this population. APWV was not a predictor of all-cause mortality in this population. When APWV was divided into classes, applying either a threshold of 17.7 m/s (according to the upper decile) or 20 m/s (5% of the population), adjusted odds ratios were 4.60 (1.4–15.7) and 8.8 (1.5–50.9), respectively, for being in the class of subjects with APWV above the threshold.

Cruickshank et al. suggested in a paper published in 2002 [7] that APWV was an integrated index of vascular risk factors (e.g., duration of hypertension or diabetes), which could precede the development of cardiovascular disease. He studied a cohort mixed of 397 patients with known type 2 diabetes selected from an outpatient's clinic and 174 subjects randomly selected from the population. All subjects from the population sample were given a glucose tolerance test and afterward divided into those with normal and with glucose intolerance. Mean age in the total population was 60 [95% confidence interval (CI) 59–61] years. Information on mortality was obtained after a median follow-up around 10 years, and the endpoint considered was all-cause mortality. Subjects with ECG changes coded by Minnesota coding as ischemic heart disease were included.

In a model including other cardiovascular risk factors, APWV remained a significant risk factor [relative risk: 1.08 (1.03–1.14), $p = .001$ per 1 m/s increase], and it displaced systolic blood pressure ($p = .34$) as a marker of risk. This indicates that when measurement of APWV is present, then measurement of systolic blood pressure does not provide any further information about risk of cardiovascular disease. The interpretation of this observation could be that aortic stiffness is the cause of systolic hypertension, but another interpretation could be that several risk factors, such as high cholesterol, smoking, diabetes, and high blood pressure, damage the aorta over time, and an increased aortic stiffness then represents real subclinical vascular disease, such as an increased intima–media thickness, and therefore APWV comes out as a stronger risk factor for cardiovascular disease than does systolic blood pressure.

4.3. STUDIES IN SUBJECTS FROM THE GENERAL POPULATION

All studies conducted in the general population have been published since 2005.

The first study, from 2005, was conducted in a small cohort of 492 Japanese inhabitant of Hawaii [8]. The sample included an almost equal number of women and men, and the mean age was 63.7 ± 8.8 years. Subjects with ECG abnormality were included in the analyses. The cohort was followed for around 10 years, but only information on mortality was collected. From a total number of 43 deaths just 14 were classified as attributable to a cardiovascular cause.

APWV was handled both as a categorical and as a continues variable. The cutoff point for the categorical analyses was 9.9 m/s according to the receiver operating characteristic (ROC) curve. On the basis of unadjusted survival curves, the risk of all-cause mortality was higher in subjects with APWV above the cutoff point, but after adjustment for other risk factors APWV lost its significance when analyzed as both a categorical and as a continuous variable.

According to cardiovascular mortality, APWV analyzed as dichotomized variable was a significant predictor also after adjustment for traditional cardiovascular risk factors including systolic blood pressure, but APWV was not a predictor when analyzed as a continuous variable. However, because of the few subjects and number of events, the power to detect a significant prediction was limited in this study.

The next paper [9] included subjects from the Health, Aging, and Body Composition (Health ABC) Study. A total of 2488 elderly subjects aged 70–79 years randomly requited from Pittsburgh and Memphis were included. All participants were without life-treating illness but 642 patients with known cardiovascular disease (25.8%) were included. Median follow-up was 4.6 years, and information on mortality as well as morbidity was collected. The endpoints considered were all-causes mortality, cardiovascular mortality, fatal and nonfatal coronary heart disease, stroke, or congestive heart failure. The Kaplan–Meier survival curves indicated that the risk sharply increased between quartiles 1 and 2, particularly in relation to cardiovascular events. APWV was thus analyzed divided into gender-specific quartiles. In adjusted analyses, including systolic blood pressure, age, sex, site, and race, the relative risk for subjects belonging to the highest quintile compared to subjects belonging to the lowest quintile was significant for coronary heart disease and stroke, but not for congestive heart failure. After further adjustment for smoking, physical activity, hemoglobin A_{1c}, and heart rate, the risk was significant only for stroke [relative risk for highest vs. lowest quintile was 2.76 (1.33–5.74)]. Inclusion of mean arterial pressure or pulse pressure instead of systolic blood pressure did not change the results. APWV was not a predictor of congestive heart failure, not even in unadjusted analyses. Pulse pressure was, however, a predictor of congestive heart failure also in adjusted analyses.

The limitations of this study were risk-of-survival bias due to the older age in the population and the fact the subjects with previous cardiovascular disease were included. The present of prior cardiovascular disease might interfere with the results due to changes in blood pressure in relation to the cardiovascular disease.

In the same issue of *Circulation* from 2006, the next two population-based studies were published. One was from Rotterdam [10] and the other, from Copenhagen [11]. The Rotterdam study [10] included 2835 randomly recruited women and men. All the participants were older than 55 years and mean age was 71.7 ± 6.7 years. Patients with a history of coronary heart disease and stroke were excluded. During a mean follow-up of 4.1 years, 101 events of fatal or nonfatal coronary heart disease were recorded; and during a mean of 3.2 years, 63 subjects developed fatal or nonfatal stroke. APWV was studied in gender-specific tertiles, and there was a significantly higher risk for all of the endpoint except for all-causes mortality in the third tertile compared to the first tertile in adjusted models, including age, gender, mean arterial pressure, and heart rate. However, in the fully adjusted model also including other cardiovascular risk factors, carotid IMT, ankle–arm index, and pulse pressure, APWV lost significance for stroke ($p = .06$), but remained significant for the combined cardiovascular endpoint ($p = .04$) and for coronary heart disease ($p = .02$). The area under the ROC curve for the combined cardiovascular endpoint increased from 0.70 to 0.72 when APWV was added to a model including established cardiovascular risk factors, carotid IMT, ankle–arm index, and pulse pressure.

In the study from Copenhagen [11], a randomly recruited cohort of 1678 women and men free from previous myocardial infarction or stroke were followed for a median of 9.4 years. Information on fatal as well as nonfatal events was recorded. The endpoints considered were a combination of cardiovascular events ($n = 154$), coronary heart disease ($n = 101$), and cardiovascular mortality ($n = 62$). Mean age was 54.8 ± 10.6 years. In this cohort, information on ambulatory blood pressure was available. Ambulatory blood pressure monitoring is by far superior to conventional blood pressure measurement in the prediction of cardiovascular events and risk stratification [12–14]. In analyses adjusted for other cardiovascular risk factors and mean arterial pressure measured in the office, APWV was a significant predictor of the combined endpoint ($p = .01$), cardiovascular mortality ($p = .03$), and coronary heart disease ($p = .05$). For each standard deviation (SD) increment in APWV (3.4 m/s), the risk of an event increased by 16–20%. With similar adjustment applied, the office and 24-h pulse pressure lost their prognostic value with the exception of office pulse pressure in relation to coronary heart disease. When the above model was adjusted for 24-h mean arterial pressure instead of the office measurement, APWV was still a predictor of the combined endpoint ($p = .02$); however, APWV lost significance for cardiovascular mortality ($p = .12$), and coronary heart disease ($p = .09$), due to a widening of the confidence intervals.

4.4. CONCLUSIONS

The progression of atherosclerosis can be slowed by a number of pharmacological agents and possibly with lifestyle modifications. Thus, markers that can recognize the vascular disease in asymptomatic individuals could facilitate suitable intervention. The results summarized in this chapter clearly demonstrate that APWV is a promising risk marker and that it probably adds information on future cardiovascular events above traditional risk factors. However, some important issues have to be mentioned. First, validated normal values applicable to the individual patient have to be established. Also, because of the inherent relation between distending blood pressure and APWV, it is important to standardize APWV to the present blood pressure. Next, since changes in APWV are influenced mainly by long-term structural modifications in the arterial wall, it is not a sensitive measure of short-term changes in relation to intervention. Finally, and very importantly, intervention studies are required to determine whether a reduction in APWV is connected with a concomitant reduction in cardiovascular events, independently of the normalization of traditional cardiovascular risk factors.

REFERENCES

1. Blacher J, Guerin AP, Pannier B, Marchais SJ, Safar ME, London GM: Impact of aortic stiffness on survival in end-stage renal disease, *Circulation* **99**:2434–2439 (1999).
2. Blacher J, Safar M, Guerin AP, Pannier B, Marchais SJ, London GM: Aortic pulse wave velocity index and mortality in end-stage renal disease, *Kidney Int* **63**:1852–1860 (2003).
3. Laurent S, Boutouyrie P, Asmar R, Gautier I, Laloux B, Guize L, Ducimetière P, Benetos A: Aortic stiffness is an independent predictor of all-cause and cardiovascular mortality in hypertensive patients, *Hypertension* **37**:1236–1241 (2001).
4. Boutouyrie P, Tropeano AI, Asmar R, Gautier I, Benetos A, Lacolley P, Laurent S: Aortic stiffness is an independent predictor of primary coronary events in hypertensive patients. A longitudinal study, *Hypertension* **39**:10–15 (2002).
5. Laurent S, Katsahian S, Fassot C, Tropeano AI, Gautier I, Laloux B, Boutouyrie P: Aortic stiffness is an independent predictor of fatal stroke in essential hypertension, *Stroke* **34**:1203–1206 (2003).

6. Meaume S, Rudnichi A, Lynch A, Bussy C, Sebban C, Benetos A, Safar ME: Aortic pulse wave velocity as a marker of cardiovascular disease in subjects over 70 years old, *J Hypertens* **19**:871–877 (2001).

7. Cruickshank K, Riste L, Anderson SG, Wright JS, Dunn G, Gosling RG: Aortic pulse-wave velocity and its relationship to mortality in diabetes and glucose intolerance: An integrated index of vascular function? *Circulation* **106**:2085–2090 (2002).

8. Shokawa T, Imazu M, Yamamoto H, Toyofuku M, Tasaki N, Okimoto T, Yamane K, Kohno N: Pulse wave velocity predicts cardiovascular mortality: Findings from the Hawaii-Los Angeles-Hiroshima study, *Circ J* **69**:259–264 (March 2005).

9. Sutton-Tyrrell K, Najjar SS, Boudreau RM, Venkitachalam L, Kupelian V, Simonsick EM, Havlik R, Lakatta EG, Spurgeon H, Kritchevsky S, Pahor M, Bauer D, Newman A: For the health ABC study: Elevated aortic pulse wave velocity, a marker of arterial stiffness, predicts cardiovascular events in well-functioning older adults, *Circulation* **111**:3384–3390 (2005).

10. Mattace-Raso F, van der Cammen T, Hofman A, van Poppel NM, Bos ML, Schalekamp MADH, Asmar R, Reneman RS, Hoeks APG, Breteler M, Witteman JCM: Arterial stiffness and risk of coronary heart disease and stroke, *Circulation* **113**:657–663 (2006).

11. Hansen TW, Staessen AJ, Torp-Pedersen C, Rasmussen S, Thijs L, Ibsen H, Jeppesen J: Prognostic value of aortic pulse wave velocity as index of arterial stiffness in the general population, *Circulation* **113**:664–670 (2006).

12. Hansen TW, Jeppesen J, Rasmussen S, Ibsen H, Torp-Pedersen C: Ambulatory blood pressure and mortality: A population based study, *Hypertension* **45**:499–504 (2005).

13. Clement DL, De Buyzere ML, De Bacquer DA, de Leeuw PW, Duprez DA, Fagard RH, Gheeraert PJ, Missault LH, Braun JJ, Six RO, Van der Niepen P, O'Brien E: For the Office versus Ambulatory Pressure Study Investigators: Prognostic value of ambulatory blood-pressure recordings in patients with treated hypertension, *N Engl J Med* **348**:2407–2415 (2003).

14. Dolan E, Stanton A, Thijs L, Hinedi K, Atkins N, McClory S, Den Hond E, McCormack P, Staessen JA, O'Brien E: Superiority of ambulatory over clinic blood pressure measurement in predicting mortality. The Dublin Outcome Study, *Hypertension* **46**:156–161 (2005).

CHAPTER 5

Closed-Loop Modeling of the Circulatory System

CAROL L. LUCAS and RANDALL COLE

Department of Biomedical Engineering and Surgery, University of North Carolina at Chapel Hill, Chapel Hill, North Carolina

AJIT YOGANATHAN

Department of Biomedical Engineering, Georgia Institute of Technology, Atlanta, Georgia

Abstract. The history of modern medicine begins with William Harvey's 1628 advancement of the revolutionary theory that blood circulates repeatedly throughout the body in a unidirectional manner within a closed loop system, with the heart acting as a pump and with flow reversal impeded by one way valves. While Harvey's work provided the conceptual framework for closed loop models of the circulatory system, quantitative models were relatively slow to develop, with earliest efforts being advanced by the work of Hales (1711) and Otto Frank (1899), who envisioned the systemic circulation as a fireman's water pump or an air kettle (*windkessel*), respectively. Both concepts can be modeled by a capacitor (mimicking the compliance of large arterial walls) acting in paralle with a resistor (mimicking the downstream resistance). The goal of this chapter is to provide a wide variety of examples in which a closed loop model has been developed to address a particular physiological problem. Models range in complexity from those combining a single ventricle with a simple windkessel-type load to those that add the right ventricle, artia and separate vascular beds (e.g., head, coronary, legs, etc.). Additional features include the effects of interacting ventricles, respiration, gravity, and pleural pressures. Coverage is limited to models that have electrical analogs and can be described mathematically with ordinary differential equations. Though advances in computer technologies enable investigators to generate models with an unlimited number of parameters, the best model is the simplest that will promote understanding of the problem of interest.

Vascular Hemodynamics: Bioengineering and Clinical Perspectives, Edited by Peter J. Yim
Copyright © 2008 John Wiley & Sons, Inc.

5.1. INTRODUCTION

When writing about the history of modern medicine, historians usually begin with the work of William Harvey, an English physician, who in 1628 was the first to publicly advance the theory that blood circulates repeatedly throughout the body in a unidirectional manner within a closed-loop system, with the heart acting as a pump and with flow reversal impeded by one-way valves [1,2]. Harvey's theory was revolutionary and initially quite controversial, as the accepted concept at that time was still based on the teachings of an ancient Greek physician, Galen (Galenos of Pergamon, 129–200 AD), who believed that blood was made from food by the liver, consumed by the organs and flowed from one ventricle to the other through tiny pores, with the ventricles "sucking" rather than "pumping" [3]. Acceptance of Harvey's theory was advanced in 1660, when the Italian anatomist Malpighi, with the use of a microscope, discovered the capillaries that connect the arteries to the veins, a connection that was assumed by Harvey but that he could not explain [4].

While Harvey's work provided the conceptual framework for closed-loop models of the circulatory system, quantitative models were relatively slow to develop. Nearly 100 years later (1711), Stephen Hales, a clergyman and English naturalist, observed that the relationship between the relatively steady blood flow at the tissue level and the pulsatile flow exiting the beating heart was similar to that observed when firefighters were able to produce a steady jet by hand-pumping water into a high-pressure air chamber [5]. In addition to his pioneering work in plant physiology and the famous experiment in which he was the first to measure blood pressure by measuring the vertical height of a fluid column originating from a pipe placed in the crural artery of a supine horse, Hales pioneered the concept of peripheral resistance in tiny blood vessels [5–7].

In 1899, the German physiologist Otto Frank expanded the neglected work of Stephen Hale and the air cushion Hale used to describe the buffering within the fire engines became an air kettle or *windkessel* [8]. In its simplest form, the windkessel theory considers the impedance of the systemic circulation (afterload) against which the heart pumps to consist of a lumped compliance element (cushion of air) and a lumped resistance (the downstream hose). Frank's research with the isolated frog heart enabled him to recognize that the amount of ventricular filling and the downstream load against which the ventricle pumps each affect the contractility of the ventricle. Ernest Starling later expanded this view in a statement of the Frank–Starling law of the heart, which says that "within physiological limits, the larger the volume of the heart, the greater are the energy of its contraction and the amount of chemical change at each contraction" [2].

Although the contributions of Harvey, Hale, Frank, and Starling are highlighted above, the efforts of numerous scientists provided the quantitative tools that are fundamental to today's circulatory system modelers, including the Hagen–Poiseuille equation relating resistance to laminar flow and the Moens–Korteweg and Newton–Young equations for relating pulse-wave velocity to vessel wall properties [9]. Modelers are likewise indebted to advances made concurrently by nonphysiologists who developed equations to describe fluid flow, such as the transmission line equations attributed to Maxwell, Kelvin, and Heaviside and the Navier–Stokes equations that are applicable to all fluid flow situations.

The goal of this chapter is to provide the reader with a wide variety of examples in which a closed-loop model of the circulatory system was developed to address a particular physiological problem. Models will range in complexity from those combining a single ventricle with a simple windkessel-type load, termed a "closed-loop model of the systemic circulation," to those that isolate individual vessel segments and vascular beds. Coverage will be limited to models that have electrical analogs and can be described mathematically with ordinary differential equations. Although advances in computer technologies enable investigators to generate models with an unlimited number of parameters, the best model is the simplest one that will promote understanding of the problem of interest.

Examples will be presented in increasing order of complexity. The framework presented in Table 5.1 will serve as a checklist when considering model features.

Readers interested in following an instructional development of lumped-parameter models of increasing complexity to mimic the circulatory system are encouraged to refer to the textbook by Rideout entitled *Mathematical and Computer Modeling of Physiological Systems* [10].

5.2. CLOSED-LOOP MODELS OF THE SYSTEMIC CIRCULATION

Closed-loop models of the systemic circulation designed to study the coupling of the left ventricle to the peripheral circulation commonly share four features: (1) a windkessel-type load, (2) a beating ventricle, (3) representations of the mitral and/or aortic valves, and (4) flow return through some representation of the venous pool.

The Vascular Load

The original windkessel (Figure 5.1a) can be represented in open-loop configurations as a resistor and a capacitor acting in parallel. The resister represents the resistance of small arteries and arterioles, and the capacitor represents the elastic properties of the large arteries. The original windkessel has undergone several modifications.

The first, attributed to Westerhof and sometimes termed the "westkessel" (Figure 5.1b), positioned a resistor between the ventricle and the RC parallel circuit [11,12]. This element, termed *characteristic impedance* (Z_0), is based on wave transmission theory, in which Z_0 is defined as the impedance of a line in the absence of wave reflections and is routinely estimated by averaging modulus values at high frequencies. The added impedance accounts for the local inertia and local compliance of the proximal ascending aorta. This configuration addressed the two major shortcomings of the original two-element windkessel in matching

TABLE 5.1. Checklist for Closed-Loop Model of the Circulatory System

---

Closed-loop Configuration
    Systemic circulation
      Original windkessel afterload
      Modified windkessel afterload
    Systemic and pulmonary circulations in series
      Systemic vascular beds
        Single bed
        Body and head
          Lumped body
          Gastrointestinal tract and legs
          Splanchnic, renal, and legs
        Coronary bed
      Pulmonary vascular beds
        Single bed
        Right lung and left lung

Heart Representation
    Beating
      Time-varying elastance
      Model based on Starling principles
      Modifications based on work of others, such as Suga and Sagawa
    Chambers modeled
      Left ventricle
        Right atrium
      Left ventricle and right ventricle
        No interaction between ventricles
        Interaction between ventricles
      Right and left atria
    Nonbeating, considered as a constant pressure/flow source

Other Features
    Respiration effects
    Pleural pressure effects
    Gravitational effects
    Subjects for which parameter sets apply
      Humans: adults versus children
      Animals: dogs, sheep, pigs, and so on

---

the characteristics of physiologically measured systemic input impedance at high frequencies: (1) the model amplitude settled at high frequencies to Z_0 compared to the zero value mandated by the two-element model and (2) the model phase delay settled at high frequencies to $0°$ compared to $-90°$ as mandated by the two-element model.

Other modifications have added an inertial term to improve model performance. A four-element model (Figure 5.1c), originated by Burattini and Gnudi

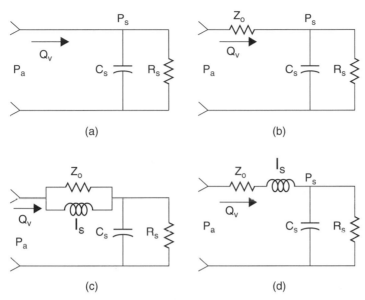

Figure 5.1. Commonly used ventricular afterload configurations [18]: (a) the original two-element windkessel [large-vessel compliance (c) in parallel with peripheral vascular resistance (R)]; (b) three-element westkessel [with the addition of characteristic impedance (Z_0)]; (c) four-element system adding an inertial term in parallel with Z_0; (d) four-element system adding an inertial term in series with Z_0.

[13] and further developed by Campbell et al. [14] and Stergiopulos et al. [15], placed the inertial term in parallel with the characteristic impedance. The element represented the inertia of the entire arterial system and, because of its parallel position, came into play at low frequencies, with Z_0 continuing to dominate at mid–high frequencies. This parallel arrangement of Z_0 and the inertial element was shown to be superior in matching many details of the arterial pressure waveforms.

Placing the inertial term in series with characteristic impedance (Figure 5.1d) [16], likewise has the desired effect at low frequencies but dominates the spectrum at high frequencies, with the impedance modulus increasing linearly and the phase angles approaching $+90°$. Although this has not been observed in vivo, the configuration is applicable to hydraulic systems in which the outflow from the pumping mechanism, whether it is a pulsatile pump, an isolated heart preparation, or an artificial heart, is mechanically coupled to a hydraulic load [17].

The input impedance of the preceding models using the equations below and parameter values obtained from Cole et al. [18] are illustrated in Figure 5.2.

Original windkessel:

$$H(f) = \frac{R_s}{R_s C_s (j2\pi f) + 1} \tag{5.1}$$

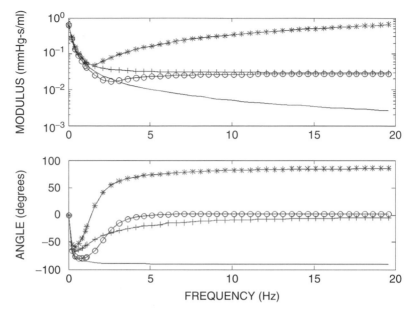

Figure 5.2. Input impedance spectra calculated for the four afterloads illustrated in Figure 5.1: (a) equation (5.1) (--------), (b) equation (5.2) (-+-+-+-), (c) equation (5.3) (-o-o-o-), and (d) equation (5.4) (-*-*-*-). Upper panel: Modulus in mmHg·s/mL. Lower panel: phase shifts in degrees. (Values for model parameters were taken from Cole et al. [18].)

Westkessel:

$$H(f) = Z_0 + \frac{R_s}{R_s C_s (j2\pi f) + 1} \tag{5.2}$$

Burattini four-element:

$$H(f) = \frac{Z_0 L_s (j2\pi f)}{L_s (j2\pi f) + Z_0} + \frac{R_s}{R_s C_s (j2\pi f) + 1} \tag{5.3}$$

Waldman four-element:

$$H(f) = Z_0 + L_s (j2\pi f) + \frac{R_s}{R_s C_s (j2\pi f) + 1} \tag{5.4}$$

Other configurations introducing inertial terms have also been found useful in modeling the load on the right ventricle. Engelberg and DuBois replaced the characteristic impedance with an inertial term [19]. Shaw split the compliance into near and distal components and placed the inertial term in the middle [20]. Neither match high-frequency components well, with the inertial term dominating in the Engelberg model as in the Cole model and with the large artery compliance term dominating in the Shaw model as in the original windkessel.

The Ventricle

In the models considered in this chapter, pulsatile pressure and flow were created by one of two mechanisms: (1) a time-varying elastance or (2) a pressure source. Both techniques produce realistic results and have been used extensively. As will be obvious from the following examples, the two mechanisms, although considered philosophically different, yield almost identical results once implemented.

Pulsatile pressure is generated in time-varying elastance models via functions that alternate between systolic (stiff) and diastolic (relaxed) ventricular elastances. Three examples are illustrated in Figure 5.3.

The first, attributed to Rideout, is shaped by two sinusoidal harmonics [10]. Heart period (T) and systolic time (T_s) are independent model variables:

$$E(t) = E_{syst} \min\left(1.0, \, 0.9 \sin\left(\frac{\pi t}{T_s}\right) - 0.3 \sin\left(\frac{2\pi t}{T_s}\right)\right) \quad 0 \leq t \leq T_s$$

$$= E_{diast} \quad\quad\quad\quad\quad\quad\quad\quad\quad\quad\quad T_s < t < T \quad (5.5)$$

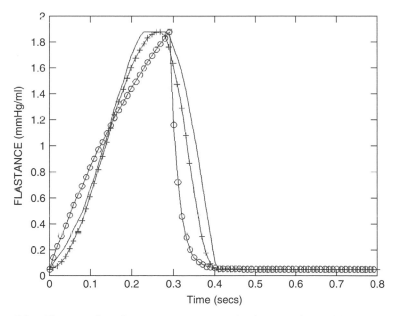

Figure 5.3. Time-varying elastance curves created using equations (5.5) (--------) [10], (5.6) (-+--+--+-) [21] and (5.7) (-o-o-o-) [22]. Parameters were selected to obtain identical maximum (1.88 mm Hg/mL) and minimum (0.05 mmHg/mL) values for the three models.

The second, attributed to Heldt, achieves a similar waveform using cosine functions [21]. The heart period is divided into three segments: T_s is calculated from the heart period via the Bazett formula, $T_s(n) = 0.3\sqrt{T(n-1)}$; $T(n)$ is the heart period of the nth beat.

$$
\begin{aligned}
E(t) &= E_{\text{diast}} + \frac{E_{\text{syst}} - E_{\text{diast}}}{2}\left(1 - \cos\left(\frac{\pi t}{0.3\sqrt{T(n-1)}}\right)\right) & 0 \le t \le T_s \\
&= E_{\text{diast}} + \frac{E_{\text{syst}} - E_{\text{diast}}}{2}\left(1 + \cos\left(\frac{2\pi t - 0.3\sqrt{T(n-1)}}{0.3\sqrt{T(n-1)}}\right)\right) & T_s < t \le \tfrac{3}{2}T_s \\
&= E_{\text{diast}} & \tfrac{3}{2}T_s < t < T
\end{aligned}
$$

$$(5.6)$$

where $T(n-1) = $ length of previous beat.

The third example, attributed to Sun et al. [22], achieves a somewhat different shape with exponential functions with different time constants before (τ_c) and after (τ_R) peak elastance is reached, reflecting the different elastances of the ventricle during systole and diastole respectively:

$$
\begin{aligned}
E(t) &= E_{\text{diast}} + E_{\text{syst}}\left(1 - e^{-t/\tau_c}\right) & 0 \le t \le T_s \\
&= E_{\text{diast}} + (E(T_s) - E_{\text{diast}})e^{-(t-T_x)/\tau_r} & T_s < t \le T
\end{aligned}
\qquad (5.7)
$$

Comparable to the time-varying elastance models, pressure source models, which have been attributed to Frank's observation that ventricular pressure in the isovolumic frog heart increased with volume, incorporate diastolic and systolic components. The diastolic component P_d is a function of volume, while the systolic component P_s depends on time and volume; P_s functions are typically separated into the product of a volume dependent component and a time-varying, volume-independent activation function F. Expressions typically are of the form

$$
P(t, V_v) = P_d(V) + P_s(t, V) = P_d(V) + P_{\text{sv}}(V)F(t) \qquad (5.8)
$$

Pressure $P_d(v)$ is represented by equations that attempt to fit the diastolic portion of the chamber's pressure–volume loop. Parabolic and exponential fits have been used, for example [23–25]

$$
P_d(V) = a(V_v - b)^2 \qquad (5.9)
$$

$$
= \gamma + \beta e^{\alpha V(t)} \qquad (5.10)
$$

$$
= A(e^{\lambda(V-b)} - 1) \qquad (5.11)
$$

where b represents an unstressed volume. Likewise, the volume-dependent component of the P_s segment has an elastance component and an offset; for example,

$$
P_{\text{sv}}(V) = cV - d \qquad (5.12)
$$

The optimal form of the activating function, which is a bell-shaped function that varies between 0 and 1, has been the object of much attention. One widely used $F(t)$ configuration, attributed to Mulier, Palladino, and colleagues, is the product of two exponentials that have time constants related to contraction and relaxation [26]

$$F(t) = \frac{\left(1 - e^{-(t/\tau_r)^\alpha}\right)\left(e^{-((t-t_h)/\tau_r)^\alpha}\right)}{\left(1 - e^{-(t_p/\tau_c)^\alpha}\right)\left(e^{-((t_p-t_b)/\tau_r)^\alpha}\right)} \tag{5.13}$$

where t_p is the time chosen for peak activation; t_b is then calculated by obtaining $F'(t)$ and setting the value equal to zero:

$$t_b = t_p \left(1 - \left(\frac{\tau_r}{\tau_c}\right)^{\alpha/(\alpha-1)} \left(\frac{e^{-(t_p/\tau_c)^\alpha}}{1 - e^{-(t_p/\tau_c)^\alpha}}\right)^{1/(\alpha-1)}\right) \tag{5.14}$$

The total pressure source was then modeled as

$$P(t, V_v) = a(V_v - b)^2 + (cV_v - d)F(t) \tag{5.15}$$

Ottesen and colleagues, after critically evaluating a wide range of possibilities, including the Mulier model, found that the best match to experimental data was obtained with a polynomial activation function of the form [27]

$$F(t) = \begin{cases} \left[\dfrac{(t-\alpha)^n (\beta-t)^m}{n^n m^m \left(\dfrac{\beta-\alpha}{m+n}\right)^{m+n}}\right] & \alpha \le t \le \beta(H) \\[20pt] 0 & \beta(H) \le t \le t_h \text{ (period)} \end{cases} \tag{5.16}$$

where m and n are constants that alter the speed of the relaxation and contraction phases, respectively; H is the heart rate in cycles per second; and t_h is the length of one cardiac cycle.

Ottesen and colleagues then expanded F, adding features associated with heart period variability (H) and aortic flow Q_v. The expanded model is summarized as follows [27]

$$P_v(t, V_v, Q_v, H) = a(V_v - b)^2 + (cV_v - d)F(t, Q_v, H) \tag{5.17}$$

$$F(t, Q_v, H) = f(t, H) - k_1 Q_v + k_2 Q_v^2(t - \tau) \tag{5.18}$$

where $f(t, H)$ is a normalized activation function [equation (5.19)] and $\tau = \kappa t$ (time variable, time delay) and

$$
f(t, H) = \begin{cases} P_p(H)\left[\dfrac{(t-\alpha)^n(\beta(H)-t)^m}{n^n m^m \left(\dfrac{\beta(H)-\alpha}{m+n}\right)^{m+n}}\right] & \alpha \le t \le \beta(H) \\[4ex] 0 & \beta(H) \le t \le t_h \text{ (period)} \end{cases}
$$

$$(5.19)$$

Peak ventricular pressure as a function of heart rate frequency $P_p(H)$

$$
P_p(H) = P_{p\min} + \left[\frac{H^\eta}{H^\eta + \phi^\eta}\right](P_{p\max} - P_{p\min}) \tag{5.20}
$$

where ϕ is the median of the Hill function relation $t_P(H)$ and η is the steepness of $P_P(H)$.

Time for onset of ventricular relaxation as a function of heart rate frequency $\beta(H)$:

$$
\beta(H) = \frac{n+m}{n} t_p(H) - \frac{\alpha m}{n} \tag{5.21}
$$

Time for peak ventricular pressure as a function of heart rate frequency $t_p(H)$:

$$
t_p(H) = t_{p\min} + \left[\frac{\theta^\upsilon}{H^\upsilon + \theta^\upsilon}\right](t_{p\max} - t_{p\min}) \tag{5.22}
$$

where θ is the median of the Hill function relation $P_p(H)$ and υ is the steepness of $t_p(H)$.

As a third example, Smith et al. developed a "minimal model" in which the activating function was a sum of symmetric exponentials [25]

$$
F(t) = \sum_{i=1}^{N} A_i e^{-B_i(t-C_i)^2} \tag{5.23}
$$

with the entire chamber pressure model having the form

$$
P_d(t) = A(e^{\lambda(V-V_0)} - 1) + (E_s(V - V_d) - A(e^{\lambda(V-V_0)} - 1))F(t) \tag{5.24}
$$

Comparison of waveforms calculated using equations (5.16), (5.19), and (5.23) and parameter values provided by Ottesen et al. are shown in Figure 5.4.

Other implementations can be found in the literature. For example, Martin et al. used time-varying elastance for modeling the "active" component of the cardiac cycle, but a pressure–volume relationship to model the "passive" component [24]:

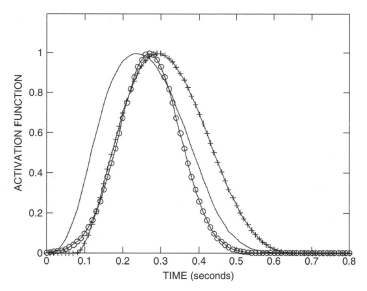

Figure 5.4. Activation function curves created using equations (5.13) (--------) [26], (5.16) (-+-+-+-) [27], and (5.23) (-o-o-o-) [25]. Parameter values were obtained from referenced articles.

During the passive phase:

$$P_p(t) = \gamma + \beta e^{\alpha V(t)} \tag{5.25}$$

During the active phase:

$$P_a(t) = (V(t) - DS(t))E(t), \tag{5.26}$$

where $DS(t)$ is the unstressed volume and

$$E(t) = 0.5E_{\text{syst}}\left(1 - \cos(\frac{2\pi t}{T_{\text{active}}})\right) \tag{5.27}$$

$$DS(t) = DS_{\text{max}} - 0.5(DS_{\text{max}} - DS_{\text{min}})\left(1 - \cos\left(\frac{2\pi t}{T_{\text{active}}}\right)\right) \tag{5.28}$$

The Valves

When using electrical analogs of the circulatory system, valves are represented naturally as diodes, components that effectively conduct current in one direction and block it in the other. The concept is simply implemented mathematically by not allowing flow reversal. In practice, however, to obtain more physiological waveforms, the valves are usually modeled using limited integraters in series with a resistance and/or inertance. Rather than expressing the usual linear relationship between pressure and flow, $\Delta P = RQ$, resistances across valves may be modeled as Bernoulli resistances that effect a quadratic relationship between pressure and flow

$$\Delta P = B Q^2, \text{ where } B = \frac{\rho A}{2666} \text{mmHg} \cdot \text{s} \cdot \text{mL}^{-1} \tag{5.29}$$

and A is the cross-sectional area of the valve.

The Feedback/Preload

The simplest closed-loop models connect the systemic resistance of a modified windkessel directly to a venous pressure reservoir that feeds into the ventricular compartment through a resistance and a valve. More complex models include features such as dividing the peripheral vascular load into multiple compartments, such as arterial, venous and capillary, and/or a beating atrium.

Some Examples

This section looks more closely at several of the models that have been developed using the approaches described above; Figures 5.5a and 5.5b illustrate models with identical loads but with pulsations caused by time-varying elastance versus pressure source [28]. The constant venous pressure reservoir is considered to include the right heart and the pulmonary circulation. Both models have been used successfully to study ventricular dynamics; for instance, Ottesen et al. showed that their model matched ventricular pressure tracings recorded in dog hearts over a wide range of heart rates with respect to shape, peak pressures, and time of peak pressures [27].

Figures 5.5c and 5.5d illustrate the next stage of complexity. Figure 5.5c illustrates a cardiovascular model, originally developed by Martin et al. [24] and later used by Woodruff et al. to demonstrate the physiological effect of four frequently titrated cardiovascular drugs: sodium nitroprusside (SNP), nitroglycerin (NTG), dobutamine (DBT), and dopamine (DOP) [29]. The compartments consisted of a left atrium, left ventricle, arterial pool, capillary pool, and venous pool. Pulsatility for the ventricle and atrium was provided by the time-varying elastance equations (5.25)–(5.28). A baroreceptor model was in place to maintain homeostatic pressure by adjusting arterial resistance, venous tone, ventricular contractility, and heart rate. Extensive studies in dogs were performed to determine timing and concentrations of drug infusion and dispersion in the different compartments. The vasodilator effects of SNP and NTG were modeled to decrease preload and afterload by varying arterial resistance and venous dead space. The vasopressor effects of DBT and DOB were modeled to increase heart rate and left ventricular contractility and decrease arterial resistance.

Figure 5.5d illustrates a model that was developed by Cole et al. as part of a plan to build a mechanical afterload for Langendorff preparations [18]. The compartments consisisted of the left ventricle [pressure source model of Ottesen, equations (5.17)–(5.22)], systemic arteries, systemic veins, left atrium,

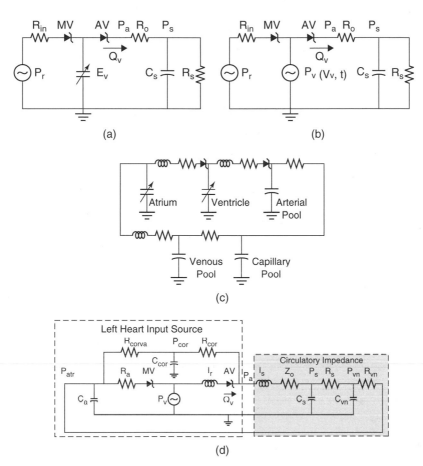

Figure 5.5. Examples of closed-loop models of the systemic circulation coupled to simple afterloads. (a) A pressure source model coupled to a three-element modified wind-kessel arterial load and a venous pressure reservoir p_r (the mitral and aortic valves are represented as diodes) (re-created from Danielsen and Ottesen [28]; (b) comparable to Figure 5.5a, but the ventricle is described by a time-varying elastance (E) (the mitral and aortic valves are represented as diodes) (re-created from Danielsen and Ottesen; [28]); (c) time-varying elastance model configuration, including a beating left atrium, developed to demonstrate the effects of frequently used cardiovascular drugs [29] (re-created from Martin et al. [24]); (d) pressure source model developed as part of a plan to build a mechanical afterload for Langendorff preparations (re-created from Cole et al. [18]).

and coronary circulation. The model was tested successfully against a wide range of aortic pressure and flow tracings representing different age groups and different cardiovascular pathologies.

Figure 5.6 illustrates a model of the closed-loop systemic circulation (Olufsen et al.) that has pumping characteristics based on the pressure source model of Ottesen expanded to include a pulsatile atrium and a separation of the vascular

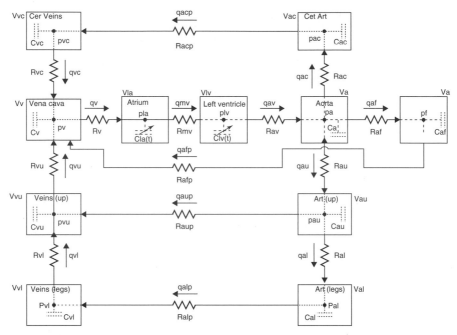

Figure 5.6. Example of a closed-loop model of the systemic circulation with a divided vascular bed (qxx, pxx, and vxx refer to flow, pressure, and volume, respectively, in each compartment; see text for more detail). (Reproduced with permission from Olufsen et al. [30].)

load into cerebral, fingers, upper body, and lower body pathways [30]. With the exception of the "fingers," which were modeled with a single resistance, the pathways were modeled with arterial and venous capacitances separated by resistances, specifically, expanded westkessels. The nonlinear resistances were pressure-dependent [see equation (5.34)]. The model was developed to predict dynamic changes in beat-to-beat arterial blood pressure and middle cerebral artery blood flow velocity during a postural change from sitting to standing. A physiologically based submodel was used to describe effects of gravity on venous blood pooling during postural changes. An autonomic control mechanism mediated by sympathetic and parasympathetic responses affected heart rate, cardiac contractility, resistance, and compliance. An autoregulation control mechanism mediated by responses to local changes in myogenic tone, metabolic demand, and CO_2 concentration affected cerebrovascular resistance. The model was successfully validated using physiological data obtained from a young subject.

5.3. CLOSED-LOOP MODELS OF THE ENTIRE CIRCULATION

In a development similar to that used for closed-loop models of the systemic circulation, the features of models of the entire circulation can be allocated to three component types: (1) modified windkessel-type representations of vascular beds, (2) pulsating chambers (left and right ventricles that may interact and possibly left and right atria), and (3) representations of up to four valves (mitral, aortic, tricuspid, and pulmonic). As the modeling requirements of pulsating chambers and valves are the same as for the models featured above (closed-loop models of the systemic circulation), the focus below is on different representations of vascular beds and possible ventricular interactions.

Vascular Beds

The simplest representation of a bed is a resistance. This may be all that is needed if only the pressure drop across the bed is of interest. But model compartments usually have resistive and compliance terms, may have inertial terms, and, particularly if vessels are large, have resistive terms in series with the compliance components to incorporate the effects of viscoelastic walls. Vessels subject to external forces, such as those associated with respiration, will have a pressure source representation in series with the compliance terms. Figure 5.7 illustrates four common configurations used for vascular beds or segments of vascular beds. For completeness, resistance (R), compliance (C), inertance (I), viscoelasticity (R_w) and external pressure terms ($\varnothing$) are shown in each example, although many of the complete models reviewed at the end of this section include only resistance and compliance terms. Arrows have been drawn across components to indicate the possibility of nonlinearities; for example, investigators may wish to include

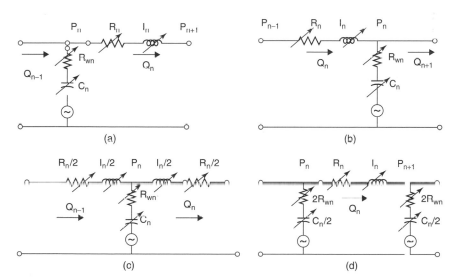

Figure 5.7. Commonly used configurations for vascular beds, to be used singularly or in series, as indicated by $n-1$, n, and $n+1$ subscripts, and/or branching patterns. (a) $\mathcal{L}$ section; (b) inverted $\mathcal{L}$ section; (c) T section; (d) π section.

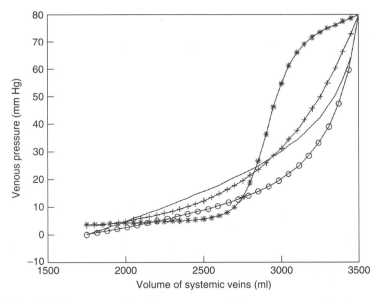

Figure 5.8. Nonlinear systemic vein pressure–volume curves created using equations (5.31) (--------) [22], (5.32) (-+-+-+-) [31]; (5.33) (-o-o-o-) [21], and (5.34) (-*-*-*-) [32]. Values were selected to match equation (5.31) at 2000 and 3500 mL.

the possibility of vessel collapse at low volumes [31]

$$\text{If } V \geq V_0, \text{ then } P(V) = D_1 + K_1(V - V_0)$$
$$\text{If } V < V_0, \text{ then } P(V) = D_2 + K_2 e^{V/V_{\min}}$$
(5.30)

or vessel stiffening at high volumes, particularly of large veins, as illustrated by the equations below and in Figure 5.8. [21,22,31,32]

$$P(V) = P_0 e^{V/\theta} \tag{5.31}$$

or

$$P(V) = -K_1 \log\left(\frac{V_{\max}}{V_v} - K_2\right) \tag{5.32}$$

$$= \frac{2E_0 V_{\max}}{\pi} \tan \frac{\pi V}{2 V_{\max}} \tag{5.33}$$

$$P(V) = \left(\frac{E_{\min} + E_{\max} e^{((V - V_{\text{off}})/K_v)^5}}{1 + e^{((V - V_{\text{off}})/K_v)^5}}\right) V \tag{5.34}$$

from which $E(v)$ can be calculated as $E(v) = dP/dV$.

Likewise, resistances have been modeled to vary inversely with volume through equations of the form [31]

$$R = K \left(\frac{V_{\max}}{V} \right)^2 + R_0 \tag{5.35}$$

Resistances may also be pressure-dependent; for instance, in the postural study described above, large-vessel resistances varied between a minimal and maximal value via a sigmoidal pressure dependent function of the form [30]

$$R = (R_{\max} - R_{\min}) \frac{\alpha^k}{P^k + \alpha^k} + R_{\min} \tag{5.36}$$

Equations pertinent for simulating pressure and flow in Figure 5.7a, commonly referred to as the "$\mathcal{L}$ configuration," are given below:

$$P_n = [\text{compliance term}] + [\text{viscoelastic term}] + [\text{external or bias term}]$$

$$= \left[\frac{V_n - V_{nU}}{C_n} \right] + [R_{W_n} * (Q_{n-1} - Q_n)] + [P_{E/B}] \tag{5.37}$$

With inertance:

$$Q_n = \int \frac{(P_n - P_{n+1} - R_n^* Q_n)}{L_n} dt \tag{5.38}$$

Without inertance:

$$Q_n = \frac{P_n - P_{n+1}}{R_n} \tag{5.39}$$

$$V_n = \int (Q_{n-1} - Q_n) dt + V_{n \text{ init}} \tag{5.40}$$

Figure 5.7b, comparable to Figure 5.7a, is an inverted $\mathcal{L}$. Figures 5.7c and 5.7d are commonly referred to as a "T section" and a "π section," respectively. With proper halving of the RLC terms, one can envision the T section as an inverted $\mathcal{L}$ cascaded with an $\mathcal{L}$ section and the π section as an $\mathcal{L}$ section cascaded with an inverted $\mathcal{L}$ section. The $\mathcal{L}$ sections are particularly useful for modeling individual vessels, such as following branching patterns.

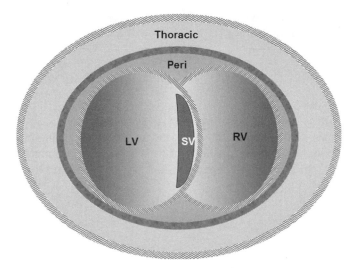

Figure 5.9. Schematic of volumes involved in ventricular interaction models: LV (volume contained by left ventricle freewall, RV (volume contained by right ventricle freewall, SV (volume in left ventricle controlled by the septal wall), Peri (pericardial fluid) and Thoracic (thoracic cavity).

Ventricular Interactions

Models that include ventricular interactions often refer to the 1987 isolated heart experiments of Maughan, Sunagawa, and Sagawa [33]. Studies were performed to measure elastances and volumes using a three-volume framework as illustrated in Figure 5.9: left ventricular freewall volume (V_{LVF}), right ventricular freewall (V_{RVF}) volume, and septal volume (V_S) as represented by the portion of the volume of the left ventricle controlled through septal movement

Volume of left ventricle:

$$V_{LV} = V_{LVF} + V_S \qquad (5.41)$$

Volume of right ventricle:

$$V_{RV} = V_{RVF} - V_S \qquad (5.42)$$

Elastances were measured for the freewalls (E_{LVF} and E_{RVF}) and the septum (E_S). Left and right ventricular pressures (P_{LV} and P_{RV}) were then computed via

$$P_{LV} = \frac{E_S E_{LVF}}{E_S + E_{LVF}} (V_{LV} - V_{0LV}) + \frac{E_{LVF}}{E_S + E_{LVF}} P_{RV} \qquad (5.43)$$

$$P_{RV} = \frac{E_S E_{RVF}}{E_S + E_{RVF}} (V_{RV} - V_{0RV}) + \frac{E_{RVF}}{E_S + E_{RVF}} P_{LV} \qquad (5.44)$$

The original work focused on end-systolic pressure–volume relationships. The work has been expanded by others to include the entire cardiac cycle and the in vivo situation in which the heart is further constrained by the pericardial sac and other external pressures.

Sun et al. added pericardial pressure (P_{PC}) to the chambers of the heart by assuming that pericardial volume (V_{PC}) was the sum of the heart volume and the pericardial fluid (V_{PE}) and that the pericardial pressure and volume were related in an exponential fashion comparable to that used for ventricles during diastole [22]

$$V_{PC} = V_{heart} + V_{PE} \tag{5.45}$$

$$V_{heart} = V_{LV} + V_{RV} + V_{LA} + V_{RA} \tag{5.46}$$

$$P_{PC} = K e^{(v_{PC} - v_{0PC})/\theta_{PC}} \tag{5.47}$$

where θ_{PC} is a pericardial volume constant. Pulsatility was achieved by applying time-varying elastance waveforms to all four heart chambers.

Chung et al. added thoracic (P_{TC}) and body surface pressures (P_{BS}) and thus the pressure balance equations could be expressed as [34]

$$P_{LV} = P_{LVF} + P_{PE} \tag{5.48}$$

$$P_{RV} = P_{RVF} + P_{PE} \tag{5.49}$$

$$P_{PE} = P_{CD} + P_{TC} \tag{5.50}$$

$$P_{TC} = P_{TH} + P_{BS} \tag{5.51}$$

$$P_S = P_{LV} - P_{RV} = P_{LVF} - P_{RVF} \tag{5.52}$$

where P_{LVF}, P_{RVF}, P_{CD}, P_{TH}, and P_s represent transmural pressures across the left ventricular freewall, the right ventricular freewall, the pericardial sac, the thoracic cavity, and the septal wall, respectively. Pulsatility was achieved by time-varying pressure–volume relationships for ventricular freewalls and the septum. Three different septal characterizations were considered: (1) a rigid, nondeformable septum; (2) a passive, compliant septum; and (3) an active septum with a time-varying pressure–volume relationship similar to those used for the ventricular freewalls.

Some Examples

Lumped Systemic and Pulmonary Vascular Beds. This section looks at several models in which the vascular bed representations are limited to lumped systemic and pulmonary vascular beds.

The first example, illustrated in Figure 5.10, is an eight-compartment model based on the expansion of the pressure source model developed by Palladino et al., described above [equations (5.13)–(5.15)], to the four chambers of the heart

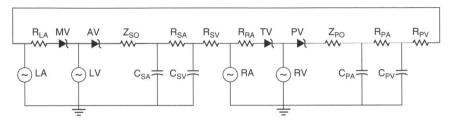

Figure 5.10. Closed-loop model of the entire circulation incorporating systemic (S) and pulmonary (P) vascular beds and four pulsating heart chambers. The model was developed to realisticly simulate the human circulation in the classroom. Please see original article for details. (Re-created from Palladino et al. [35].)

[35]. Systemic and pulmonary vascular beds were modeled with westkessels with added terms for venous compliance and resistance. The model, whose parameters were matched to human measurements and produced realistic pressure and flow waveforms for both the aorta and main pulmonary artery, was initially developed for teaching purposes

The second example, illustrated in Figure 5.11, is a six-compartment model, very similar componentwise to the model in Figure 5.10, without beating atria and with pulsatility created by time-varying elastance rather than pressure source. This model, developed by Mukkamala and Cohen [36], was part of a system identification effort to study five physiological coupling mechanisms relating heart rate (HR), arterial blood pressure (ABP), and instantaneous lung volume (ILV): (1) circulatory mechanics, (2) baroreflex response, (3) ILV coupling to HR, (4) ILV coupling to ABP, and (5) sinoatrial (SA) node. For example, the baroflex response was implemented through changes in HR, ventricular contractility, systemic venous unstressed volume, and systemic arterial resistance. Other features of the model included low-frequency "noise" superimposed on HR and ABP signals, intrathoracic pressures that were modulated with respiration, and a mathematical relationship between HR and respiration rate. The model was successfully validated on the basis of data obtained from 12 healthy subjects breathing at a fixed rate.

The third example, illustrated in Figure 5.12, with the exception of inertial terms associated with the aortic and pulmonary valves, has the same six compartments as the model shown in Figure 5.11. This model, developed by Smith et al., was the basis for simulating the interaction between right and left ventricles within a minimal cardiovascular system [25]. Equations similar to those originally developed by Chung et al. [equations (5.45)–(5.52) without thoracic and body surface pressures], were based on relationships determined by assuming that the ventricles were constrained within a relatively stiff pericardial sac. Pulsating pressures across the freewalls were computed using equations in the form of equation (5.24). The model was shown to be quite robust under a wide range of perterbations, with those showing effects of thoracic pressure and septal wall effects being of most interest.

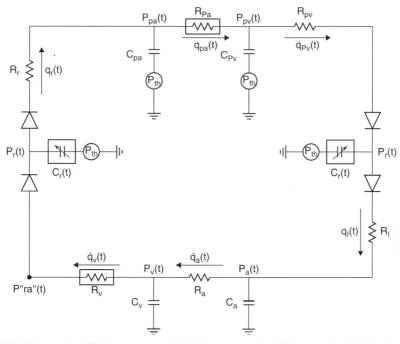

Figure 5.11. Closed-loop model of the entire circulation incorporating systemic and pulmonary vascular beds with two pulsating chambers. Nonlinear elements are enclosed in boxes. Pulmonary and ventricular pressures were referenced to intrathoracic pressure (th). The model was developed to study various physiological coupling mechanisms. Please see original article for details. (Reproduced with permission from Mukkamala and Cohen [36].)

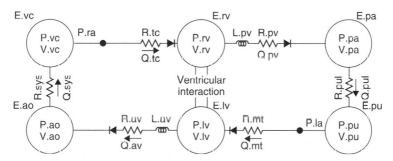

Figure 5.12. Closed-loop model of the entire circulation incorporating systemic and pulmonary vascular beds, two pulsating chambers, and ventricular interaction. The minimal model was designed to simulate the interaction between right and left ventricles within a minimal cardiovascular system. Please see original article for details. (Reproduced with permission from Smith et al. [25].)

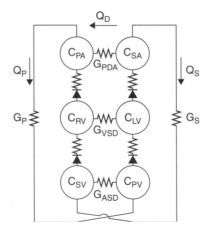

Figure 5.13. Closed-loop model of the entire circulation incorporating systemic and pulmonary vascular beds, two pulsating chambers, and conduits between chambers. The use of "G" in resistor names indicates that admittance rather than resistance ($G = 1/R$) was used in developing model equations. The minimal model was designed to study the effects of increased pulmonary vascular resistance on flow shunted through various cardiac defects. Please see original article for details. (Re-created from Peskin and Tu [37].)

   The fourth example, illustrated in Figure 5.13, is a minimal closed-loop system developed by Peskins and Tu to study the effects of various congenital heart defects [37]. The model consisted of components almost identical to those shown in Figure 5.12: two heart chambers with inflow and outflow valves and systemic and pulmonary beds each modeled as two compliances (arteries and veins) separated by a resistance. Pulsatility was created with time-varying elastance. Congenital heart defects were modeled by inserting connections (modeled as resistors) between relevant compartments, for example, between systemic and pulmonary veins (considered to include right and left atria) for atrial septal defects (ASD), between right and left ventricles for ventricular septal defects (VSD), and between systemic and pulmonary arteries for patent ductus arteriosus (PDA). The series resistances in the valves could be increased to simulate stenosis and a parallel resistance could be added (not shown) to simulate a leaky valve. The focus of the initial study using the model was to examine the influence of increasing pulmonary vascular resistance on the shunt flow through an ASD or a PDA. Results indicted that, compared to the PDA, the ASD shunt flow was more time-independent and less sensitive to pulmonary vascular resistance.

   The fifth example, illustrated in Figure 5.14, was developed by Pekkan et al. to guide preliminary design studies for a pediatric ventricular assist device (VAD) [38]. The basic circulation model was adapted from the Peskins–Tu model described above. Various pump characteristics, including continuous versus pulsatile flow, were considered. Of particular interest was the patient with a single-ventricle physiology who had undergone a surgical repair to separate the

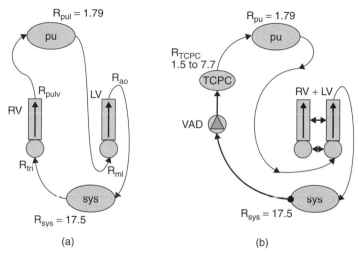

Figure 5.14. Closed-loop model adapted from the model illustrated in Figure 5.13 to guide preliminary studies in designing pediatric ventricular assist devices (VADs): (a) schematic of a normal circulation with right and left ventricles; (b) schematic of a patient with a univentricular heart physiology (single-ventricle circulation) and a total cavopulmonary (TCPC) repair in whom a VAD was implanted between the systemic and pulmonary circulations. Please see original article for details. (Reprinted with permission from Pekkan et al. [38].)

pulmonary and systemic circuits and place them in series with the univentricular pump. The numerous variations of these right heart bypass operations are referred to as "Fontan repairs," in deference to one of the surgeons credited with having the first clinical success [39]. The focus of the initial study was the patient in whom the repair was accomplished by directly connecting the blood returning from the systemic circulation to the pulmonary circulation, a modification termed a *total cavopulmonary connection* (TCPC). The TCPC was modeled as a nonlinear resistance in which the resistance was determined through detailed finite element models of different connection geometries and their responses to varying pulmonary vascular resistances and flows. One potential problem of a TCPC repair is systemic hypertension and pulmonary hypotension. Coupling the circulation with a continuous VAD brought the pulmonary and systemic venous pressures back to manageable levels. Studies of the pulsatile operation mode with rotational speed regulation highlighted the importance of TCPC and pulmonary artery compliances.

Multiple Vascular Beds. This section considers several models in which systemic and/or pulmonary vascular beds were divided into two or more systems acting in parallel. The first five examples refer to published models. The last example illustrates work in progress.

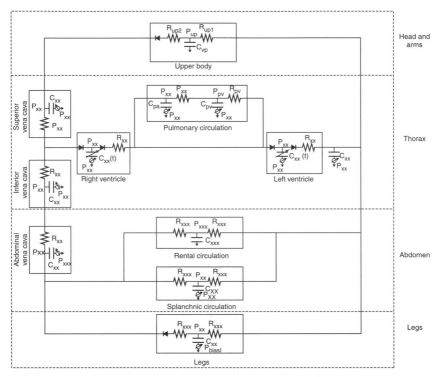

Figure 5.15.   Closed-loop model of the entire circulation incorporating a single-pathway pulmonary vascular bed, multiple systemic pathways and two pulsating chambers. The model was designed to investigate the effects of postspaceflight orthostatic intolerance. Please see original article for details. (Reproduced with permission from Heldt et al. [21].)

Examples from the Literature.   In the first example (Figure 5.15), Heldt et al. used an 11-compartment/5-pathway model based on the work of Davis and Mark [40] to simulate the short-term (<5 min) responses to head-up tilt and lower body negative pressure [21]. The systemic circulation was divided into upper body, renal, splanchnic, and lower extremity sections that were represented with T-type resistance and compliance segments. The aorta, intrathoracic superior and inferior venae cavae, and extrathoracic (abdominal) vena cava were separately identified and each represented with a resistance and a compliance. The pulmonary bed was represented with two T-type *RC* segments. Pulsatility was provided by applying time-varying compliances to right and left ventricles [equation (5.6)]. The pressure–volume relationships of the venous compartments of the legs, the splanchnic circulation, and the abdominal venous compartments were modeled with the tangential relationship shown in Figure 5.8 and equation (5.33). The total hemodynamic model was modeled with 12 differential equations. A time-varying source simulated the effects of respiration-induced pressure changes across the intrathoracic compartments. Pressure (bias) sources at the abdominal venous, the splanchnic, and the leg compartments were used to simulate changes in venous transmural pressure due to head-up tilt or lower body negative pressure. The circulatory model was connected to setpoint models of the arterial and cardiopulmonary baroreflexes. The goal of the arterial reflex model was to maintain a constant mean arterial blood pressure by adjusting heart rate, peripheral resistance, venous zero-pressure filling volume, and right and left end-systolic cardiac capacitances. The cardiopulmonary reflex affected venous zero-pressure filling volume and systemic arteriolar resistance. Orthostatic stress simulations and the transient response characteristics of heart rate and stroke volume to tilt compared well with reported data. The model was to be used for future investigation of the effects of postspaceflight orthostatic intolerance.

In the second example (Figure 5.16), Olansen et al. developed a 16-compartment/5-pathway model of the canine circulation that included ventricular interaction similar to that shown in Figure 5.9 and described by equations (5.45)–(5.52) [41]. The vascular model, however, was more complex: (1) the systemic vascular bed was divided into coronary, cerebral, and systemic load pathways; (2) the pulmonary vascular bed had a shunt between the pulmonary arteries and veins; (3) inertance and viscoelastic terms were added in areas of large arteries; and (4) pulsatile left and right atria were included. Cerebral and coronary beds and the pulmonary shunt were represented by simple resistances. Model parameters were altered to study (1) the effects of modification of septal contraction and pericardial

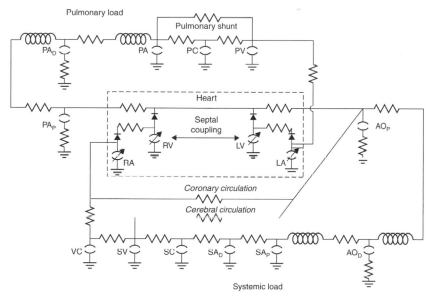

Figure 5.16. Closed-loop model of the entire circulation incorporating a pulmonary vascular bed with shunt; a systemic vascular bed with head, leg, and coronary pathways; four pulsating chambers; and ventricular interaction. Please see original article for details. (Reproduced with permission from Olansen et al. [41].)

mechanics on ventricular pump function, (2) the effects of changes in afterload on ventricular wall motion and pump function, (3) the quantification of *series* and *direct* forms of ventricular interaction and the assessment of their importance in a more global context, and (4) the effects of timing on ventricular pump function. A Labview™-based software package entitled CardioPV was developed to integrate the complete model with data acquisition tools and a graphical user interface. The software package was the basis of a virtual laboratory textbook.

In the third example (Figure 5.17), Lu et al. expanded on the circulatory model described above (still 16 compartments and 5 pathways) and in Figure 5.14 to simulate the cardiovascular response of humans to a wider variety of perturbations [31]. Venous compliances were nonlinear [equations (5.30) and (5.32)]; Baroreflex control influenced heart rate, myocardial contractility, and vasomotor tone; an airways mechanics model was coupled with the pulmonary circulation component to characterize gas exchange at the alveolarcapillary membrane. The model was shown to predict the hemodynamic response to the increased intrathoracic pressures during the Valsalva maneuver.

In the fourth example (Figure 5.18), Noordergraaf et al. [43] developed a 13-compartment/6-pathway model, termed "Donder's model," in deference to

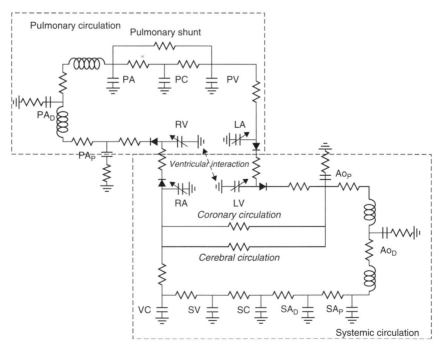

Figure 5.17. Closed-loop model of the entire circulation very similar to that shown in Figure 5.14 but used to simulate a wider range of perturbations, including the effects of the Valsalva maneuver. Please see original article for details. (Reproduced with permission from Lu et al. [31].)

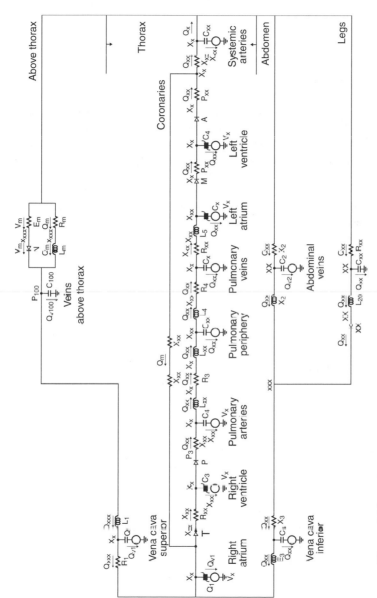

Figure 5.18. Closed-loop model of the entire circulation incorporating a pulmonary vascular bed, a systemic vascular bed with above-thorax, coronary, abdominal, and leg pathways and four pulsating chambers. The model was developed specifically to model the effects of cardiac resuscitation. Please see original article for details. (Reproduced with permission from Noordergraaff et al. [43].)

the 1856 work of Franciscus Donders [42], who proposed that the respiratory system could aid in venous return, thus concurring with the Harvey critics that the heart was too weak to be the only pump supporting the circulatory system [43]. With the goal of developing a model that was specifically suitable for cardiopulmonary resuscitation, emphasis was placed on the position of the vascular beds relative to four categories: above-thorax cavity, thoracic cavity, abdominal, and extraabdominal. The "above-thorax cavity" limb included separate pathways for the head and arms. Compartments within the thoracic and abdominal cavities could be influenced by respiratory or other external pressures as if they were intrapleural effects. The thoracic cavity housed the four chambers of the heart and the pulmonary (two pathways) and coronary circulations. Pulsations were created in all four chambers using variations of equations (5.13)–(5.15). Sections were of the T type with single resistance, compliance, and inertial terms. Cardiac output could be influenced by five controls: sympathetic stimulation operating on the contractile properties of the cardiac chambers, neural stimulation of heart rate, respiratory influences, baroreceptor control of systemic and pulmonary resistances, and pumping by small muscular venules (venomotion) possibly under metabolic control. Although venomotion was not implemented in the version of the model used in the results section of the paper, the authors did present the idea of impedance generated flow as the result of the time-varying compliance and resistance of contracting and relaxing muscular venules. Simulations were run for a wide range of physiological conditions, from rest to exercise to cardiac arrest. The results implied that increases in heart and respiratory rate tended to inhibit cardiac output, while depth of respiration, sympathetic stimulation of cardiac contractile properties, and baroreceptor activity tended to have a stimulating effect. The model was also used to demonstrate the limitations of cardiopulmonary resuscitation attempted by applying external force to intrathoracic structures. Applied high pressures limited effective cardiac output through "collapse and sloshing."

The fifth example (Figure 5.19), a 29-compartment/6-pathway model developed by Liang and Liu, provides more detail pertaining to vascular beds than do the models described above [32]. In addition to the four-chamber heart and pulmonary circulation, vascular beds were identified as (1) cerebral and upper limb (arms), (2) renal, (3) splanchnic, and (4) lower limb (legs) beds. Beds were modeled with four complete L-type segments—resistance, inertance, capacitance, and viscoelasticity—which represented the artery, arteriole, capillary, and venous beds, respectively. The ascending aorta and vena cava were modeled as separate compartments. Time-varying elastance curves, similar to those illustrated in (equation (5.7)), were used to provide pulsatility to the four heart chambers. The Maughan model [equations (5.41)–(5.44)] was used to model ventricular interactions with the addition of an equation to vary the time of peak elastance during a cardiac cycle. Particular attention was paid to modeling venous compliance, incorporating volume-dependent elastance terms in the form of equation (5.34) for systemic veins and the vena cavae and in the form of equation (5.31) otherwise. Likewise, resistances in large veins varied inversely with volume as

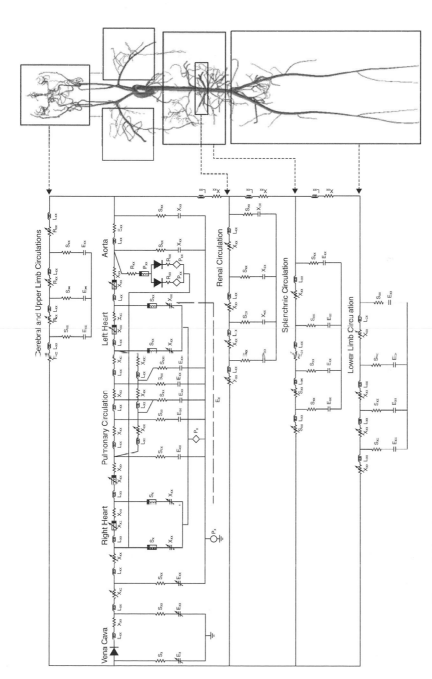

Figure 5.19. Closed-loop model of the entire circulation incorporating a pulmonary vascular bed; a systemic vascular bed with cerebral and upper limb, renal, splanchnic, and lower limb pathways; four pulsating chambers and ventricular interaction. The model was developed to include vascular detail and study the effects of diastolic dysfunction. Please see original article for details. (Reproduced with permission from Liang and Liu [32].)

expressed in equation (5.35). Hemodynamic waveforms and volume values were shown to be physiologically realistic. Diastolic dysfunction was modeled by varying the duration of relaxation and stiffness of the myocardium. Parameters were altered to mimic the three dysfunctional levels, grades I, II, and III, and the results were consistent with Doppler velocity recordings obtained in comparable patients.

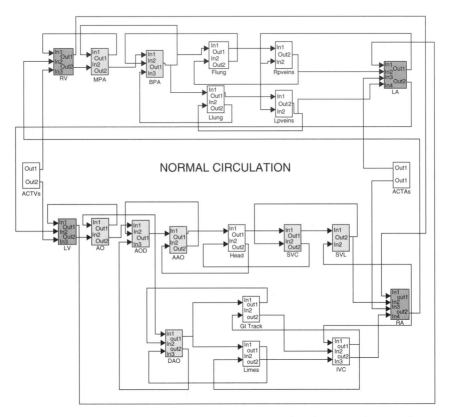

Figure 5.20. Closed-loop model of the entire circulation incorporating a pulmonary vascular bed separating right and left lungs; a systemic vascular bed with head, GI, and lower limb pathways; and four pulsating chambers. The model is being developed to study the effects of creating Fontan circulations in lambs. Darkly shaded blocks represent pulsating chambers. Lightly shaded blocks represent specific vessel segments. White boxes include up to three $\mathcal{L}$ sections or inverted $\mathcal{L}$ segments representing arterial, capillary, and venous beds of the pathway as illustrated in Figures 5.7a and 5.7b and implemented in Simulink by blocks similar to that shown in Figure 5.21. ACTV and ACTA boxes house the generation of the time-varying elastance curves as illustrated in Figure 5.3 for the ventricles and atria, respectively. The aorta and main pulmonary artery were represented with proximal and distal segments: AO and AOD for the aorta, MPA and BPA for the main pulmonary artery. Proximal segments of the ascending aorta (AAO) and descending aorta (DAO) were also modeled separately.

Work in Progress. The final example is this section, illustrated in Figures (5.20)–(5.24), is a model under development in our lab to aid in the understanding of the changes observed in lambs that have undergone a right heart bypass operation to create a Fontan circulation [44], as was illustrated in Figure 5.14. The original model was adapted from that used by Blackstone et al. [45] to simulate a one-year-old child undergoing a Mustard's operation for transposition of the great arteries. Atrial contractions were added in the manner suggested by Lau and Sagawa [46]. Chamber pulsatility was created with time-varying elastance [equation (5.5)]. Circulatory pathways included right and left lungs, head, legs, and GI vascular beds. Respiration effects were added by creating a nonlinear pulmonary resistance based on the transmural pressure between airways and vessels and by altering large vessel and heart chamber dynamics via the external/thoracic pressure source term at the end of equation (5.37). Airway pressure waveforms

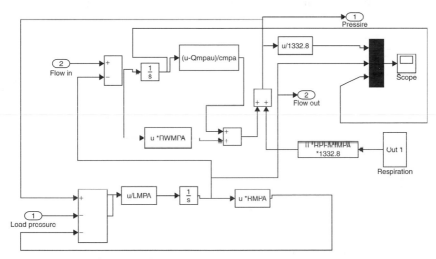

Figure 5.21. Block diagram of the Simulink configuration of the proximal section of the main pulmonary artery (MPA), including all the features of equations (5.37), (5.39), and (5.40): viscoelastic walls, inertia, and thoracic pressures resulting from respiration. Explanation of operations and terms: rectangular boxes with + and − signs are summers and signals entering are added or subtracted as indicated; square boxes with 1/s are integrators; the black square rectangle is a mux (multiplexer) that channels the three entering signals to a scope for viewing and data storage; the remaining rectangular boxes represent mathematical manipulations for which "u" is understood to be the input signal. Example 1: (u-QMPAU)/CMPA takes the input (u = volume of main pulmonary artery as determined by integrating the difference between the input and output flows) and subtracts the unstressed volume (QMPAU) and divides the result by the compliance (CMPA) to determine the compliance-related pressure term. Example 2: u*RWMPA multiplies the input (u = difference between input and output flows) times the resistance that accounts for the viscous properties of the wall. Example 3: u/1332.8 converts pressure measurements to mmHg units. (Other terms: RMPA = resistance of the MPA, LMPA = inductance of the MPA.)

were generated using rising and decaying exponentials to mimic inspiration and expiration.

The current version is implemented in Simulink, and the block diagram of the model is shown in Figure 5.20. Darkly shaded blocks represent the heart chambers. Lightly shaded blocks represent specific vessel segments with subsystem block diagrams comparable to that shown in Figure 5.21, which is an implementation of equations (5.37), (5.39), and (5.40). White boxes include up to three $\mathcal{L}$ sections or inverted $\mathcal{L}$ segments representing arterial, capillary, and venous beds of the indicated pathway.

The model can mimic the different Fontan repairs by bypassing the right ventricle and/or the right atrium. A version of the TCPC connection, referred to as TCPY, is illustrated in Figure 5.22. The superior and inferior venae cavae are both connected to a shunt that carries the blood to the main pulmonary artery. This modification, which has been used in humans [47], is particularly appropriate for the anatomy of a lamb and is described in detail by Ketner [48]. The model has

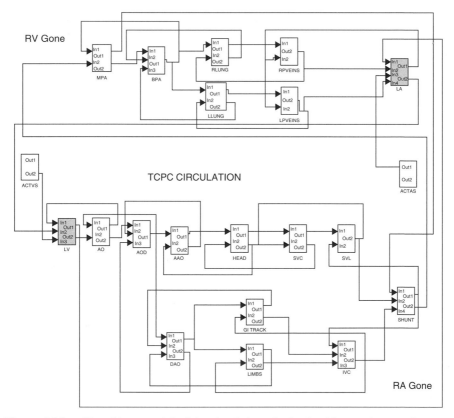

Figure 5.22. Closed-loop model of the circulation of a lamb with a total cavopulmonary circulation (TCPC). The right ventricle (RV) has been removed, and the right atrium (RA) has been replaced by a shunt between the cavae and the main pulmonary artery.

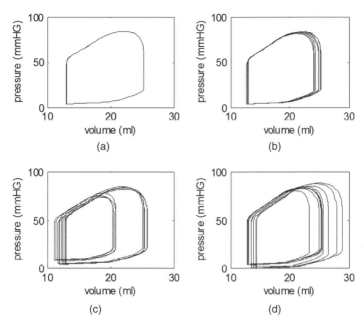

Figure 5.23. Left ventricle pressure–volume loops under four different respiration assumptions: (a) respiration has no influence on the circulation; (b) respiration influences resistance of pulmonary arterioles; (c) pulmonary resistance as in (b) with positive respiratory influence on thoracic pressures; (d) pulmonary resistance as in (b) with negative respiratory influence on thoracic pressures.

yielded valuable insights into the response of the entire cardiovascular system to a Fontan circulation assuming that the atria and left ventricle continue to have the same enervation curves.

An "average" form of the model is being used to determine parameter sensitivity and to test hypotheses about how interventions may affect and/or be affected by the global circulation. Of particular interest has been the influence of respiration on involved vessels, as respiratory effects gain in importance in the Fontan circulation. Figure 5.23 illustrates the effects on left ventricular pressure volume curves under four different respiration assumptions: (a) that respiration has no effect; (b) that respiration impacts the system only by varying pulmonary vascular resistance; (c) that in addition to increasing pulmonary vascular resistance, inspiration creates a positive thoracic pressure, thus decreasing diastolic volumes; and (d) that, in addition to increasing pulmonary vascular resistance, inspiration imposes a negative thoracic pressure, thus increasing systolic volumes and pressures. Assumption (b) works quite well for modeling the changes observed in pressure and flow waveforms in the pulmonary arteries in our acute/open-chest lamb studies in which pressure increases and flow decreases during inspiration. For several studies, however, assumption (d) is needed to model the increased

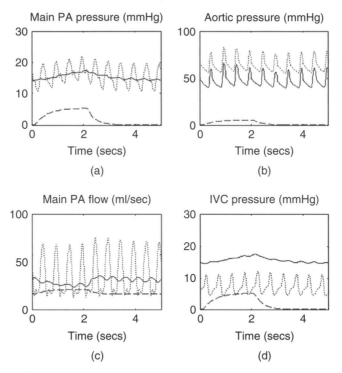

Figure 5.24.   Changes in representative waveforms as a result of creating the Fontan circulation. Normal waveforms were obtained from model illustrated in Figure 5.20. Fontan waveforms were obtained from model illustrated in Figure 5.22. Airway pressures were the same for both models. [Airway pressure (– — –); normal circulation (- - - -); Fontan circulation) (--------).] (a) Main pulmonary artery pressure; (b) aortic pressure, (c) main pulmonary artery blood flow; (d) inferior vena cava pressure.

aortic pressure and flow observed during inspiration. Explaining the wide variation in responses seen in aortic pressure and flow waveforms in our lamb models is a goal of current research, which includes fitting model parameters to animal data to determine inter-animal variability.

Selected waveforms from the "normal" (dotted line) and "Fontan" (solid line) circulations are shown in Figure 5.24. Each panel represents one respiratory cycle (dashed line). Waveform shape and amplitude changes are consistent with our animal data: loss of pulsatility in the caval veins and pulmonary arteries and increased caval pressures after the Fontan circulation is imposed.

5.4. CONCLUDING REMARKS

The models described above by no means exhaust the number of illustrative closed-looped models of the circulatory system that can be found in the literature.

Models with similar level of detail include those of Thomas et al. [49], Barnea [50], Conlon et al. [51], and Ursino [52]. Very ambitious models that attempt to include multiscale detail, such as ventricle behavior based on cardiac myocyte activity and/or sarcomere mechanics [53] or the 364-block systems analysis of circulatory regulation assembled by Guyton [54], have not been considered. Nor have models that include distributed segments [55], such as transmission line equivalents [56] or detailed 3D segments with finite-element solutions [57] been included, although such models are useful when detailed information is needed about wave reflections, turbulence, velocity profiles, energy losses, and other properties. The goal, as stated in the beginning of the chapter, has been to provide the reader with a knowledgeable framework when evaluating the nuances and capabilities of closed-loop models that can be illustrated with electrical analogs. Such models continue to be extremely useful in examining the whole-body response to a physiological change or insult. Additional detail would often only add parameters that cannot be measured and require unnecessary computational overhead.

REFERENCES

1. Harvey W: *Exercitatio Anatomica, De Motu Cordis et Sanguinis in Animalibus*, William Fitzer, Frankfurt, Germany, 1628.

2. Palladino JL, Noordergraaf A: The changing view of the heart through the centuries, *Stud Health Technol Inform* **71**:3–11 (2000).

3. Lubitz SA: Early reaction to Harvey's circulation theory, *Mt Sinai J Med* **71**:274–280 (2004).

4. Cassedy JH: The microscope in American medical science, 1840–1860, *Isis* **67**:76–97 (1976)

5. Hales S: *Statistical Essays. Containing Haemastaticks*, Hafner, New York, 1733.

6. Timmons WD: Cardiovascular models and control, in Bronzino JD, ed, *The Biomedical Engineering Handbook*, CRC Press, Boca Raton, FL, and IEEE Press, 1995, pp 2386–2403.

7. Nichols WW, O'Rourke MF, Hartley C: *McDonald's Blood Flow in Arteries: Theoretical, Experimental and Clinical Principles*, 4th ed, Arnold, London, 1998.

8. Frank O: Die grundform des artiellen pulses. Erste abhandlung. Mathemataische analyse, *Z Biol* **37**:483–526 (1899).

9. Milnor WR: *Hemodynamics*, 2nd ed, Williams & Wilkins, Baltimore, 1989.

10. Rideout VC: *Mathematical and Computer Modeling of Physiological Systems*, Prentice-Hall, Englewood Cliffs, NJ, 1991.

11. Westerhof N, Sipkema P, van den Bos GC, Elzinga G: Forward and backward waves in the arterial system, *Cardiovasc Res* **6**:648–656 (1972).

12. Westerhof N, Elzinga G, Sipkema P: An artificial arterial system for pumping hearts, *J Appl Physiol* **31**:776–781 (1971).

13. Burattini R, Gnudi G: Computer identification of models for the arterial tree input impedance: Comparison between two new simple models and first experimental results, *Med Biol Eng Comput* **20**:134–144 (1982).

14. Campbell KB, Ringo JA, Peterson NS: Informational analysis of left ventricle—systemic arterial interaction, *Ann Biomed Eng* **12**:209–231 (1984).

15. Stergiopulos N, Westerhof BE, Westerhof N: Total arterial inertance as the fourth element of the windkessel model, *Am J Physiol* **276**:H81–H88 (1999).

16. Beneken JEW: Some computer models in cardiovascular researach, in Bergel DH, ed, *Cardiovascular Fluid Dynamics*, Academic Press, New York, 1972, p 173.

17. Cole RT: Design and implementation of a fluid mechanical dynamic afterload for use in an isolated heart apparatus, PhD Dissertation, University of North Carolina at Chapel Hill, 2006.

18. Cole RT, Lucas CL, Cascio WE, Johnson TA: A LabVIEW model incorporating an open-loop arterial impedance and a closed-loop circulatory system, *Ann Biomed Eng* **33**:1555–1573 (2005).

19. Engelberg J, DuBois AB: Mechanics of pulmonary circulation in isolated rabbit lungs, *Am J Physiol* **242**:H154 (1982).

20. Shaw DB: Compliance and inertance in the pulmonary arterial system, *Clin Sci* **25**:181 (1963).

21. Heldt T, Shim EB, Kamm RD, Mark RG: Computational modeling of cardiovascular response to orthostatic stress, *J Appl Physiol* **92**:1239–1254 (2002).

22. Sun Y, Beshara M, Lucariello RJ, Chiaramida SA: A comprehensive model for right-left heart interaction under the influence of pericardium and baroreflex, *Am J Physiol* **272**:H1499–H1515 (1997).

23. Mulier JP: *Ventricular Pressure as a Function of Volume and Flow*, PhD dissertation, University of Leeuven, Belgium, 1994.

24. Martin JF, Schneider AM, Mandel JE, Prutow RJ, Smith NT: A new cardiovascular model for real-time applications, *Trans Soc Comput Simul* **3**:31–66 (1986).

25. Smith BW, Chase JG, Nokes RI, Shaw GM, Wake G: Minimal haemodynamic system model including ventricular interaction and valve dynamics, *Med Eng Phys* **26**:131–139 (2004).

26. Palladino JL, Mulier JP, Noordergraaf A: Closed-loop circulation model based on the Frank mechanism, *Surv Math Indust* **7**:177–186 (1997).

27. Ottesen JT, Danielsen M: Modeling ventricular contraction with heart rate changes, *J Theor Biol* **222**:337–346 (2003).

28. Danielsen M, Ottesen JT: Describing the pumping heart as a pressure source, *J Theor Biol* **212**:71–81 (2001).

29. Woodruff EA, Martin JF, Omens M: A model for the design and evaluation of algorithms for closed-loop cardiovascular therapy, *IEEE Trans Biomed Eng* **44**:694–705 (1997).

30. Olufsen MS, Ottesen JT, Tran HT, Ellwein LM, Lipsitz LA, Novak V: Blood pressure and blood flow variation during postural change from sitting to standing: Model development and validation, *J Appl Physiol* **99**:1523–1537 (2005).

31. Lu K, Clark JW, Ghorbel FH, Ware DL, Bidani A: A human cardiopulmonary system model applied to the analysis of the Valsalva maneuver, *Am J Physiol Heart Circ Physiol* **281**:H2661–H2679 (2001).

32. Liang F, Liu H: A closed-loop lumped parameter computational model for human cardiovascular system, *Jpn Soc. Mech. Eng. Int J Ser C* **48**:484–493 (2005).

33. Maughan WL, Sunagawa K, Sagawa K: Ventricular systolic interdependence: Volume elastance model in isolated canine hearts, *Am J Physiol* **253**:H1381–H1390 (1987).

34. Chung DC, Niranjan SC, Clark JW Jr, Bidani A, Johnston WE, Zwischenberger JB, Traber DL: A dynamic model of ventricular interaction and pericardial influence, *Am J Physiol* **272**:H2942–H2962 (1997).

35. Palladino JL, Ribeiro LC, Noordergraaf A: Human circulatory system model based on Frank's mechanism, in Ottesen JT, Danielsen M, eds, IOP Press, Netherlands, 2000, pp 29–40.

36. Mukkamala R, Cohen RJ: A forward model-based validation of cardiovascular system identification, *Am J Physiol Heart Circ Physiol* **281**:H2714–H2730 (2001).

37. Peskin CS, Tu C: Hemodynamics in congenital heart disease, *Comput Biol Med.* **16**:331–359 (1986).

38. Pekkan K, Frakes D, De Zelicourt D, Lucas CW, Parks WJ, Yoganathan AP: Coupling pediatric ventricle assist devices to the Fontan circulation: Simulations with a lumped-parameter model, *ASAIO J* **51**:618–628 (2005).

39. Fontan F, Baudet E: Surgical repair of tricuspid atresia, *Thorax* **26**:240–248 (1971).

40. Davis N, Mark RG: Teaching physiology through simulation of hemodynamics, *Comput Cardiol* **17**:649–652 (1990).

41. Olansen JB, Clark JW, Khoury D, Ghorbel F, Bidani A: A closed-loop model of the canine cardiovascular system that includes ventricular interaction, *Comput Biomed Res* **33**:260–295 (2000).

42. Donders FC: *Physiologie des Menschen*, Hirzel, Leipzig, 1856.

43. Noordergraaf GJ, Ottesen JT, Kortsmit WJ, Schilders WH, Scheffer GJ, Noordergraaf A: The donders model of the circulation in normo- and pathophysiology, *Cardiovasc Eng* **6**:51–70 (2006).

44. Lucas C, Ketner M, Steele B, Mill MR, Sheridan B, Lucas WJ, Pekkan K, Yoganathan A: Importance of respiration and graft compliance in Fontan circulations: Experimental and computational studies, *J Biomech* **39**:S207 (2006).

45. Blackstone EH, Rideout VC, Beduhn DL: Simulation analysis of interatrial transposition of venous return (Mustard's operation), *Ann Biomed Eng* **10**:193–218 (1982).

46. Lau VK, Sagawa K: Model analysis of the contribution of atrial contraction to ventricular filling, *Ann Biomed Eng* **7**:167–201 (1979).

47. Okano T, Yamagishi M, Shuntoh K, Yamada Y, Hayashida K, Shinkawa T, Kitamura N: Extracardiac total cavopulmonary connection using a Y-shaped graft, *Ann Thorac Surg* **74**:2195–2197 (2002).

48. Ketner ME: Hemodynamics, ventilation effects, energetics, and time offsets in various modified Fontan circulations, PhD dissertation, University of North Carolina at Chapel Hill, 2006.

49. Thomas JD, Zhou J, Greenberg N, Bibawy G, McCarthy PM, Vandervoort PM: Physical and physiological determinants of pulmonary venous flow: Numerical analysis, *Am J Physiol* **272**:H2453–H2465 (1997).

50. Barnea O: Mathematical analysis of coronary autoregulation and vascular reserve in closed-loop circulation, *Comput Biomed Res* **27**:263–275 (1994).

51. Conlon MJ, Russell DL, Mussivand T: Development of a mathematical model of the human circulatory system, *Ann Biomed Eng* **34**:1400–1413 (2006).

52. Ursino M: Interaction between carotid baroregulation and the pulsating heart: A mathematical model, *Am J Physiol Heart Circ Physiol* **275**:H1733–H1747 (1998).

53. Arts T, Delhaas T, Bovendeerd P, Verbeek X, Prinzen FW: Adaptation to mechanical load determines shape and properties of heart and circulation: The CircAdapt model, *Am J Physiol Heart Circ Physiol* **288**:H1943–H1954 (2005).

54. Guyton AC, Coleman TG, Granger HJ: Circulation: Overall regulation, *Annu Rev Physiol* **34**:13–46 (1972).

55. Quarteroni A, Ragni S, Veneziani A: Coupling between lumped and distributed models for blood flow problems, *Comput Visual Sci* **4**:111–124 (2001).

56. Chen CW, Shau WR, Wu CP: Analog transmission line model for simulation of systemic circulation, *IEEE Trans Biomed Eng* **44**:90–94 (1997).

57. Kerckhoffs RC, Neal ML, Gu Q, Bassingthwaighte JB, Omens JH, McCulloch AD: Coupling of a 3D finite element model of cardiac ventricular mechanics to lumped systems models of the systemic and pulmonic circulation, *Ann Biomed Eng* **35**:1–18 (2007).

■■■■■■■ CHAPTER 6

Artery Wall Mechanics Determined by Ultrasound

ARNOLD P. G. HOEKS and EVELIEN HERMELING

Department of Biophysics, Cardiovascular Research Institute Maastricht, Maastricht University, The Netherlands

ROBERT S. RENEMAN

Departments of Biophysics, Cardiovascular Research Institute Maastricht, Maastricht University, The Netherlands

Abstract. The mechanical properties of the arterial wall play an important role in reducing the heart load and conveying blood pressure and blood volume to the periphery. Because aging and cardiovascular disorders strongly impact the conduit function of the arterial system, the relevant parameters, such as lumen size, wall thickness, local blood pressure, distensibility, compliance, elasticity coefficient, and pulse wave velocity have been measured. In this chapter we will address the relevant noninvasive techniques, based mostly on ultrasound, used to assess the parameters in the normal population as well as in specific subject groups, such as hypertensives and diabetics. We will also discuss the mathematical and physical interrelationships between those parameters. It will be shown that the assumptions applied to derive these relationships inherently lead to approximations. Some characteristics are difficult to measure directly, such as local pulse pressure, prompting suggestions for alternatives to assess the mechanical properties of arterial walls.

6.1. INTRODUCTION

Many decades ago Strandness and colleagues [1] realized that Doppler techniques could be used to noninvasively identify atherosclerotic lesions in arteries accessible to ultrasound. Since then noninvasive vascular ultrasound, generally combining anatomic and flow information, has gradually been developed and is now routinely used to diagnose these lesions clinically [2]. Noninvasive vascular

Vascular Hemodynamics: Bioengineering and Clinical Perspectives, Edited by Peter J. Yim
Copyright © 2008 John Wiley & Sons, Inc.

ultrasound is also used to measure intima–media thickness (IMT), a parameter commonly employed in epidemiological [3,4] and intervention studies [5] as a possible indicator of atherosclerotic disease [6–9].

More recently, the focus of noninvasive vascular ultrasound has been extended to the assessment of artery wall properties, in terms of distension, circumferential strain, distensibility, compliance, and Young's modulus [10–13]. Understanding these mainly dynamic parameters is of utmost importance in patient management, because loss of elastic properties of elastic arteries, as in aging [14,15] and in borderline [16,17] and essential hypertension [18,19], contributes substantially to the increase in systolic arterial and pulse pressure, known independent risk factors [20,21]. Ultrasonic techniques are now available to noninvasively determine lumen diameter, distension (pulsatile changes in diameter due to changes in blood pressure during the cardiac cycle), circumferential strain, and IMT with great detail. Because these parameters can be determined with one and the same ultrasound system [22], their interrelation at a particular site along the arterial tree can be investigated. Moreover, these parameters, in combination with blood pressure, can be used to quantify the storage capacity of arteries and the stress–strain relation of arterial walls.

This chapter addresses the most important achievements in the noninvasive assessment of artery wall dynamics in humans. The focus is on the interrelationship between parameters describing the mechanical characteristics of the arterial wall. These relationships are subsequently used to derive parameters that are generally difficult to measure noninvasively (e.g., local pulse pressure and local pulse wave velocity). A special point of concern will be the noninvasive determination of the elasticity coefficient (Young's modulus) of wall material. This leads automatically to a discussion of techniques currently used to measure the relevant parameters: local blood pressure, lumen diameter, and wall thickness. Since the mid-1990s specific age and patient groups have been subjected to a detailed examination of vascular condition. Here we will discuss the changes observed in aging and in essential and borderline hypertension. The changes in artery wall properties in atherosclerosis and diabetes will be discussed as well. Although most of the data presented are derived from clinical studies; observations made in epidemiological and pharmacological studies are included where relevant.

6.2. BASIC PROPERTIES OF VASCULAR DYNAMICS

Lumen Diameter and Wall Thickness

Let us consider a circular cross section of an artery with an initial lumen diameter d and wall thickness h. Let us assume that the wall material is incompressible (conservation of volume) but can deform. The change in lumen diameter Δd due to a change in transmural pressure requires a change in wall thickness Δh to maintain the wall volume πdh:

$$\pi dh = \pi(d + \Delta d)(h + \Delta h) \quad \Rightarrow \varepsilon_h = \frac{\Delta h}{h} = \frac{-\Delta d}{d} \tag{6.1}$$

To arrive at the expression for the relative change in wall thickness ε_h (radial wall strain), second-order effects are ignored ($\Delta d << d$, $\Delta h << h$, $h << d$). The relative change in wall thickness is the inverse of the relative change in diameter. Now let us consider the displacement Δx of the outside wall as function of wall thickness for an imposed change in lumen diameter:

$$\Delta x = \frac{\Delta d}{2} + \Delta h = 0.5\Delta d(1 - 2h/d) \tag{6.2}$$

Because of the assumed conservation of volume, a gradient in radial displacement occurs over the artery wall, which increases with relative wall thickness (h/d). The displacement of the outside wall will be 20% down with respect to that of the wall–lumen interface for an h/d of 10%. Consequently at the outer wall the circumferential strain, that is, the relative change in circumference, will be down by 10% for an $h/d = 10\%$:

$$\text{Strain} = \frac{\pi(\Delta d + 2\Delta h)}{\pi(d + 2h)} = \frac{\Delta d(1 - 2h/d)}{d(1 + 2h/d)} \tag{6.3a}$$

This equation leads to a first-order estimate for the average circumferential wall strain ε_c:

$$\varepsilon_c = \frac{\Delta d(1 - h/d)}{d(1 + h/d)} \tag{6.3b}$$

It can be concluded from the expressions above that a change in lumen diameter primarily affects the inner layers of the wall, while the outer layer (i.e., the tunica adventitia) will be exposed to a lower radial strain and a considerably lower circumferential strain.

Distensibility and Compliance

Parameters that characterize the elastic behavior of arteries are distensibility and compliance, defined as the observed relative ($\Delta V/V$) and absolute (ΔV) change in arterial lumen volume (V) for an imposed change in pressure (Δp), respectively. The distensibility reflects the mechanical load of the artery wall, while the compliance reflects the ability to store temporarily blood volume, thereby reducing blood pressure increase during ventricular ejection.

Distensibility and compliance are generally expressed as changes in lumen cross-sectional area A during the cardiac cycle rather than changes in lumen volume. This is allowed, because artery length hardly changes during the cardiac cycle due to longitudinally tethering of arteries at their in vivo length [23,24]. Moreover, if the volume of wall material is indeed constant, then theoretically the wall strain in the longitudinal direction of a rotation symmetric artery will be zero and there will be no change in length regardless of whether the artery is tethered. The expression for distensibility coefficient (DC), that is, the distensibility per unit of artery length, in terms of a reference lumen diameter d (usually the end-diastolic diameter) and the change in diameter Δd (distension) due to a change in pressure Δp, assuming a circular lumen cross section, is

$$\text{DC} = \frac{\Delta A / A}{\Delta p} = \frac{((d + \Delta d)^2 - d^2)/d^2}{\Delta p} \approx \frac{2\Delta d}{d\,\Delta p} \quad (\text{Pa}^{-1}) \qquad (6.4)$$

The approximation induces an error of 5% in DC for a relative change in lumen diameter of 10% which is quite a normal value for the common carotid artery of a young healthy subject. Small animals may exhibit a considerably larger strain [25] and the approximation should then be avoided. The compliance coefficient (CC) can be rewritten as

$$\text{CC} = \frac{\Delta A}{\Delta p} = \frac{\pi((d + \Delta d)^2 - d^2)}{4\Delta p} \approx \frac{\pi d \Delta d}{2\Delta p} \, (\text{m}^2/\text{Pa}) \qquad (6.5)$$

Elasticity

The elasticity coefficient E, also known as *Young's modulus*, is defined as the change in circumferential stress S_c (force divided by area) divided by the circumferential strain (relative change in circumference). This definition may be confusing since a high value indicates a stiff (less elastic) artery. Assuming that the stress gradient over the wall is negligible (thin-walled tube), the circumferential wall stress follows from the Lamé equation, which can be easily obtained by considering a plane through the axis of an arterial segment with length l. In equilibrium the forces in the wall counterbalance the downward force pld on the plane caused by the transmural blood pressure p:

$$2S_c hl = pld \quad 2S_c h = pd \qquad (6.6)$$

Using a first-order Taylor series expansion the change in stress $\sigma_c = \Delta S_c$ due to a change in pressure Δp can be approximated with:

$$2\Delta S_c = 2\sigma_c = \frac{d}{h}\Delta p + p\frac{\Delta d}{h} - p\frac{d\Delta h}{h^2} = \frac{dp}{h}\left(\frac{\Delta p}{p} + \frac{2\Delta d}{d}\right) (\text{Pa}) \qquad (6.7)$$

In this approximation the relative change in wall thickness is approximated by the relative change in diameter [equation (6.1)]. Let Δp be the pulse pressure (systolic minus diastolic blood pressure); then the fractional change in blood pressure will be about 0.3, while the corresponding fractional change in artery diameter is generally less than 0.1. To neglect the latter with respect to the fractional change in blood pressure, it should even be less than 0.01, which would presume very stiff arteries. For a small h/d the relative change in circumference at the lumen–wall interface [equation (6.3)] can be approximated by $\Delta d/d$, and the ratio of wall stress and circumferential strain (elasticity coefficient) transfers into

$$E = \frac{\sigma_c}{\Delta d/d} = \frac{\Delta pd}{2h\,\Delta d/d} = \frac{d}{h\mathrm{DC}} \tag{6.8a}$$

$$E = \frac{\Delta pd}{2h\,\Delta d/d} = \frac{\Delta pd^2 d}{2hd\,\Delta d} = \frac{2\Delta p R_i^2}{(R_o^2 - R_i^2)}\frac{R_i}{\Delta R_i}\,\text{(Pa)} \tag{6.8b}$$

Expression (6.8b), with R_i and R_o denoting the inner and outer radius of the artery, respectively, is a conversion from equation (6.8a) to reveal the similarity with the expressions as they appear in textbooks.

The nonlinear variation in strains with radial position complicates a theoretical derivation of wall properties based on observed transmural blood pressure and diameter values, even if the situation is simplified (see below) to rotation symmetry and a homogeneously incompressible wall [26–31]. In its simplest form the expression for a minor perturbation σ_c around S_c for an imposed change in blood pressure corresponds to the Lamé equation [equation (6.6)]. However, the simplification discards the pressure-dependent term [last term in equation (6.7)], which would otherwise render the result nonlinear. If we maintain this term and rearrange the expression for the elasticity coefficient [equation (6.8)], we obtain

$$E = \frac{d^2 p}{2h\,\Delta d}\left(\frac{\Delta p}{p} + \frac{2\Delta d}{d}\right) = \frac{d^2\Delta p}{2h\,\Delta d} + \frac{dp}{h} \tag{6.9}$$

Clearly the elasticity coefficient E increases with transmural pressure due to the contribution of the last term.

In the derivation of the Young's modulus E [equation (6.8)], the contribution of wall thickness is only partly accounted for. Moreover, the mutual interaction between radial, circumferential and longitudinal (incremental) strains is ignored. Let us denote the strains in axial, circumferential, and radial directions by ε_z, ε_c, and ε_h, respectively, while the corresponding incremental stresses are given by σ_z, σ_c, and σ_h. Then, the stress–strain relations in either direction due to a pressure increase Δp are given by

$$\varepsilon_z E = \sigma_z - \mu(\sigma_h + \sigma_c)$$
$$\varepsilon_h E = \sigma_h - \mu(\sigma_z + \sigma_c) \tag{6.10}$$
$$\varepsilon_c E = \sigma_c - \mu(\sigma_h + \sigma_z)$$

In concordance with the assumed material property of volume incompressibility, the Poisson ratio $\mu = 0.5$, while the longitudinal strain ε_z will be zero. Isolating

σ_z gives

$$\varepsilon_c E = \tfrac{3}{4}(\sigma_c - \sigma_h) \tag{6.11}$$

This last expression indicates that the circumferential strain depends not only on the circumferential stress but also on the transmural stress. The circumferential strain ε_c follows from equation (6.3b), the incremental circumferential stress σ_c is provided by equation (6.7), while the incremental radial stress σ_h equals the change in transmural pressure Δp:

$$
\begin{aligned}
E &= \frac{3d(d+h)}{4\Delta d(d-h)}\left(\frac{dp}{2h}\left(\frac{\Delta p}{p} + \frac{2\Delta d}{d}\right) - \Delta p\right) \\[2mm]
&= \frac{3d(d+h)}{4\Delta d(d-h)}\left(\Delta p\left(\frac{d}{2h} - 1\right) + \frac{\Delta dp}{h}\right) \\[2mm]
&= \frac{3d(d+h)\Delta p}{4\Delta d(d-h)}\left(\frac{d}{2h} - 1 + \frac{\Delta dp}{\Delta ph}\right)
\end{aligned}
\tag{6.12}
$$

For a small wall thickness with respect to the diameter ($h<<d$) and stiff arteries (Δd small for a given Δp), the first term within parentheses will dominate and equation (6.12) can be simplified to

$$E = \frac{3d^2\Delta p}{8h\Delta d} = \frac{1.5\Delta p R_i^2}{(R_o^2 - R_i^2)} \frac{R_i}{\Delta R_i} = \frac{3d}{4h\mathrm{DC}} \tag{6.13}$$

Comparing equations (6.13) and (6.8) shows the effect of the mutual interaction of the orthogonal stresses; it lowers the estimate for E by 25%. To appreciate the effect of the assumptions made to convert equation (6.12) to equation (6.13) (estimated elasticity coefficient), let us consider an artery with a lumen diameter of 6 mm and a mean transmural pressure of 100 mmHg (13 kPa), subjected to a change in transmural pressure (pulse pressure) of 40 mmHg ($=5$ kPa). Then, the relative error in the estimated E will be only 4.8% for an $h/d = 0.01$ and a relative diameter change of $\Delta d/d = 0.01$, but will increase dramatically to 37% if both quantities assume realistic values ($h/d = 0.1$; $\Delta d/d = 0.1$) and to 41% for an increase in mean pressure to 120 mmHg. Equation (6.12), instead of equation (6.13), does not solve all the problems, because its derivation assumes that the stresses within the wall do not depend on the radial position. However, the most serious limitation of this derivation is the implicit assumption about a finite wall thickness; it seems that the artery is isolated from its environment. In reality it is embedded in tissue that can be considered as part of the wall, causing stiffer wall behavior [32].

Pulse Wave Velocity

The derivation for the pulse wave velocity c_p is based on Newton's law, applied to a thin cross-sectional slice of an artery, bounded by planes I and II with an area A, an incremental thickness δz, and a specific mass ρ, and the law of conservation of mass (Figure 6.1). The blood velocity is v_z with a velocity gradient δv_z while the pressure is p_z with a pressure gradient δp_z, both along the axis of the artery.

In the incremental time interval δt, mass $\rho A v_z \delta t$ and $\rho A(v_z + \delta v_z)\delta t$ enters and leaves the slice, respectively, resulting in an increase of the mass of the slice of $\delta m = \rho A \delta v_z \delta t$. Let us assume that blood is incompressible and the contribution of a possible longitudinal gradient in diameter is negligible since the slice thickness is very small with respect to the wavelength. Using the relationship $\rho A = m/\delta z$ (specific mass is mass divided by volume) results in

$$\frac{\delta m}{m\delta t} = -\frac{\delta v_z}{\delta z} \tag{6.14}$$

The force exerted by the pressure on plane I is $p_z A$, while on plane II it is $(p_z + \delta p_z)A$. Assuming that the contribution of a possible gradient of the velocity is negligible, the pressure gradient $-\delta p_z A$ causes an acceleration $\delta v_z/\delta t$ of the mass $\rho A \delta z$:

$$\frac{\delta p_z}{\delta z} = -\rho \frac{\delta v_z}{\delta t} \tag{6.15}$$

The final step is to link the change in volume to the change in pressure on the basis of the material properties. For an elastic artery, the distensibility D of a segment with initial volume V is defined as [cf. equation (6.4)]

$$D = \frac{\delta V}{V\delta p_z} = \frac{\delta(m/\rho)}{(m/\rho)\delta p_z} = \frac{\delta m}{m\delta p_z} \tag{6.16}$$

Substitution of equation (6.16) in (6.14) results in

$$\frac{D\delta p_z}{\delta t} = -\frac{\delta v_z}{\delta z} \tag{6.17}$$

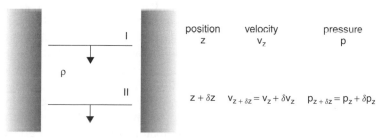

	position	velocity	pressure
	z	v_z	p
	$z + \delta z$	$v_{z+\delta z} = v_z + \delta v_z$	$p_{z+\delta z} = p_z + \delta p_z$

Figure 6.1. Definition of basic parameters for derivation of the pressure wave velocity.

Differentiation of equations (6.17) and (6.15) with respect to t and z, respectively, and elimination of v results in the following familiar wave equation:

$$\frac{\delta^2 p_z}{\delta t^2} = \frac{1}{\rho D} \frac{\delta^2 p_z}{\delta z^2} \tag{6.18}$$

Substitution of a general harmonic solution $p_z = \hat{p} \cos(2\pi f t - 2\pi z/\lambda)$ with $c_p = \lambda f$, λ the wavelength, f the frequency, and c_p the propagation speed of the wave results in the Bramwell–Hill equation:

$$-\hat{p} 4\pi^2 f^2 \cos 2\pi f t - \frac{2\pi z}{\lambda} = \frac{-\hat{p} 4\pi^2}{\rho D \lambda^2} \cos 2\pi f t - \frac{2\pi z}{\lambda} \tag{6.19}$$

$$c_p = \sqrt{\frac{1}{\rho D}} = \sqrt{\frac{1}{\rho \mathrm{DC}}}$$

Equation (6.19) also offers the opportunity to express the pulse-wave velocity c_p as function of pressure p and flow Q by using the notion of characteristic impedance Z [33]. In the absence of wave reflections, Z can be expressed by either a pressure–flow relationship or the mean cross-sectional area A and distensibility [34]:

$$Z = \sqrt{\frac{\rho}{\bar{A}^2 \cdot \mathrm{DC}}} = \frac{dp}{dQ} = \frac{dp}{dA} \frac{dA}{dQ} = \frac{1}{A \cdot \mathrm{DC}} \frac{dA}{dQ} \tag{6.20}$$

In this conversion, equation (6.16) is employed. Solving equation (6.20) for dQ/dA and using equation (6.19) result in

$$\frac{dQ}{dA} = \sqrt{\frac{1}{\rho \mathrm{DC}}} = c_p \tag{6.21}$$

6.3. MEASUREMENT AND PROCESSING OF KEY PARAMETERS

To calculate the key parameters describing the dynamic mechanical characteristics of arterial segments [35,36], that is, the distensibility and compliance coefficients and Young's modulus, we need wall thickness and local diameter and blood pressure waveforms. Since the local blood pressure waveform in, for example, the carotid artery is difficult to acquire, the pulse pressure (difference between systolic and diastolic pressure) measured elsewhere (brachial artery) is substituted for the pressure increment Δp. However, tapering and peripheral pressure wave reflections cause the systolic blood pressure in the brachial artery, but not the diastolic pressure, to be substantially higher than that in the carotid artery. Consequently the pulse pressure is overestimated and the mechanical parameters (DC and CC) are underestimated. The difference in pulse pressure at both locations depends on the age of the subject and the cardiovascular condition [36,37].

An alternative to acquire pulse pressure is provided by a tonometer [38], a pencil-like probe, containing a high-fidelity micromanometer. It is used to flatten an artery transcutaneously against a bony structure, thereby balancing the circumferential stresses in the artery wall. If the probe can be maintained in a steady position, the time-dependent change in blood pressure is accurately recorded. However, the recording requires calibration of the diastolic blood pressure. In diastole, because the pressure drop over the central arteries is negligible if measured at heart level, any accessible location can be selected for the calibration procedure, such as, the brachial artery. Under steady-state conditions the diastolic blood pressure exhibits only minor fluctuations, allowing for an incidental reference measurement, for example, with a conventional sphygmomanometer or an oscillometric blood pressure meter. Likewise, assuming that mean arterial pressure (MAP) is also the same in the major arteries, the average of the tonometer waveform over a cardiac cycle can be equated to the MAP derived in another way. Unfortunately, there is no physically sound algorithm to estimate MAP from oscillometric blood pressure readings. The reported values for MAP, but also for the recorded systolic and diastolic blood pressures, may vary considerably [39]. Since diastolic pressure and MAP are used to calibrate the tonometer readings, any error in the reference values will equally emerge in the tonometer blood pressure values.

The approach as outlined above assumes that the tonometer is held firmly in position, meaning that the applied force should vary in accordance with the blood pressure to be measured. This requirement is difficult to comply with, resulting in distorted pressure registrations especially in late systole. The other prerequisite is that a solid background supports the artery of interest. This is true for the radial, brachial, and femoral arteries, but not for the carotid artery. That is why blood pressure results for this artery are subject to dispute, especially since, for ethical reasons, verification measurements are scarce and virtually absent for the normal population.

Diastolic diameter and its pulsatile change over the cardiac cycle can be measured accurately and reliably with modern echo-tracking systems [40], using a two-dimensional B-mode imager attached to a vessel wall moving detector system [10]. The displacement detection algorithm is based on radiofrequency (RF) correlation tracking rather than narrowband Doppler processing [41]. Processing in the RF domain has the advantage that the high depth resolution offered by the echo mode (wideband RF signals) is maintained. A fine depth resolution is essential since the displacement gradient over the wall can be substantial [cf. (equation (6.2)]. On the other hand, for a wideband RF signal the frequency-dependent attenuation causes a significant downward shift in the mean RF frequency depending on depth location and intervening tissues. That is why displacement detection based on echo-mode RF processing involves the estimation of both the phase shift over subsequent observations and the underlying mean RF frequency. This is readily achieved for RF signals with a specific spectral shape, such as a Gaussian distribution (or at least a symmetric distribution). Then, the shape of the cross-correlation function of the RF signals, converted to a complex representation using the Hilbert transform, is well defined [22, 42–44]. Only three complex coefficients are required (autocorrelation, correlation at depth, and time lag 1, respectively) to estimate the local carrier frequency (phase at depth lag 1), displacement (phase at time lag 1), signal level (autocorrelation), and the RF bandwidth and signal-to-noise ratio (amplitude of the coefficients).

Displacement detection using echo-mode RF signals has a good precision [45], even when extremely short (few ms) temporal estimation windows are used. This is because the random appearance of reflections, that is, its random phase, is maintained while processing the signal [41]. Moreover, the signal segment considered for displacement detection [43], as set at the onset of registration, is automatically repositioned according to the observed displacement, ensuring that throughout the cardiac cycle the same wall segment is tracked despite wall displacements of more than 2 times the resolution of the echo system. The same procedure is followed for both the anterior and posterior wall; the difference between both gives the change in lumen diameter over time (distension waveform), while the initial distance between the selected segments is used as an estimate for the end-diastolic lumen diameter. In more recent systems, artery wall–lumen transitions at end diastole are identified automatically, allowing beat-to-beat acquisition and presentation of the end-diastolic diameter and distension waveform. The end-diastolic diameter is not the true lumen diameter since the identification algorithm locks onto the large ultrasound echo transient of the media–adventitia interface. Hence, the estimated diameter is the adventitia–adventitia distance minus one resolution of the echo system (trailing edge of anterior wall echo).

To get the true lumen diameter, algorithms have been developed that, starting from an arbitrary position within the lumen, looks for transients in echo level. If they are consistent in time or in position and the change in echo level is substantial, then the transient is quite likely caused by the lumen–intima boundary. Again an error is made because the distance between the trailing echo edge of the anterior intima–lumen interface and the leading edge of the posterior interface is considered.

Once the positions of the adventitia–media and intima–lumen boundaries are established, it is a small step to derive the intima–media thickness (IMT). However, at the anterior artery wall, large trailing echoes from the adventitia extend into the media and may even partially cover the media–intima transition, especially for young subjects or for echo systems with an inadequate resolution [46]. That is why generally only the IMT measured at the posterior wall is considered [47]. IMT should not be confused with wall thickness because the latter also includes the adventitia layer, whose outer boundary cannot reliably be distinguished with present ultrasound techniques.

The use of IMT rather than whole-wall thickness in assessing artery wall dynamics is acceptable, because the media is the most important determinant of these dynamics, at least under normal circumstances and in hypertension. In atherosclerosis, however, the intima is the layer most affected. Ever since the first IMT measurements by Pignoli et al. [48], a variety of automated techniques have been developed [49,50]. All these techniques provide a mean IMT extracted from B–mode images over a length of 10–20 mm, thereby reducing the obscuring effect of ultrasound speckle. In the past, the end-diastolic images were selected from videorecordings according to a standard TV format with only 25 frames per second and thus a limited temporal resolution. Nowadays real-time B-mode display is decoupled from the TV standard, allowing a considerable increase in image quality and image update rate. However, the B-mode image stream, and thus the image threshold level, remains susceptible to the settings for gain and amplitude compression [46,51].

The local relative dynamic amplitude characteristics of RF signals are inherently insensitive for gain settings and are not modified by nonlinear processing techniques, such as amplitude thresholding and dynamic range compression. That is why it is logical to extend the RF system for the measurement of end-diastolic diameter d and relative change in diameter $\Delta d/d$ with an automated method to derive the local IMT from the recorded RF signals. If the RF signals have been recorded in M mode, then the final IMT estimate will be the mean of subsequent observations [47,52]. For RF signals recorded in B-mode the spatial mean over a short image segment length provides an instantaneous estimate of wall thickness [53].

6.4. PRESSURE AND DIAMETER WAVEFORMS

As stated before, the estimation of mechanical parameters requires that both pressure and diameter waveforms be obtained at the same location and preferably simultaneously. For the carotid artery, a predilection site for atherosclerotic disease and, hence, a site of clinical interest, local pressure measurements are quite difficult. Substitution of the carotid pulse pressure by the pulse pressure obtained from the nearby brachial artery is not an option because of an unpredictable difference between both pulse pressures [37].

In Section 6.2 attempts were made to develop a theoretical expression for the pressure–diameter relationship of an artery. Because of the interrelation between pressure, diameter, wall thickness, and stresses, only an approximation could be obtained under quite rigid constraints (stiff artery). For the physiological pressure range, experimental measurements confirmed an exponential relationship between the time-dependent pressure $p(t)$ and cross-sectional area $A(t) = \pi d^2/4$ [54–57]:

$$p(t) = p_0 e^{\gamma A(t)} \tag{6.22}$$

The unknown constant γ can be derived if the local blood pressure and lumen area are known. This is the case for the diastolic pressure p_d and area A_d; and for the systolic pressure p_s and area A_s. Solving the resulting set of two equations gives

$$p(t) = p_d e^{\alpha((A(t)/A_d)-1)} \tag{6.23}$$

with

$$\alpha = \frac{A_d \ln(p_s/p_d)}{A_s - A_d} \tag{6.24}$$

Since the wall rigidity index α (dimensionless) is pressure independent, equation (6.24) is valid over a large physiological pressure range [54–57]. The rigidity index as used here is the reciprocal of the stiffness parameter defined earlier [54].

Equation (6.24) requires that the local diastolic and systolic blood pressures be known, but generally this is not the case. However, equation (6.23) offers the opportunity to derive the local pressure waveform, in conjunction with the local diameter waveform, using blood pressures recorded elsewhere. It is based on the assumption that for the major arteries, diastolic blood pressures and MAP do not vary with location. This assumption is reasonable since in the brachial artery mean wall shear stress, and hence friction loss, is low; the mean pressure drop over the major arteries is about 1 mmHg. Suppose that the area (diameter) waveform were recorded in the common carotid artery and the blood pressure waveform with a tonometer in the radial artery. Starting with an initial guess for α, based on the diastolic and systolic blood pressures observed elsewhere [equation (6.24)], provides a first estimate of the local pressure waveform. The observed difference between its time average and the peripheral MAP subsequently initiates an iterative adaptation procedure for α until the carotid and peripheral MAPs are equal [58]. For the final value of α, equation (6.23) describes the pressure waveform in the carotid artery, linked to the local area (diameter) waveform.

Given equation (6.23), it is now possible to estimate the distensibility and compliance coefficients and pulse wave velocity at any pressure, for example, at 100 mmHg [59]:

$$DC = \left.\frac{\delta A}{A \delta p}\right|_{p=100} = \left.\frac{A_d}{\alpha A(p) p}\right|_{p=100} = \frac{A_d}{100 \alpha A_{100}}$$

$$PWV = \sqrt{\frac{1}{\rho DC}} = \sqrt{\frac{100 \alpha A_{100}}{\rho A_d}} \tag{6.25}$$

$$CC = \left.\frac{\delta A}{\delta p}\right|_{p=100} = \frac{A_d}{100 \alpha}$$

The value A_{100} follows from equation (6.23) by substituting $p = 100$ mmHg ($= 13.3$ kPa) and solving the equation. Indeed, for an exponential relationship between lumen area and pressure, the mechanical parameters turn out to be pressure-dependent, complicating direct comparison of subject groups with different blood pressures. Equation (6.25), in combination with equation (6.23), offers convenient ways to circumvent the problems associated with local blood pressure measurements. The diastolic pulse wave velocity provides a direct estimate for the rigidity index α. Then, the local pressure waveform is known without the iteration procedure or assumption about a possible drop in MAP. Its combination with the diameter waveform provides isobaric estimates for distensibility and compliance. Because the latter are now based on derivatives rather than large increments (pulse pressure and associated pulsatile change in lumen diameter), the effect of the nonlinear relationship is inherently suppressed.

For elastic arteries, such as the common carotid artery, the above approach can be simplified by assuming for the physiological pressure range a linear relationship between pressure and area [60]. Again, the mean of the pulsatile pressure waveform ($\text{MAP} - p_d$) is now directly related to the mean of the pulsatile area waveform ($\bar{A} - A_d$):

$$\text{MAP} - p_d = \zeta(\bar{A} - A_d)$$

$$\zeta = \frac{\text{MAP} - p_d}{\bar{A} - A_d} \qquad (6.26)$$

$$p(t) = \frac{\text{MAP} - p_d}{\bar{A} - A_d} A(t)$$

6.5. WHAT WE HAVE LEARNED

Across mammals the blood pressure is of the same order [61,62], although the orthostatic contribution to transmural pressure will vary with size. Hence, the arteries are subjected to the same load, which has to be borne primarily by the vascular smooth muscular fibers. Then Young's modulus, the circumferential wall stress, and the relative change in diameter, and thus the distensibility, will be of the same order across species. This consideration does not apply for the compliance, which increases with mammal size (absolute change in vessel cross section).

The general statement above is not intended to stimulate generalization and extrapolation. Within species individual and interarterial variations of a factor of 5 are quite likely. That dynamic wall behavior of elastic arteries (ascending and descending aorta, carotid artery) differs from that of muscular arteries (coronary femoral, and brachial arteries) is not surprising, but that their properties adapt differently to, for example, aging and hypertension was unknown until the introduction of dynamic vascular ultrasound [35,36,63]. Carotid IMT also increases substantially as a function of age at an estimated rate of 7–10 μm/year [64–68] or varies within a relatively short arterial segment [69].

Proper interpretation of the data is hampered by the various methods in use to acquire and process the basic data (diameter, wall thickness, blood pressure). In a large number of studies the adventitia–adventitia diameter is used as a substitute for the lumen diameter. Because the carotid artery IMT increases considerably with age, the involved error is confounding the statistical analysis. There is still no consensus about the expression to use for Young's modulus, and it is quite unlikely that a universal solution will be found (see Section 6.2). Finally, the issue of artery properties is clouded by the indiscriminate use of distensibility and compliance. Especially the English literature uses compliance where distensibility is intended [70,71].

Aging

Under normal circumstances distensibility and compliance of the elastic carotid artery decrease linearly with age from the third decade onward, with the reduction of compliance less steep than the reduction of distensibility [15,63]. The latter can be explained by the increase in diameter with increasing age [12,14,15] (Table 6.1) [72]. In this way elastic arteries counteract the reduction of their ability to store volume and, hence, the increase in systolic arterial and pulse pressure, with increase in age. In our analysis end-diastolic diameter is considered. When mean diameters were considered, the difference in reduction between distensibility and compliance would have been quantitatively different but qualitatively similar. Distension and circumferential strain also decrease with age (Figure 6.2; Table 6.1).

The loss of dynamic properties along the arterial tree is inhomogeneous. At older age distensibility of the muscular common femoral artery is reduced, but the distensibility of the deep and superficial muscular femoral arteries [73] and the compliance of the muscular brachial artery are not [74,75]. Similarly, in the elastic carotid artery bifurcation, distensibility of the bulb, where predominantly the baroreceptors are located, is more severely affected by age than the distensibility of the common carotid artery [14,17].

Hypertension

In patients with essential hypertension, arterial stiffening [63,76,77] is not a generalized phenomenon along the arterial tree. In untreated hypertensive patients, at ambient mean arterial pressure, distensibility and compliance of the elastic carotid artery, but not of the radial artery [78], are significantly reduced [18]. In

TABLE 6.1. Diameter (d) and Percentage Systolic Circumferential Strain ($\Delta d/d * 100\%$) as Function of Age per Decade in Right Common Carotid Artery in Females ($n = 55$) and Males ($n = 56$); Mean $\pm$ SD

Age (years)	Females			Males		
	n	d (mm)	$\Delta d/d$ (%)	n	d (mm)	$\Delta d/d$ (%)
10–19	10	5.9 ± 0.3	13 ± 2	8	6.0 ± 0.3	14 ± 3
20–29	12	6.0 ± 0.3	10 ± 1	12	6.5 ± 0.6	10 ± 2
30–39	15	6.2 ± 0.5	8 ± 2	18	6.5 ± 0.5	9 ± 2
40–49	10	6.4 ± 0.6	7 ± 2	10	6.5 ± 0.4	6 ± 2
50–59	8	6.3 ± 0.3^a	6 ± 2^a	7	6.4 ± 0.5^a	5 ± 2^a

^{a}Significantly different from second age decade.

Source: After Samijo et al. [72].

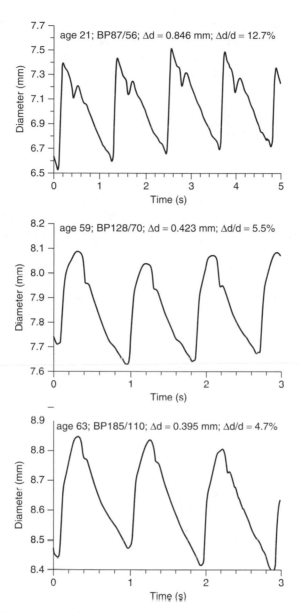

Figure 6.2. Distension waveforms as recorded in the common carotid artery of a young (top) and an older normotensive volunteer (middle), and an older hypertensive patient (bottom). During the recordings the volunteers and the patient were fully relaxed. Note the reduced distension (Δd) and circumferential strain ($\Delta d/d$; d = diameter), at an even higher blood pressure, in normotensive volunteer at older age, reflecting increased arterial stiffness. In hypertension arterial stiffness is further increased, as indicated by the slightly reduced distension and the substantially reduced circumferential strain at a significantly higher blood pressure. (After Reneman et al. [35]).

the latter the Young's modulus was found to be similar in essential hypertensive patients and in age-matched control subjects [79].

It is still incompletely understood whether in essential hypertension the reduction of artery wall distensibility and compliance of the elastic arteries (see Table 6.2) is caused by the increase in blood pressure or whether intrinsic changes in the wall contribute to this process [63]. The observation by Laurent et al. [18,80] favors a dominant role of increased arterial pressure, but our observations in borderline hypertensives [17,81] indicate that the reduction of dynamic artery wall properties cannot be fully explained by increased blood pressure. This is in line with the observation that blood pressure reduction in hypertensive patients by nitroglycerine does not normalize artery stiffness [82]. In young spontaneously hypertensive rats the reduced dynamic artery wall properties are independent of elevated blood pressures [83], which agrees with the more recent finding that in younger essential hypertensives, intrinsic changes in the artery wall contribute to increased stiffness of the arteries [84]. Therefore, in the treatment of patients with essential and borderline hypertension, not only reduction of blood pressure but also enhancement of compliance of elastic arteries has to be considered, especially because the loss of compliance and distensibility strongly correlates with left ventricular hypertrophy [85]. Compliance and distensibility of elastic arteries can be increased substantially by pharmacological intervention (increases up to 16%), but one should bear in mind that not all antihypertensive drugs improve artery wall compliance, despite their blood pressure–lowering effect [86,87].

Diabetes

In cross-sectional studies, elastic and muscular arteries are generally found to be stiffer in diabetic patients than in age-matched control subjects [63], although

TABLE 6.2. Carotid Artery Diameter, Distensibility, and Compliance in Patients with Essential Hypertension (HT; 54 ± 15 years) and in Age-Matched Normotensives

Parameters	HT $n = 15$	NT $n = 14$
At mean arterial pressure		
Diameter (mm)	7.3 ± 0.3	6.9 ± 0.2
Distensibility (MPa^{-1})	7.8 ± 0.7^a	11.7 ± 1.7
Compliance (mm^2/kPa)	0.6 ± 0.1^b	0.9 ± 0.1
At 100 mmHg		
Diameter (mm)	7.5 ± 0.3	7.3 ± 0.2
Distensibility (MPa^{-1})	10.0 ± 1.0	9.0 ± 1.1
Compliance (mm^2/kPa)	0.8 ± 0.1	0.7 ± 0.1

[a](NT; 48 ± 15 years). Data in the table are mean $\pm$ standard error of the mean.
[b]Significantly different from NT.

Source: After Laurent et al. [18].

TABLE 6.3. Percentage Peak Systolic Circumferential Strain ($\Delta d/d * 100\%$; Mean $\pm$ SD) in Common Carotid Artery (CCA) and Proximal (B_p) and Distal (B_d) Parts of Carotid Artery Bulb and at Level of Its Maximum Diameter (B_{max}) in Normotensive Young (NTY; 24 ± 3 years) and Older (NTO; 38 ± 5 years) Volunteers, and in Borderline Hypertensives (BHT; 38 ± 3 years); Mean $\pm$ SD

Subject	n	CCA	B_p	B_{max}	B_d
BHT	16	6.3 ± 1.3	3.8 ± 1.4^a	$5.1 \pm 1.4^{a,b}$	$5.4 \pm 1.6^{a,b}$
NTO	15	7.5 ± 1.9	5.7 ± 2.3^a	7.0 ± 1.9	$5.4 + 2.3^a$
NTY	18	9.5 ± 2.2	9.2 ± 2.4	9.9 ± 2.3	8.7 ± 2.6

[a] Significantly different from CCA.
[b] Significantly different from B_p

Source: After Van Merode et al. [17].

the findings in insulin-dependent diabetes mellitus (IDDM; type I diabetes) are inconsistent. For example, in patients with uncomplicated IDDM, Kool et al. [88] did not find an obvious reduction of wall properties of elastic and muscular arteries in young patients, while Hu et al. [89] observed increased stiffness of the descending aorta in children and adolescents. The observations in non-insulin-dependent diabetes mellitus (NIDDM; type 2 diabetes) are far more consistent in the studies published so far. In cross-sectional [90] and population-based studies [91,92] NIDDM was shown to be associated with loss of distensibility and compliance of both elastic and muscular arteries. Distensibility of the carotid artery is even reduced in healthy, nondiabetic subjects with an insulin resistance syndrome [91,93], indicating that artery stiffening is an early marker of pathology in this disorder.

Atherosclerosis

Relatively little is known about arterial dynamic properties in atherosclerosis [63]. In hypertensive patients arterial stiffness is associated with the presence and extent of atherosclerosis [94]. Population-based studies demonstrate that both aortic and common carotid artery stiffness have a strong positive association with carotid IMT and severity of plaque in these vessels [95]. The carotid–femoral pulse wave velocity, but not the carotid distensibility, provides additional predictive value for coronary events [96].

6.6. CONCLUSIONS

An important shortcoming in the noninvasive assessment of dynamic vascular properties is the lack of a direct method to reliably determine pulse pressure non-invasively at the site of measurement. Using brachial pulse pressure as a substitute for carotid pulse pressure is not ideal because disease processes affect brachial and carotid artery wall properties, and, hence, pulse pressure, differently [37]. There is no pulse pressure substitute for the femoral artery. Reliable noninvasive acquisition of the pulse pressure waveform is also necessary to adequately compare normotensives and hypertensives at isobaric pressures, requiring the construction and comparison of full pressure–diameter relations. A direct approach is feasible only for radial and brachial arteries [79] because these arteries allow (simultaneous) acquisition of pressure and diameter waveforms. For the carotid artery a simple approach allows the derivation of the local pressure waveform from the diameter waveform assuming a linear relationship [60]. This can be extended to an exponential pressure–area relationship [54], with the rigidity coefficient as a single parameter [58], allowing a more general approach for the characterization of the mechanical behavior of arteries. However, its implementation requires knowledge about the mean arterial pressure, which is quite susceptible for measurement artifacts. This problem can be avoided if techniques become available to acquire the local pulse wave velocity [97]. Then, it will be possible to fully explore the effects of age and risk factors on the mechanical properties of both elastic and muscular arteries locally. This may eventually settle the current dispute about possible associations between central (carotid–femoral pathway) or carotid arterial stiffness on one hand and coronary or cerebral vascular disease on the other hand [96].

REFERENCES

1. Strandness DE, Jr., McCutcheon EP, Rushmer RF: Application of a transcutaneous Doppler flowmeter in evaluation of occlusive arterial disease, *Surg Gynecol Obstet* **122**: 1039–1045 (1966).
2. Polak JF: Peripheral arterial disease. Evaluation with color flow and duplex sonography, *Radiol Clin North Am* **33**:71–90 (1995).
3. Bots ML, Hofman A, Grobbee DE: Increased common carotid intima-media thickness. Adaptive response or a reflection of atherosclerosis? Findings from the Rotterdam study, *Stroke* **28**:2442–2447 (1997).
4. O'Leary DH, Polak JF, Kronmal RA, Manolio TA, Burke GL, Wolfson SK: Carotid artery intima and media thickness as a risk factor for myocardial infaction and stroke in older adults, *N Engl J Med* **340**:14–22 (1999).
5. Boutouyrie P, Bussy C, Hayoz D, Hengstler J, Dartois N, Laloux B, Brunner H, Laurent S: Local pulse pressure and regression of arterial wall hypertrophy during long-term antihypertensive treatment, *Circulation* **101**:2601–2606 (2000).
6. Simon A, Gariepy J, Chironi G, Megnien JL, Levenson J: Intima-media thickness: A new tool for diagnosis and treatment of cardiovascular risk, *J Hypertens* **20**:159–169 (2002).
7. Bots ML, Grobbee DE, Hofman A, Witteman JC: Common carotid intima-media thickness and risk of acute myocardial infarction: The role of lumen diameter, *Stroke* **36**:762–767 (2005).
8. Lorenz MW, von Kegler S, Steinmetz H, Markus HS, Sitzer M: Carotid intima-media thickening indicates a higher vascular risk across a wide age range: prospective data from the Carotid Atherosclerosis Progression Study (CAPS), *Stroke* **37**:87–92 (2006).

9. Staub D, Meyerhans A, Bundi B, Schmid HP, Frauchiger B: Prediction of cardio-vascular morbidity and mortality: Comparison of the internal carotid artery resistive index with the common carotid artery intima-media thickness, *Stroke* **37**:800–805 (2006).

10. Hoeks APG, Brands PJ, Smeets FAM, Reneman RS: Assessment of the distensibility of superficial arteries, *Ultrasound Med Biol* **16**:121–128 (1990).

11. Tardy Y, Meister JJ, Brunner HR, Arditi M: Non-invasive estimate of the mechanical properties of peripheral arteries from ultrasonic and photoplethysmographic measurements, *Clin Phys Physiol Meas* **12**:39–54 (1991).

12. Riley WA, Barnes RW, Evans GW, Burke GL: Ultrasonic measurement of the elastic modulus of the common carotid artery. The atherosclerosis risk in communities (ARIC) study, *Stroke* **23**:952–956 (1992).

13. Hoeks APG, Brands PJ, Willigers JM, Reneman RS: Non-invasive assessment of mechanical properties of arteries in health and disease, *Proc Inst Mech Eng* **213**:195–202 (1999).

14. Reneman RS, Van Merode T, Hick P, Hoeks APG: Flow velocity patterns in and distensibility of the carotid artery bulb in subjects of various ages, *Circulation* **71**:500–509 (1985).

15. Reneman RS, Van Merode T, Hick P, Muytjens AMM, Hoeks APG: Age-related changes in carotid artery wall properties in man, *Ultrasound Med Biol* **12**:465–471 (1986).

16. Van Merode T, Hick PJJ, Hoeks APG, Rahn KH, Reneman RS: Carotid artery wall properties in normotensive and borderline hypertensive subjects of various ages, *Ultrasound Med Biol* **14**:563–569 (1988).

17. Van Merode T, Brands PJ, Hoeks APG, Reneman RS: Faster ageing of the carotid artery bifurcation in borderline hypertensive subjects, *J Hypertens* **11**:171–176 (1993).

18. Laurent S, Caviezel B, Beck L, Girerd X, Billaud E, Boutouyrie P, Hoeks A, Safar M: Carotid artery distensibility and distending pressure in hypertensive humans, *Hypertension* **23**:878–883 (1994).

19. Laurent S: Arterial wall hypertrophy and stiffness in essential hypertensive patients, *Hypertension* **26**:355–362 (1995).

20. Menotti A, Seccareccia F, Giampaoij S, Giuli B: The predictive role of systolic, diastolic and mean blood pressure on cardiovascular and all causes of death, *J Hypertens* **7**:595–599 (1989).

21. Safar ME, Levy BI, Struijker-Boudier H: Current perspectives on arterial stiffness and pulse pressure in hypertension and cardiovascular diseases, *Circulation* **107**:2864–2869 (2003).

22. Brands PJ, Hoeks APG, Willigers J, Willekes C, Reneman RS: An integrated system for the non-invasive assessment of vessel wall and hemodynamic properties of large arteries by means of ultrasound, *Eur J Ultrasound* **9**:257–266 (1999).

23. Patel DJ, Fry DL: Longitudinal tethering of arteries in dogs, *Circ Res* **19**:1011–1021 (1966).

24. L'Italien GJ, Chandrasekar NR, Lamuraglia GM, Pevec WC, Dhara S, Warnock DF, Abbott WM: Biaxial elastic properties of rat arteries in vivo: influence of vascular wall cells on anisotropy, *Am J Physiol* **267**:H574–H579 (1994).

25. Van Gorp A, Van Ingen Schenau DS, Willigers J, Hoeks AP, De Mey JG, Struijker Boudier HA, Reneman RS: A technique to assess aortic distensibility and compliance in anesthetized and awake rats, *Am J Physiol* **270**:H780–H786 (1996).

26. Taylor LA, Gerrard JH: Pressure-radius relationships for elastic tubes and their application to arteries: Part 1—Theoretical relationships, *Med Biol Eng Comput* **15**:11–17 (1977).

27. Taylor LA, Gerrard JH: Pressure-radius relationships for elastic tubes and their applications to arteries: Part 2—A comparison of theory and experiment for a rubber tube, *Med Biol Eng Comput* **15**:18–21 (1977).

28. Demiray H: Incremental elastic modulus for isotropic elastic bodies with application to arteries, *J Biomech Eng* **105**:308–309 (1983).

29. Fung YC: *Biodynamics: Circulation*, Springer-Verlag, New York, 1984.

30. Nichols WW, O'Rourke MF: *McDonald's Blood Flow in Arteries*, Edward Arnold, London, 1998.

31. Zamir M: *The Physics of Blood Flow*, Springer-Verlag, New York, 2000.

32. Zhang X, Greenleaf JF: The stiffening of arteries by the tissue-mimicking gelatin, *IEEE Trans Ultrason Ferroelectr Freq Control* **53**:1534–1539 (2006).

33. Westerhof N: Arterial haemodynamics, in Strackee J, Westerhof N, eds, *The Physics of Circulation*, Inst Physics Publ, Bristol, UK, 1993.

34. Rabben SI, Stergiopulos N, Hellevik LR, Smiseth OA, Slordahl S, Urheim S, Angelsen B: An ultrasound-based method for determining pulse wave velocity in superficial arteries, *J Biomech* **37**:1615–1622 (2004).

35. Reneman RS, Meinders JM, Hoeks AP: Non-invasive ultrasound in arterial wall dynamics in humans: What have we learned and what remains to be solved, *Eur Heart J* **26**:960–966 (2005).

36. Laurent S, Cockcroft J, Van Bortel L, Boutouyrie P, Giannattasio C, Hayoz D, Pannier B, Vlachopoulos C, Wilkinson I, Struijker-Boudier H: Expert consensus document on arterial stiffness: Methodological issues and clinical applications, *Eur Heart J* **27**:2588–2605 (2006).

37. Waddell TK, Dart AM, Medley TL, Cameron JD, Kingwell BA: Carotid pressure is a better predictor of coronary artery disease severity than brachial pressure, *Hypertension* **38**:927–931 (2001).

38. Kelly R, Hayward C, Avolio A, O'Rourke M: Noninvasive determination of age-related changes in the human arterial pulse, *Circulation* **80**:1652–1659 (1989).

39. Amoore JN, Geake WB, Scott DHT: Oscillometric non-invasive blood pressure measurements: The influence of the make of instruments on readings? *Med Biol Eng Comput* **35**:131–134 (1997).

40. Kool MJF, Van Merode T, Reneman RS, Hoeks APG, Struijker Boudier HAJ, Van Bortel LMAB: Evaluation of reproducibility of a vessel wall movement detector system for assessment of large artery properties, *Cardiovasc Res* **28**:610–614 (1994).

41. Hoeks APG, Arts TGJ, Brands PJ, Reneman RS: Comparison of the performance of the cross correlation and Doppler autocorrelation technique to estimate the mean velocity of simulated ultrasound signals, *Ultrasound Med Biol* **19**:727–740 (1993).

42. Brands PJ, Hoeks APG, Ledoux LAF, Reneman RS: A radio frequency domain complex cross-correlation model to estimate blood flow velocity and tissue motion by means of ultrasound, *Ultrasound Med Biol* **23**:911–920 (1997).

43. Meinders JM, Brands PJ, Willigers JM, Kornet L, Hoeks AP: Assessment of the spatial homogeneity of artery dimension parameters with high frame rate 2-D B-mode, *Ultrasound Med Biol* **27**:785–794 (2001).

44. Hoeks APG, Reneman RS: Do Doppler systems color arteries red? in Kowalewski TA et al, eds, *Blood Flow Modelling and Diagnostics*, Polish Academy of Sciences, Warsaw, 2005, pp 243–271.

45. Bennett MJ, McLaughlin S, Anderson T, McDicken WN: Error analysis of ultrasonic tissue Doppler velocity estimation techniques for quantification of velocity and strain, *Ultrasound Med Biol* **33**:74–81 (2007).

46. Touboul PJ, Hennerici MG, Meairs S, Adams H, Amarenco P, Bornstein N, Csiba L, Desvarieux M, Ebrahim S, Fatar M, Hernandez Hernandez R, Jaff M, Kownator S, Prati P, Rundek T, Sitzer M, Schminke U, Tardif JC, Taylor A, Vicaut E, Woo KS, Zannad F, Zureik M: Mannheim Carotid Intima-Media Thickness Consensus (2004–2006). An update on behalf of the Advisory Board of the 3rd and 4th Watching the Risk Symposium 13th and 15th European Stroke Conferences, Mannheim, Germany, 2004, and Brussels, Belgium, 2006, *Cerebrovasc Dis* **23**:75–80 (2006).

47. Willekes C, Hoeks AP, Bots ML, Brands PJ, Willigers JM, Reneman RS: Evaluation of off-line automated intima-media thickness detection of the common carotid artery based on M-line signal processing, *Ultrasound Med Biol* **25**:57–64 (1999).

48. Pignoli P, Tremoli E, Poli A, Oreste P, Paoletti R: Intimal plus medial thickness of the arterial wall: A direct measurement with ultrasound imaging, *Circulation* **74**:1399–1406 (1986).

49. Selzer RH, Hodis HN, Kwong-Fu H, Mack WJ, Lee PL, Liu CR, Liu CH: Evaluation of computerized edge tracking for quantifying intima-media thickness of the common carotid artery from B-mode ultrasound images, *Atherosclerosis* **111**:1–11 (1994).

50. Graf S, Gariepy J, Massonneau M, Armentano RL, Mansour S, Barra JG, Simon A, Levenson J: Experimental and clinical validation of arterial diameter waveform and intimal media thickness obtained from B-mode ultrasound image processing, *Ultrasound Med Biol* **25**:1353–1363 (1999).

51. Bots ML, Mulder PG, Hofman A, van Es GA, Grobbee DE: Reproducibility of carotid vessel wall thickness measurements. The Rotterdam study, *J Clin Epidemiol* **47**:921–930 (1994).

52. Hoeks APG, Willekes C, Boutouyrie P, Brands PJ, Willigers JM, Reneman RS: Automated detection of local artery wall thickness based on M-line signal processing, *Ultrasound Med Biol* **23**:1017–1023 (1997).

53. Meinders JM, Kornet L, Hoeks AP: Assessment of spatial inhomogeneities in intima media thickness along an arterial segment using its dynamic behavior, *Am J Physiol Heart Circ Physiol* **285**:H384–H391 (2003).

54. Hayashi K, Handa H, Nagasawa S, Okumura A, Moritake K: Stiffness and elastic behavior of human intracranial and extracranial arteries, *J Biomech* **13**:175–184 (1980).

55. Stettler JC, Niederer P, Anliker M: Theoretical analysis of arterial hemodynamics including the influence of bifurcations. Part I: Mathematical model and prediction of normal pulse patterns, *Ann Biomed Eng* **9**:145–164 (1981).

56. Langewouters GJ, Wesseling KH, Goedhard WJA: The static elastic properties of 45 human thoracic and 20 abdominal aortas in vitro and the parameters of a new model, *J Biomech* **17**:425–435 (1984).

57. Powalowski T, Pensko B: A noninvasive ultrasonic method for the elasticity evaluation of the carotid arteries and its application in the diagnosis of the cerebro-vascular system, *Arch Acoust* **13**:109–126 (1988).

58. Meinders JM, Hoeks AP: Simultaneous assessment of diameter and pressure waveforms in the carotid artery, *Ultrasound Med Biol* **30**:147–154 (2004).

59. Hayashi K: Experimental approaches on measuring the mechanical properties and constitutive laws of arterial walls, *J Biomech Eng* **115**:481–488 (1993).

60. Van Bortel LM, Balkestein EJ, van der Heijden-Spek JJ, Vanmolkot FH, Staessen JA, Kragten JA, Vredeveld JW, Safar ME, Struijker Boudier HA, Hoeks AP: Non-invasive assessment of local arterial pulse pressure: Comparison of applanation tonometry and echo-tracking, *J Hypertens* **19**:1037–1044 (2001).

61. West GB, Brown JH, Enquist BJ: A general model for the origin of allometric scaling laws in biology, *Science* **276**:122–126 (1997).

62. Greve JM, Les AS, Tang BT, Draney Blomme MT, Wilson NM, Dalman RL, Pelc NJ, Taylor CA: Allometric scaling of wall shear stress from mice to humans: Quantification using cine phase-contrast MRI and computational fluid dynamics, *Am J Physiol Heart Circ Physiol* **291**:H1700–H1708 (2006).

63. Cheng KS, Baker CR, Hamilton G, Hoeks AP, Seifalian AM: Arterial elastic properties and cardiovascular risk/event, *Eur J Vasc Endovasc Surg* **24**:383–397 (2002).

64. Dinenno FA, Jones PP, Seals DR, Tanaka H: Age-associated arterial wall thickening is related to elevations in sympathetic activity in healthy humans, *Am J Physiol Heart Circ Physiol* **278**:H1205–H1210 (2000).

65. Kornet L, Reneman RS, Hoeks APG: Age-related increase in femoral intima-media thickness in healthy humans [Letter], *Arterioscler Thromb Vasc Biol* **20**:2172 (2000).

66. Homma S, Hirose N, Ishida H, Ishii T, Araki G: Carotid plaque and intima-media thickness assessed by b-mode ultrasonography in subjects ranging from young adults to centenarians, *Stroke* **32**:830–835 (2001).

67. Tanaka H, Dinenno FA, Monahan KD, DeSouza CA, Seals DR: Carotid artery wall hypertrophy with age is related to local systolic blood pressure in healthy men, *Arterioscler Thromb Vasc Biol* **21**:82–87 (2001).

68. Yanase T, Nasu S, Mukuta Y, Shimizu Y, Nishihara T, Okabe T, Nomura M, Inoguchi T, Nawata H: Evaluation of a new carotid intima-media thickness measurement by B-mode ultrasonography using an innovative measurement software, intimascope, *Am J Hypertens* **19**:1206–1212 (2006).

69. Willekes C, Brands PJ, Willigers JM, Hoeks APG, Reneman RS: Assessment of local differences in intima-media thickness in the human carotid artery, *J Vasc Res* **36**:222–228 (1999).

70. Lehmann ED, Hopkins KD, Gosling RG: Multiple definitions of "compliance", *Clin Sci* (Colch) **90**:433–434 (1996).

71. Gosling RG, Budge MM: Terminology for describing the elastic behavior of arteries, *Hypertension* **41**:1180–1182 (2003).

72. Samijo SK, Willigers JM, Barkhuysen R, Kitslaar PJEHM, Reneman RS, Hoeks APG: Wall shear stress in the common carotid artery as function of age and gender, *Cardiovasc Res* **39**:515–522 (1998).

73. Van Merode T, Brands PJ, Hoeks APG, Reneman RS: Different effects of ageing on elastic and muscular arterial bifurcations in men, *J Vasc Res* **33**:47–52 (1996).

74. Benetos A, Laurent S, Hoeks AP, Boutouyrie PH, Safar ME: Arterial alterations with aging and high blood pressure, *Arterioscler Thromb* **13**:90–97 (1993).

75. Van der Heijden-Spek JJ, Staessen JA, Fagard RH, Hoeks AP, Boudier HA, Van Bortel LM: Effect of age on brachial artery wall properties differs from the aorta and is gender dependent: A population study, *Hypertension* **35**:637–642 (2000).

76. Green MA, Friedlander R, Boltax AJ, Hadjigeorge CG, Lustig GA: Distensibility of arteries in human hypertension, *Proc Soc Exp Biol Med* **121**:580–585 (1966).

77. Gribbin B, Pickering TG, Sleight P: Arterial distensibility in normal and hypertensive man, *Clin Sci* **56**:413–417 (1979).

78. Hayoz D, Rutschmann B, Perret F, Niederberger M, Tardy Y, Mooser V, Nussberger J, Brunner HR: Conduit artery compliance and distensibility are not necessarily reduced in hypertension, *Hypertension* **20**:1–6 (1992).

79. Laurent S, Girerd X, Mourad JJ, Lacolley P, Beck L, Boutouyrie P, Mignot JP, Safar M: Elastic modulus of the radial artery wall material is not increased in patients with essential hypertension, *Arterioscler Thromb* **14**:1225–1231 (1994).

80. Laurent S, Lacolley P, Girerd X, Caviezel B, Beck L, Challande P, Safar M: Isobaric arterial compliance is not reduced in essential hypertensives, *Arch Mal Coeur Vaiss* **87**:1069–1072 (1994).

81. Reneman RS, Hoeks AP: Noninvasive vascular ultrasound: An asset in vascular medicine, *Cardiovasc Res* **45**:27–35 (2000).

82. Stewart AD, Jiang B, Millasseau SC, Ritter JM, Chowienczyk PJ: Acute reduction of blood pressure by nitroglycerin does not normalize large artery stiffness in essential hypertension, *Hypertension* **48**:404 410 (2006).

83. Van Gorp AW, Schenau DS, Hoeks AP, Boudier HA, de Mey JG, Reneman RS: In spontaneously hypertensive rats alterations in aortic wall properties precede development of hypertension, *Am J Physiol Heart Circ Physiol* **278**:H1241–H1247 (2000).

84. Bussy C, Boutouyrie P, Lacolley P, Challande P, Laurent S: Intrinsic stiffness of the carotid arterial wall material in essential hypertensives, *Hypertension* **35**:1049–1054 (2000).

85. Boutouyrie P, Laurent S, Girerd X, Benetos A, Lacolley P, Abergel E, Safar M: Common carotid artery stiffness and patterns of left ventricular hypertrophy in hypertensive patients, *Hypertension* **25**(Pt1):651–659 (1995).

86. Van Bortel LMAB, Kool MJF, Spek JJ: Disparate effects of antihypertensive drugs on large artery distensibility and compliance in hypertension, *Am J Cardiol* **76**:46E 49E (1995).

87. Giannattasio C, Mancia G: Arterial distensibility in humans. Modulating mechanisms, alterations in diseases and effects of treatment, *J Hypertens* **20**:1889–1899 (2002).

88. Kool MJ, Lambert J, Stehouwer CD, Hoeks AP, Struijker Boudier HA, Van Bortel LM: Vessel wall properties of large arteries in uncomplicated IDDM, *Diabetes Care* **18**:618–624 (1995).

89. Hu J, Wallensteen M, Gennser G: Increased stiffness of the aorta in children and adolescents with insulin-dependent diabetes mellitus, *Ultrasound Med Biol* **22**:537–543 (1996).

90. Emoto M, Nishizawa Y, Kawagishi T, Maekawa K, Hiura Y, Kanda H, Izumotani K, Shoji T, Ishimura E, Inaba M, Okuno Y, Morii H: Stiffness indexes beta of the common carotid and femoral arteries are associated with insulin resistance in NIDDM, *Diabetes Care* **21**:1178–1182 (1998).

91. Henry RM, Kostense PJ, Spijkerman AM, Dekker JM, Nijpels G, Heine RJ, Kamp O, Westerhof N, Bouter LM, Stehouwer CD: Arterial stiffness increases with deteriorating glucose tolerance status: The Hoorn Study, *Circulation* **107**:2089–2095 (2003).

92. Van Popele NM, Elizabeth Hak A, Mattace-Raso FU, Bots ML, van der Kuip DA, Reneman RS, Hoeks AP, Hofman A, Grobbee DE, Witteman JC: Impaired fasting glucose is associated with increased arterial stiffness in elderly people without diabetes mellitus: The Rotterdam study, *J Am Geriatr Soc* **54**:397–404 (2006).

93. Van Popele NM, Westendorp ICD, Bots ML, Reneman RS, Hoeks APG, Hofman A, Grobbee DE, Witteman JCM: Variables of the insulin resistance syndrome are associated with reduced arterial distensibility in healthy non-diabetic middle-aged women, *Diabetologia* **43**:665–672 (2000).

94. Blacher J, Asmar R, Djane S, London GM, Safar ME: Aortic pulse wave velocity as a marker of cardiovascular risk in hypertensive patients, *Hypertension* **33**:1111–1117 (1999).

95. Van Popele NM, Grobbee DE, Bots ML, Asmar R, Topouchian J, Reneman RS, Hoeks AP, van Der Kuip DAM, Hofman A, Witteman JCM: Association between arterial stiffness and atherosclerosis: The Rotterdam study, *Stroke* **32**:454–460 (2001).

96. Mattace-Raso FU, van der Cammen TJ, Hofman A, van Popele NM, Bos ML, Schalekamp MA, Asmar R, Reneman RS, Hoeks AP, Breteler MM, Witteman JC: Arterial stiffness and risk of coronary heart disease and stroke: the Rotterdam Study, *Circulation* **113**:657–663 (2006).

97. Meinders JM, Kornet L, Brands PJ, Hoeks AP: Assessment of local pulse wave velocity in arteries using 2D distension waveforms, *Ultrason Imag* **23**:199–215 (2001).

CHAPTER 7

Plaque Mechanics

ZHI-YONG LI

Departments of Radiology and Engineering, Cambridge University Hospitals
NHS Foundation Trust, Cambridge, United Kingdom

Abstract.   Atherosclerotic plaques often rupture without warning and cause acute cardiovascular syndromes such as myocardial infarction or stroke. More recent studies have shown that plaque vulnerability is associated with plaque morphology, inflammatory burden, and biomechanical stress. Plaque mechanics studies the mechanical behavior of the atherosclerotic plaque and focuses on the biomechanics of plaque rupture. The study of plaque mechanics combines computational modeling, magnetic resonance imaging (MRI), mechanical measurement, and pathological analysis to investigate plaque progression and quantify critical blood flow and plaque stress–strain conditions under which plaque rupture is likely to occur. In this chapter, vulnerable plaque morphology is first introduced. Mechanical forces, material fatigue, and plaque rupture are then discussed. Plaque imaging and in vivo MRI-based plaque stress analysis are also presented. Following this, the mechanical properties of plaque components and their measurements are reviewed. Simulations of plaque mechanics are then illustrated and a blood flow–plaque interaction model is used to demonstrate the importance of fibrous cap thickness. Finally, the progress and current problems in plaque mechanics study followed by the future challenges and trends in clinical applications are discussed. The investigation of plaque mechanics and plaque stability may be useful in the understanding of plaque progression and plaque rupture mechanism. The study of plaque mechanics may lead to a quantitative technique for accessing plaque progression and rupture, which would ultimately lead to a clinical tool aimed at improving patient management.

7.1. INTRODUCTION

Atherosclerotic vascular disease is the most common cause of morbidity and mortality in the developed countries, and acute events are often triggered by the development of plaque rupture and subsequent thrombosis formation. More

Vascular Hemodynamics: Bioengineering and Clinical Perspectives, Edited by Peter J. Yim
Copyright © 2008 John Wiley & Sons, Inc.

than 50% of cerebral ischemic events are the result of rupture of vulnerable carotid atherosclerotic plaques and subsequent thrombosis [1]. Such strokes are potentially preventable by carotid intervention, for example, endarterectomy, angioplasty and/or stenting. Luminal stenosis is commonly used in current clinical practice as an indicator for surgical intervention. The degree of luminal stenosis can be measured by angiography [whether traditional X-ray angiography, magnetic resonance angiography (MRA) with or without gadolinium, ultrasound, or computed tomography angiography (CTA)]. Carotid endarterectomy has been shown to be beneficial in patients with high-grade (70–99%) stenosis [2,3], but conclusions cannot be drawn about possible benefits for patients with moderate stenosis (30–70%). The debate continues as to whether we should be operating on asymptomatic patients with a moderate carotid stenosis despite the report from the Asymptomatic Carotid Surgery Trial (ACST) [4]. Furthermore, there is growing evidence to suggest that luminal stenosis alone may not adequately reflect disease burden due to the process of arterial remodeling [5]. Remodeling may result in normal endoluminal dimensions as measured at angiography belying a substantial volume of atheromatous plaque that may be at risk of rupture [6]. Plaque composition, activity, and plaque mechanics are thought to be more accurate predictors of future thromboembolic events [7–9]. Previous studies have suggested that plaque fibrous cap thickness and plaque biomechanical stress should also be considered as major determinants for plaque vulnerability [10]. Plaque mechanics studies the mechanical behavior of atherosclerotic plaque and focuses on the biomechanics of plaque rupture. The investigation of plaque mechanics and plaque stability may be useful in identifying vulnerable plaques for risk stratification of patients with luminal stenosis, especially for those with a moderate stenosis or in asymptomatic patient groups.

A vulnerable plaque can be described as a large, soft lipid core covered by a thin fibrous cap [11]. It is the rupture of the plaque fibrous cap that ultimately leads to a rupture of the endothelium, exposure of the lipid pool, and subsequent thrombosis and ischemic sequelae. Factors contributing to plaque rupture include not only unfavorable plaque morphologies (e.g., a thin fibrous cap and extensive lipid pool) but also inflammation burden within the plaque and biomechanical stresses on the plaque as a result of blood flow [12,13]. Structural analysis has suggested that rupture is associated with stress concentration on the thin fibrous cap, high shear stresses, turbulent flow, and high local pressure, which are assumed to be the triggers of plaque rupture [14–16]. It is assumed that when the external stresses applied on the fibrous cap exceed the intrinsic fibrous cap strength limit, the fibrous cap fails to resist the loading and fibrous cap rupture occurs.

Plaque rupture itself represents a structural failure of component(s) of the diseased vessel, and it is, therefore, reasonable to propose that the biomechanical properties of atheromatous lesions may influence their susceptibility to rupture. Recognizing which features contribute to this increased vulnerability may improve risk stratification and allow aggressive interventions to be targeted at patients with plaques who are prone to rupture. Previously, such biomechanical profiling was based on finite-element analyses utilizing ex vivo histological or imaging data to generate geometric stress maps of vessel walls [17–19]. The recent advent of high-resolution imaging techniques such as intravascular ultrasound (IVUS) and magnetic resonance imaging (MRI) has allowed detailed morphological and structural characterization of carotid plaques to be performed in vivo, and the derivation of vessel geometries from such techniques avoids the inherent problems associated with changes in plaque size and shape as a result of histological fixation and surgical trauma.

In this chapter, vulnerable plaque morphology is first introduced. Mechanical forces, material fatigue, and plaque rupture are then discussed. Following this, the mechanical properties of plaque components and their measurements are reviewed on the basis of current literature. Next, plaque imaging using MRI is described and in vivo MRI-based plaque stress analysis is presented. Examples of simulations of plaque mechanics are then illustrated and a blood flow–plaque interaction model is used to demonstrate the importance of the fibrous cap thickness. Finally, the progress and current problems in plaque mechanics study followed by the future challenges and trends in clinical applications are discussed.

7.2. VULNERABLE PLAQUE MORPHOLOGY

The vulnerable atheromatous plaque was described by Stary et al. in 1995 by defining plaque histological characteristics that made it vulnerable [20]. A number of types and characteristics were defined (see Table 7.1).

The vulnerable atherosclerotic plaque has a thin fibrous cap, extensive and necrotic lipid core, and a significant amount of associated inflammation with infiltration of T lymphocytes and activated macrophages. These cells can often be found predominantly in the shoulders of the plaque in the fibrous cap, usually at its weakest point. Once activated, they secrete proteolytic enzymes such as matrix metalloprotienases (MMPs), which degrade the collagenous extracellular matrix and serve to weaken the cap further, tending to increase its risk of rupture. Direct interactions with the vascular smooth muscle cells (VSMCs) may lead to promotion of VSMC apoptosis, further weakening the cap [21–24].

Loree et al. published a study in 1992 simulating stress on idealized eccentric atheroma [10], using finite-element analysis (FEA) to determine the changing of plaque stress when varying the overall degree of stenosis and the thickness of the fibrous cap. They postulated that the final link in the chain of plaque rupture was likely to be mechanical stress on a chronically weakened fibrous cap leading finally to rupture. Their simulations found that circumferential stress on the plaque was exquisitely linked to the thickness of the fibrous cap and degree of arterial remodeling. More evidence comes from cardiologic postmortem studies looking at culprit coronary lesions for sudden cardiac death. It has been shown that responsible lesions could be split broadly into three groups: (1) the so-called fibroatheroma, with a very thin ruptured fibrous cap and extensive lipid core with

TABLE 7.1. American Heart Association (AHA) Histological Definitions of Atherosclerosis

Lesion Type	Histological Classification	Other Terms Used for Same Lesions Often Based on Macroscopic Appearance	Progression
I	Initial lesion	—	Early lesions
IIa	Progression-prone type II lesion	Fatty dot or streak	—
IIb	Progression-resistant type II lesion	—	—
III	Intermediate lesion (preatheroma)	—	—
IV	Atheroma	Atheromatous plaque	Intermediate lesions
Va	Fibroatheroma (type V lesion)	Fibrolipid plaque, fibrous plaque, plaque	—
Vb	Calcific lesion (type VII lesion)	Calcified plaque	Advanced lesions
Vc	Fibrotic lesion (type VIII lesion)	Fibrous plaque	Raised lesions
VI	Lesion with surface defect, hematoma–hemorrhage, and/or thrombotic deposit	Complicated lesion, complicated plaque	—

Source: Stary et al. [78].

associated intraluminal thrombus formation; (2) the erosion, with no evidence of plaque rupture or intraplaque hemorrhage but a denuded fibrous cap with no overlying vascular endothelium and an associated overlying thrombus; and (3) a thrombus overlying a superficial calcified nodule. The fibroatheroma lesion with a thin fibrous cap was by far the most common one. More recently, clinical studies histologically assessing symptomatic carotid atheroma following endarterectomy have shown these patients to manifest vulnerable plaque morphologies.

7.3. PLAQUE RUPTURE

Mechanical Stress

In 1989, Richardson et al. studied the effects of mechanical stress within the fibrous cap using a finite-element method in individuals who died of acute coronary thrombosis [16]. Evaluating the different geometries of plaques that caused lethal coronary thrombosis, they observed increased levels of stress concentrating at the edges of the fibrous cap near the border. It was also observed that in those cases with very small lipid cores (<15% of the vessel circumference), the point of maximum stress was located over the center of the plaque. The concentration of mechanical stress in the fibrous cap regions is possibly due to the inability of the soft lipid core to bear the large mechanical stresses that develop during elevation of blood pressure or repetitive dynamic pressure. Supporting these results, Cheng et al. evaluated the distribution and magnitude of circumferential stress within plaques by studying lesions from patients who had died of acute coronary disease and comparing them with nonruptured lesions of individuals who died from other causes [19]. It was observed that mechanical stresses were higher in ruptured regions than nonruptured ones. Here it should be noted that the ruptured plaque was modeled at the prerupture assumption. Therefore, the high-stress region was not due to the region of rupture itself. However, it was also found that in some cases, the location of plaque rupture was not always at the area of greatest stress regions. This observation suggested that local variations in plaque material strength may also play an important role in determining the location of plaque rupture.

It is crucial to emphasize the importance of the fibrous cap thickness in plaque stability. Loree et al. determined that decreasing the thickness of the fibrous cap greatly enhanced the peak circumferential stress; increasing stenosis severity actually decreased stress [10]. These results may, in part, explain the discord between angiographic findings and clinical events, and emphasize the limitation of current methods of diagnosis in the identification of unstable plaques.

The study of mechanical stress and plaque rupture/stability is generating much interest currently, based on both histological and angiographic techniques, and using either static or dynamic analysis. Computational simulations for plaque rupture in coronary and carotid arteries have been developed by many investigators [10,17,19,25–28]. Hung et al. used histology-based 2D solid models of arterial plaque and found that thin plaque fibrous caps and large lipid pools are important determinants of increased plaque stress [17]. Cheng et al. used a finite-element model based on histology to analyze coronary lesions, and their data suggested that concentration of circumferential tensile stress in the lesion may play an important role in plaque rupture and myocardial infarction [19]. Tang et al. used an ex vivo, MRI-based, flow–structure interaction model to study the interaction between flow and plaque and suggested that large cyclic stress–strain variations in the plaque under pulsating pressure may lead to plaque fatigue and possible rupture [18]. Imoto et al. examined the longitudinal structural analysis of plaque rupture and revealed that specific effects of plaque shape, size, and remodeling may be associated with plaque rupture [29]. Li et al. used in vivo MRI-based finite-element analysis on plaque rupture and modeled blood flow–plaque interaction and demonstrated why the fibrous cap thickness is critical to plaque stability [30,31].

Material Fatigue

The biomechanical interpretation of the stress trigger event is that rupture is induced by stresses that exceed the intrinsic fibrous cap strength. Therefore, it is implied that as long as induced stresses are below the strength of the cap, rupture will not occur. However, patients are frequently exposed to potential triggers without an inevitable acute morbid event [32,33]. Furthermore, experimental studies in animals and human subjects have reported that the pressure values needed to induce plaque rupture were 2–10 times higher than the maximum pressure that clinically results in plaque rupture [34–36]. It seems that plaque rupture is not well characterized by considerations based on nominal strength or critical stress alone.

Therefore there may be more mechanical factors involved. The repetitive deformations caused by the cardiac cycle would be another important role in lesion stability. McCord and Ku evaluated the effect of cyclic mechanical tension on the morphological and mechanical changes in diseased arteries [37]. Versluis et al. simulated crack propagation in an idealized plaque model [38]. The implication of these studies is that the effect of pulse loading on plaque rupture may be acting in the same way as the repeated bending of a paper clip eventually causes it to breaks. The propagating pulsed wave induces cyclic changes in lumen size and plaque morphology. Eccentric plaques typically bend at their edges or plaque shoulders, that is, at the junction between the fibrous cap and plaque-free vessel wall. Cyclic bending may, in the long term, weaken these points, leading to unprovoked "spontaneous" fatigue disruption, and a sudden accentuated bending or stress may "trigger" the rupture at these regions. In addition, plaque rupture may occur as a result of artery collapse or arterial spasm due to the large pressure gradients at the stenosis region [39]. It is important to note that nonbiologic materials may undergo fatigue when subjected to deformation, while biologic materials may compensate under some circumstances to increase tissue strength. Quite possibly, failure to compensate adequately by the remaining cells in the atheroma is a major factor in plaque stability.

7.4. MECHANICAL PROPERTIES OF PLAQUE COMPONENTS

Currently, stenosis severity is one of the most common criteria for clinical diagnosis. This criterion has been challenged for more than 10 years by observations in vitro and in vivo. Mann and Davies studied 160 mature coronary plaques using autopsy and found no relation between plaque size or stenosis severity and the vulnerability of the lesion [40], which may explain why stenosis severity evaluated by angiography is a poor predictor for subsequent progression to occlusion and/or myocardial infarction [41–43]. Thus, angiography is not a good method to screen for vulnerable plaques, partly because of their small size and partly because of vascular remodeling. Now, as mentioned in Section 7.3, the concept that stress is crucial for plaque stability has been widely accepted. However, nowadays the mechanical simulation still cannot provide comprehensive and sufficiently accurate information for the evaluation of plaque stability because of poor understanding of the mechanical properties of plaque components. The precision of numerical simulation is dependent largely on plaque material parameters. Understanding the mechanical behavior of plaque components is the most important aspect of the study of plaque mechanics. However, it is currently the most uncertain part in plaque mechanics study. There are relatively few validated data on the mechanical properties of plaque components in the literature, and the material testing protocols have varied widely among the measurements that have been published. Future work should focus on this aspect of the problem, and a database of plaque component mechanical properties is greatly needed for plaque mechanical modeling in order to provide a useful clinical tool for risk stratification of patients with vulnerable plaques.

The first uniaxial tensile tests on ulcerated and nonulcerated thoracic plaque caps from human aortas seem to have been performed by Lendon et al. [44]. Results showed marked differences between plaques and heterogeneity within individual plaque caps. Fracture stresses ranged from 12 to 1938 kPa. The study also compared ruptured plaque caps and the caps of intact plaques [45]. Caps of ruptured aortic plaques showed a significant increase in macrophage density, an increase in extensibility, and a decrease in ultimate stress when compared with caps from intact plaques. Lee et al. performed dynamic and static uniaxial compression tests on aortic plaque caps, which were classified as cellular, hypocellular, or calcified [46,47]. All caps demonstrated an increase in stiffness with increasing frequencies of stress ranging from 0.05 to 10 Hz. Values of plaque "moduli" are presented as a function of the plaque type. McCord performed cyclic bending tests on fresh human arterial ring segments that allowed the passive collapse of an artery, which may occur downstream of a stenosis [37]. Their studies indicated that cyclic bending and compression may cause artery fatigue and plaque rupture. Lendon et al. showed preliminary results of the stress–strain relationships of four (nonulcerated and ulcerated) plaque caps of human aortas [44]. The findings for the caps were very different, and the stress–strain curves were qualitatively similar to that of the normal arterial wall. Lorce et al. investigated the uniaxial tensile behavior of circumferentially oriented samples of human aortic plaque caps with correlation of the underlying composition (cellular, hypocellular, and calcified) [48]. This seems to be the first study where the samples were preconditioned with three cycles at physiological tensile stresses followed by progressive loading until fracture occurred. The authors concluded that the static circumferential tangential modulus of the samples is not significantly affected by the degree of cellularity and calcification determined by histological characterization. Topoleski et al. studied the radial compressive behavior of different plaque compositions of human aorta–iliac artery segments [49]. Data showed that plaques exhibit composition and history-dependent nonlinear and inelastic responses under finite deformations. They also found that the area of the hysteresis loop tended to decrease with subsequent cycles. Topoleski and Salunke [50] investigated the multiple cyclic compression and stress–relaxation response of diseased and healthy specimens, and Salunke et al. demonstrated composition-dependent differences and different responses of plaques to successive relaxation tests in uniaxial compression [50]. Holzapfel et al. performed uniaxial extension tests in both axial and circumferential directions with different components in plaque and showed that tissues in plaque reveal anisotropic and highly nonlinear tissue properties as well as considerable interspecimen differences [51]. The calcification showed, however, a linear property, with about the same stiffness as observed for the adventitia in high-stress regions. The stress and stretch values at calcification fracture were smaller than those of the other tissue components. Of all intimal tissues investigated, the lowest fracture stress occurred in the circumferential direction of the fibrous cap. The adventitia demonstrated the highest, and the nondiseased media the lowest, mechanical strength on average.

A fiber-based mechanical property of fibrous cap can be used when simulating the material test. The material composition and structure need to be factored in when the experimental data are dealt with. The strain energy function developed by Holzapfel and Gasser, initially for healthy arteries, could be one of the ideal constitutive laws for the fibrous cap [52]

$$\psi = \frac{c}{2}(I_1 - 3) + \frac{k_1}{k_2}\left\{\frac{1}{2}\exp[k_2(I_4 - 1)^2] - 1\right\} \tag{7.1}$$

where c, k_1, and k_2 are material constants; I_1 is the first invariant of the Cauchy–Green deformation tensor and $I_4 = I_4(\lambda, \alpha)$; λ is the stretch ratio; and α is the fiber orientation angle. The concrete form of I_4 can be developed according to the experiments. Another, presented by Zulliger et al., could be another constitutive law, which uses distribution function to describe the fibrous orientation [53].

7.5. MAGNETIC RESONANCE IMAGING

Plaque Imaging Using MRI

Magnetic resonance imaging is an attractive noninvasive imaging modality for the assessment of plaque morphology in vivo, as it allows exquisite resolution, and using multisequence techniques, allows good discrimination between fibrous cap and lipid core [54–57]. It is usually well tolerated by patients and has few contraindications. Its disadvantages in the context of atheroma relate to relatively long imaging time and the availability of technology such as dedicated surface radiofrequency coils to maximise signal-to-noise ratio (Flick Engineering Ltd, Holland, Figure 7.1).

Different components of the plaque have inherently different signal characteristics on multispectral imaging. Using a number of different sequences including T_1-weighted, T_2-weighted, Short inversion time inversion recovery (STIR) and proton density (PD) sequences, plaque components can be distinguished from each other in axial section. These signal characteristics are outlined in Table 7.2. A number of articles have been published comparing the accuracy of this type of segmentation with histology following endarterectomy and show good correlation between the two. Yuan et al. and Trivedi et al. published the most recent papers on this topic with over 200 cases in total [55,56,58–61].

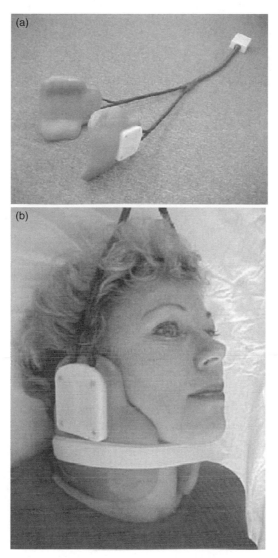

Figure 7.1. Four-channel phased-array surface coil dedicated to carotid imaging to maximize signal-to-noise ratio at a 12 × 12-cm field of view (Flick Engineering).

More recently we imaged 40 consecutive patients scheduled for endarterectomy using a multisequence high-resolution MR protocol. Fibrous cap and lipid core thicknesses were measured on MR and histology images. Bland–Altman plots were generated to determine the level of agreement between the two methods, and in all, 133 corresponding MR and histology slices were identified for analysis. MR and histology-derived fibrous cap to lipid core thickness ratios

TABLE 7.2. Signal Characteristics of Different Plaque Components in Various MR Sequences

Component	T_1 Weighted	Intermediate T_2 Weighted	Long T_2	STIR
Fibrous cap	+	++	++	+++
Lipid core	+	+/−	+/−	−
Calcium	−	−	−	−
Hemorrhage	++	+/−	+/−	+/−

^{a}*Key*: + indicates enhancement; − indicates signal loss; +/− indicates variable signal characteristics.

showed strong agreement, with a mean difference between MR and histology ratios of 0.02 (±0.04). The intraclass correlation coefficient between two readers for measurement was 0.87 (95% confidence interval, 0.73 and 0.93). Thus, multisequence imaging accurately quantified the relative thickness of fibrous cap and lipid core components of carotid atheromatous plaques.

Many methods of image segmentation have been published, including manual segmentation and fully automatic algorithms based on probabilistic analysis. These have always been shown to work well on high-resolution ex vivo data, imaging the plaque either in a microcoil on a standard 1.5-T clinical machine, or in a high-field machine (9.8 T). The semiautomated algorithms appear to be less robust when dealing with in vivo data since resolution and SNR are much less optimal in the in vivo setting.

In Vivo MRI-Based Plaque Stress Modeling

Both the linear elastic model [19,27,35] and the hyperelastic Mooney–Rivlin model [18,62] have been used in previous studies. In our more recent work, a two-term Ogden strain energy formulation was chosen to simulate the nonlinear stress–strain relation for plaque components [63]. This model was originally developed to describe large deformation isotropic elasticity in incompressible elastomeric solids. A two-term strain energy form was used as

$$W = \sum_{i=1}^{N} \frac{\mu_i}{\alpha_i} J^{-(\alpha_i/3)}(\lambda_1^{\alpha_i} + \lambda_2^{\alpha_i} + \lambda_3^{\alpha_i} - 3) + 4.5(K^{-(1/3)} - 1)^2 \qquad (7.2)$$

where N is the number of terms, which was taken to be 2 in this simulation; λ_i are the principal stretch ratios; J is the Jacobian modulus; K is the bulk modulus; μ_i are moduli constants; $\mu_1 = -\mu_2$, α_i are exponent constants; and $\alpha_1 = -\alpha_2$. In this simulation, selection of the values of carotid plaque components were based on Bank et al.'s experiment [64] and Versluis et al.'s study [38]. The values used for these parameters are reported in Table 7.3.

Plaque geometry can be obtained from multisequence MR data and compared with histology data for plaque characterization. The regions of interest (ROIs)

TABLE 7.3. Parameters Used for Plaque Components and Vessel Wall in Ogden Model

Tissue Properties	μ_1	μ_2	α_1	α_2	K (MPa)
Vessel wall	0.0008	−0.0008	30	−30	1600
Fibrous cap	0.0015	−0.0015	30	−30	3000
Lipid pool	0.0001	−0.0001	27	−27	200

are delineated manually in MR segmentation software (CMR tools v4.0) and correspond to plaque constituents of lipid core, fibrous cap, vessel wall, and lumen. These components have different signal characteristics when imaged using our multisequence protocol. For example, fibrous cap is particularly bright on STIR imaging, and lipid core is dark on intermediate T_2-weighted imaging with fat suppression. Figure 7.2 shows an example of the different signal intensities of the various components on multisequence imaging. These techniques have been validated in a previous study against the histological gold standard [55].

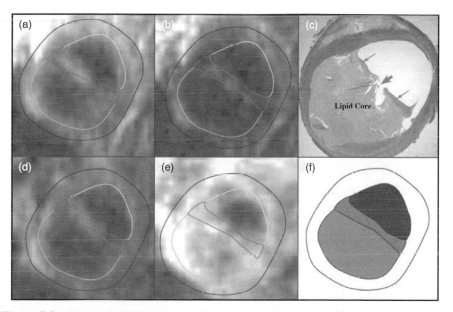

Figure 7.2. Image analysis and plaque segmentation based on multisequence in vivo MR images: (a,b) intermediate T_2-weighted imaging with short and long TEs, respectively; (d) intermediate T_2-weighted with saturated fat; (e) T_1-weighted black blood imaging; (c) H&E histology showing localized hemorrhage and a region of rupture (large, red arrow) in fibrous cap (small red arrows); (f) reconstructed geometry showing fibrous cap (red), lipid core (blue), and lumen (black). (See insert for color representation).

Once delineated, control vertices can be exported from the segmentation software and imported into a specialist engineering package (MSC Patran 2004 r2, MSC Software Corp, Santa Ana, California and ABAQUS Software v6.5, Providence, Rhode Island) where the contours were reconstructed using a closed B-spline technique to form the geometry for mesh generation.

A 2D simulation based on the geometry derived from each MR slice was performed. An internal pulse pressure waveform was measured noninvasively using a high-fidelity external pressure transducer applied to the skin overlying the pulse of the common carotid artery by Zhao et al. [65]. A standardized mean pressure was applied on the internal vessel wall in this numerical simulation. The baseline mean pressure value was chosen to be 115 mmHg and pulse pressure to be 60 mmHg. The pressure on the outside vessel surface was assumed negligible and the plaque was considered stress-free at zero pressure (no residual stress).

Numerical modeling consists of a number of components: (1) computational grid generation for the plaque and vessel wall, (2) specification of material properties and boundary conditions, and (3) simulation and results analysis. Meshes were generated with an average element dimension of 0.1 mm. Prior to the FEA, the 2D-generated mesh was viewed alongside the MR images to ensure that there were no gross dissimilarities between the two. The numerical simulation was carried out using a finite-element analysis (FEA) package ABAQUS (ABAQUS Software V6.5, Providence, Rhodes Island). Contour plots of Von Mises stress were displayed using ABAQUS postprocessing. Von Mises stress σ_v is used to estimate yield criteria for ductile materials. It is calculated by combining stresses in two or three dimensions, with the result compared to the tensile strength of the material loaded in one dimension. Stress is in general a complicated six-dimensional tensor quantity. Von Mises stress reduces this to a single number (a scalar) for the purposes of calculating yield criteria. Von Mises stress in three dimensions is:

$$\sigma_v = \sqrt{\frac{(\sigma_1 - \sigma_2)^2 + (\sigma_2 - \sigma_3)^2 + (\sigma_3 - \sigma_1)^2}{2}}$$

where $\sigma_1, \sigma_2, \sigma_3$ are the principal stresses.

7.6. PLAQUE CHARACTERIZATION

Ruptured versus Unruptrued Plaques

Figure 7.3 shows the coregistration of an MR image (STIR sequence) with histology (EVG stain) for plaque characterization in a symptomatic patient with a 60% degree of stenosis of the right internal carotid artery. The geometry was also compared with histology data for plaque component characterization. The plaque is a concentric plaque with obvious vessel remodeling, the fibrous cap surrounding the lumen completely. It is histologically vulnerable with a large lipid pool and a relatively thin fibrous cap. The computed stress contour from

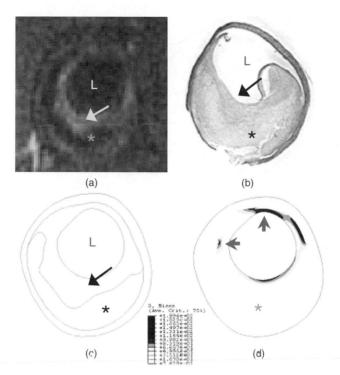

Figure 7.3. Computed Von Mises stress contour of a carotid plaque in a patient with a 60% degree of stenosis based on in vivo MRI plaque geometry: (a) registration of plaque components from in vivo carotid MRI [L—lumen; fibrous cap—yellow arrow; lipid pool—green star (*)]; (b) histology for coregistration of plaque characterization; (c) plaque geometry for FEA; (d) Von Mises stress contour shows the peak stress concentration on the shoulder of the plaque. (See insert for color representation).

FEA demonstrates the high stress concentrations localizing at the thin fibrous cap on the top and in the shoulder regions. The reason for high stress on the top of the fibrous cap is that the very thin fibrous cap resists pressure loading.

An unruptured plaque is shown in Figure 7.4. It demonstrated the correlation of the locations between maximum Von Mises stress concentration and plaque rupture. Panel (b) shows EVG and H&E stains demonstrating a complex plaque with rupture of the fibrous cap at the shoulder region that is associated with a small area of focal haemorrhage. Panels (c) and (d) show the plaque geometry used for FEA and the computed results of the stress contours showing high stress in the regions of plaque rupture and in the shoulder regions of the plaque.

Symptomatic versus Asymptomatic Plaques

Multisequence MRI studies were performed on all 40 patients (20 symptomatics and 20 asymptomatics). There was no significant difference in the severity

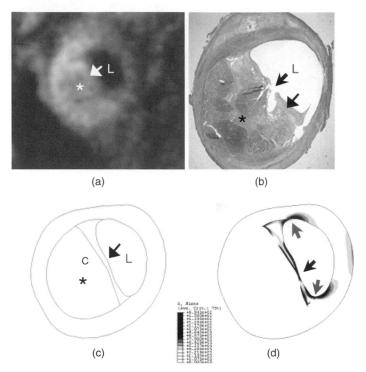

Figure 7.4. Correlation of locations between maximal Von Mises stress concentration and plaque rupture: (a) corresponding T_1-weighted MRI [L—lumen; fibrous cap—yellow arrow; lipid pool—green star (*)]; (b) EVG and H&E stains demonstrating a complex type IV plaque with rupture of fibrous cap at shoulder region (black arrow), associated with a small area of focal hemorrhage; (c) plaque geometry for FEA; (d) computed stress contour showing high stress in plaque rupture region (black arrow) and shoulder regions (thick red arrow). (See insert for color representation).

of stenosis as measured by carotid duplex, between the symptomatic (median = 73.5%, range 53.5–87.5%) and asymptomatic groups (median = 69.0%, range 51.5–82.5%) ($p = .36$). Analysis revealed that all plaques had evidence of a lipid core and a fibrous cap. However, very few foci of calcification were depicted. There were no statistically significant differences in the relative areas of fibrous cap (47.5% vs 42.0% of total plaque area, $p = .27$) or lipid core (36.5% vs. 38.5% of total plaque area, $p = .23$) between the symptomatic and asymptomatic plaques. The geometry obtained from the in vivo MR imaging required no alteration following coregistration with histology, as histological fixation was deemed likely to distort the plaque geometry and make it unsuitable as a geometric gold standard.

Stress distributions within the plaques were calculated using FEA. High stress concentrations were found at the regions of rupture and the shoulder regions of the

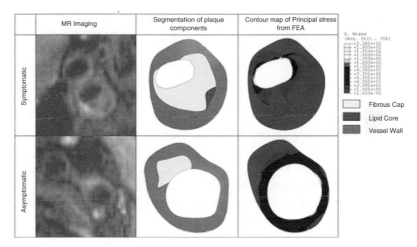

Figure 7.5. A comparison of symptomatic and asymptomatic subjects showing MR, subsequently derived plaque geometry used for FEA and stress maps for each case. (See insert for color representation).

plaque. Figure 7.5 shows a comparison between symptomatic and asymptomatic subjects. The symptomatic plaque had a much higher stress concentration than that of the asymptomatic plaque. The longitudinal stress along the stenotic vessel has been investigated, and it can be seen in Figure 7.6 that stress was higher in the maximum stenosis region.

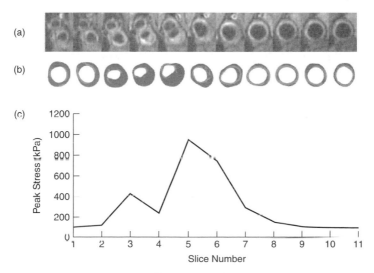

Figure 7.6. Longitudinal stress profile along a single vessel (symptomatic individual) showing MR imaging (a), stress maps (b), and longitudinal stress profile graph (c).

Following this evaluation of normality, parametric statistical analysis was undertaken using a nonpaired T test (SPSS v12.0) and considered at the 5% significance level. The maximal stresses in the plaques of symptomatic patients were significantly higher than those of asymptomatic patients. High stress concentrations were found at the shoulder regions of the plaques.

7.7. BLOOD FLOW–PLAQUE INTERACTION

We used a coupled fluid–structure interaction to demonstrate how blood flowed through a stenotic artery and deformed the plaque [31]. The model scheme is shown in Figure 7.7. The shape of the plaque was governed by a sinusoidal function

$$y_1 = \frac{D - A}{2} \times (1 + \cos x) \text{ and } y_2 = \frac{D - A}{2}(1 + \cos x) - d \qquad (7.3)$$

where D = the lumen diameter in the healthy part of the vessel ($D = 10$ mm was used), $\phi = A/D$ indicates the degree of stenosis, L is the length of the diseased artery that was studied ($L = 20$ mm was chosen), and d is the fibrous cap thickness.

The degree of stenosis was varied by changing the value of ϕ. The fibrous cap thickness was varied by changing the distance between the two curves d. The flow was assumed to be laminar, Newtonian, viscous, and incompressible. The incompressible Navier–Stokes equations in arbitrary Lagrangian–Eluerian (ALE) formulation were used as the governing equations:

$$\rho \frac{\partial \mathbf{u}}{\partial t} - \nabla \cdot \left[(-p)\mathbf{I} + \eta \left(\nabla \mathbf{u} + (\nabla \mathbf{u})^T \right) \right] + \rho((\mathbf{u} - \psi) \cdot \nabla)\mathbf{u} = \mathbf{F} \qquad (7.4)$$

$$-\nabla \cdot \mathbf{u} = 0 \qquad (7.5)$$

where ρ is the fluid density, u is the flow velocity field, p is fluid pressure, I is the unit diagonal matrix, F is the volume force affecting the fluid, and ψ is

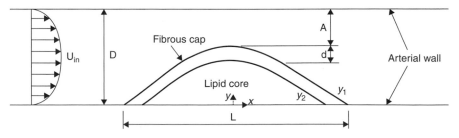

Figure 7.7. Blood flow–plaque interaction model scheme.

the mesh velocity, which was introduced to the equation by movement of the coordinate system.

Inflow was assumed to have a fully developed laminar characteristic with a parabolic velocity profile on the left boundary, but the flow's amplitude varied with time. The centerline velocity U_{in} with the steady-state amplitude U was given by the equation

$$U_{in} = \frac{U \cdot t^2}{\sqrt{(0.04 - t^2)^2 + (0.1 \cdot t)^2}} \tag{7.6}$$

where $U = 0.2$ m/s was used and t was the time.

Outflow was the right boundary with a pressure $p = 0$ on all other boundaries. The fluid was not moving with respect to the boundaries, corresponding to the no-slip boundary condition.

Plaque components were assumed incompressible and nonlinear because ideally human tissue is hyperelastic. In order to model this hyperelastic effect, a two-term Ogden strain energy formulation was chosen to simulate the nonlinear stress–strain relation for the mechanical properties of plaque components [63,64]. The parameters were chosen to be the same as our previous in vivo MRI study of plaque rupture [30].

The coupled fluid–structure interaction simulation was performed, and both fluid flow and plaque structure reached a balance at each timestep. Fluid velocity, plaque deformation, and plaque internal principal stress were calculated at each timestep. The simulation was performed using a finite-element solver (FEMLAB 3.1, COMSOL, Inc., USA). A previous in vitro study of human atherosclerotic material has shown that fibrous caps usually fracture when the static stress exceeds 300 kPa [17]. Therefore, a rupture stress of 300 kPa and above was chosen to indicate a high risk of plaque rupture.

Flow velocity arrows and stress distribution in a vessel with a 70% degree of luminal stenosis is shown in Figure 7.8a. The fibrous cap thickness is 1.0 mm. The flow velocity arrows show the flow profile across the plaque. Reverse flow can be seen distal to the plaque. The stress contours are shown in the fibrous cap and the lipid pool, and high stress concentrations can be found within the fibrous cap. The stress concentrations are found at the shoulder regions of the plaque. The streamlines of flow and flow velocities within the artery are demonstrated in Figure 7.8b (luminal stenosis is 80% and fibrous cap thickness is 0.5 mm). The plaque can be seen to be deformed (maximum deformation is 2.44 mm) because of the large luminal stenosis (80%) and thin fibrous cap (0.5 mm). Here the maximum deformation is the maximum displacement at a certain location in the plaque. Severe stenosis and 100% eccentricity lead to high flow velocity, high pressure at the throat of the stenosis, and a large recirculation region distal to this.

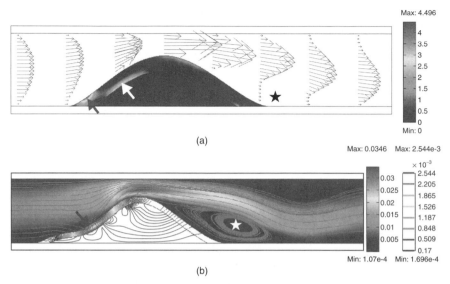

Figure 7.8. Simulation results of pulsatile flow through a stenotic carotid artery. (a) Arrow plot of flow velocity and surface plot of plaque stress (in color) showing the stress distribution within the plaque. The color scale shows the magnitude of plaque stress. In this figure carotid stenosis was 70% and the fibrous cap thickness was 1 mm. Red arrows show the stress concentrations and the star indicates the flow recirculation zone. (b) Surface plot showing the pressure distribution within the artery and streamline flow. The contour plot within the plaque shows the stress distribution. The left scale shows flow velocity, and the right scale shows plaque stress. In this figure, carotid stenosis was 80% and the fibrous cap thickness was 0.5 mm. White arrow shows the maximal plaque deformation, and star indicates the large flow recirculation zone. (See insert for color representation).

7.8. DISCUSSION AND FUTURE CHALLENGES

Atherosclerosis is a complicated disease, involving both physiological and biomechanical factors. Biomechanical analysis has been playing an important role in the analysis of hemodynamics for the initiation and progression of atherosclerosis, in the analysis of thrombotic processes, and in the analysis of arterial wall mechanics and plaque rupture mechanics. The emphasis has been on plaque mechanics for the prevention of mature plaque rupture. This is because plaque mechanics is extremely important in identifying vulnerable plaques for the risk stratification of patients with luminal stenosis. More recent advances in high-resolution imaging techniques such as intravascular ultrasound (IVUS) and MRI have allowed detailed morphological and structural characterization of carotid plaques to be performed in vivo. Plaque mechanics analysis based on in vivo imaging of atherosclerotic plaque is the new trend and may lead to establishment of new clinical tools for arterial disease assessment in the future.

Understanding which mechanical forces impacting on plaque lead to progression of plaque and which forces trigger plaque rupture is very important. The hemodynamic forces include shear stress and pressure or pressure drop across the plaque. Wall shear stresses are produced as a result of the action of blood flow against the vessel wall and are independent of plaque mechanical properties. While shear stresses may be important in the pathology of endothelial dysfunction, they are relatively small if its contribution is compared with the overall load on the plaque. Wall shear stress may play an important role in the progression of plaque, but it may not directly trigger plaque rupture. Pressure drop is relatively large across the plaque and may be an important trigger of plaque rupture. The interaction between mechanical forces and the changes in plaque morphology during plaque progression is complicated. How each develops over time is uncertain. It could be useful to investigate this process of development in order to have a better treatment strategy for the prevention of plaque rupture at an early stage.

Plaque rupture is a dynamic fatigue and repair process. Fatigue is the process of damage accumulation in a material that is subjected to cyclic loading. The artery has to suffer 39,420,000 times of periodic loading per year (heartbeat here is assumed to be 75 beats per minute). Although the damage could be repaired by living cells in normal physiologic conditions, if decompensation occurs, the failure of soft tissues can cause life-threatening events such as the rupture of an aneurysm or plaque cap, leading to a myocardial infarction or sudden cardiac death. The evidence that plaque can rupture at a stress condition that is much lower than the cap strength limit supports the hypothesis that fatigue is one of the most important rupture triggers. Although the concept of fatigue in soft tissue has been proposed for more than 10 years, very few studies have been presented on this topic. The most recent study on plaque fatigue was the simulation of crack propagation using an idealized plaque model [38]. Moreover, the reported fatigue tests of living tissue are performed mostly in a traditional protocol, either a tensile test or a bending test, rather than mimicking the loading environment in vivo, which is expansion loading. In those tests, the tissue humidity was taken into account, but not its living condition. In fact, living tissue displays a different biological behavior if the mechanical stimulus is different. Therefore, a reasonable experimental protocol is needed to study the fatigue process in more realistic conditions.

Residual stress within plaques needs to be considered. It is well known that residual stress exists in many kinds of living tissues, such as in arteries [66], the trachea [67], and the oesophagus [68]. Stress still remains when all external loadings are removed. Since almost all living tissues, including the components of the plaque, are nonlinear materials, the stress analysis should refer to their zero-stress states. When the residual stress is not taken into account, the stress concentration at the inner wall of an artery may appear to be several times higher than it should be [69]. To simulate plaque rupture, if the nonload stress is not coincident with its zero-stress state, the stress magnitude and stress distribution will result in huge error because of the complication of plaque geometry. There are no reported data available in the literature currently that address the importance of plaque residual stress–strain. Experimental work is greatly needed to clarify this issue.

Stress analysis using in vivo carotid plaque imaging to identify vulnerable plaques is an important step toward real-time clinical assessment. The first study was done by Li et al. using FEA and in vivo carotid MRI, and the relationship between local stress distribution and plaque vulnerability within diseased vessels was examined. This stress analysis predicts that the maximal stresses in the ruptured plaques are higher than those in unruptured plaque [30]. The study suggests that a high stress concentration in the thin fibrous cap may lead to plaque rupture in vulnerable plaque. The consistency in finding the peak stresses in the shoulder regions of the plaque seems to support the notion that the location of plaque rupture is associated with the location of the peak stress. This is different from previous studies using the geometry derived from histology [17,19] and ex vivo MRI [18]; this distinction is crucial as changes in the shape of vessels as a result of endarterectomy and histological fixation will have a significant impact on the predicted stress distributions [70]. Any alteration in plaque geometry as a result of these processes will have a significant impact on the stress analysis. One major advantage of determining plaque geometry from in vivo MR imaging is that luminal morphology can be best determined under physiological conditions where a flow of blood under pressure is maintaining the lumen shape. Histological analysis and derivation of geometry using this method have a number of disadvantages: (1) endarterectomy specimens do not involve the whole thickness of the artery, and the process of harvesting the plaque often involves entry into the lumen, thereby altering the morphology; (2) histological processing, including decalcification and fixation, can significantly alter plaque morphology, and specimen shrinkage of $\leq 50\%$ can be seen; and (3) finally, of course, a fixed specimen has an absence of pressure within the lumen, and thus loses shape.

Image analysis and plaque reconstruction are critical steps for the accuracy of plaque stress simulation. The in vivo noninvasive image resolution is still limited at the moment. Developing noninvasive methods for the determination of plaque components and measurement of plaque components' mechanical properties, fluid pressure, and wall shear stress remains very challenging. Plaque segmentation and reconstruction are currently done manually, and this is time-consuming. An automatic or semiautomatic image-processing tool needs to be developed for future data analysis.

Calcification is commonly found in atherosclerosis, and it has been thought to be associated with plaque disease burden. There is a debate as to the extent to which plaque calcification contributes to plaque stability. Some studies indicate beneficial effects in stabilizing the plaque [17,19,71], whereas others suggest that it has a detrimental effect and actually increases the risk of plaque rupture [72–76]. The criteria from the American Heart Association (AHA) defined the presence of superficial calcified nodules within or very close to the cap as a risk factor, albeit minor, for plaque vulnerability [77]. Calcium deposition within a thin fibrous cap would be more likely to lead to plaque rupture due to the pulsatile cyclic hemodynamic flow condition within the artery. The difference in material properties between calcium deposit and fibrous cap may cause crack propagation and lead to material fatigue failure. This suggests that calcification of the fibrous cap should be classified as a predictor of plaque vulnerability.

Clinical validation of plaque stress simulation is also crucial. As atherosclerosis is a long-term development disease, a follow-up longitudinal study would be useful in understanding the plaque prerupture stage. Tracing plaque progression and recognizing what is the most import stage in developing a vulnerable plaque can improve the treatment of arterial disease. Plaque mechanical simulation can be compared at each stage of plaque growth until plaque rupture. This can serve as a golden standard for risk stratification of patients with atherosclerotic diseases.

In summary, the investigation of plaque mechanics and combining in vivo high-resolution imaging techniques with computational modeling could help in identifying vulnerable plaques and may potentially act as a useful tool for risk stratification of patients with arterial disease. Future study should be concentrated on plaque mechanical measurement, image analysis, and fast computational modeling methods. The investigation of plaque mechanics may point out the future direction of biomechanics research as it is useful not only in the understanding of pathological processes but also in improving clinical treatment.

ACKNOWLEDGEMENTS

We would like to acknowledge the hard work carried out by the other members of the team, especially Dr. Jonathan Gillard, Mr. Martin Graves, Mr. Tjun Tang, Mr. Simon Howarth, and Mr. Tim Baynes.

REFERENCES

1. Casscells W, Naghavi M, Willerson JT: Vulnerable atherosclerotic plaque: A multifocal disease, *Circulation* **107**:2072–2075 (2003).

2. MRC European Carotid Surgery Trial: Interim results for symptomatic patients with severe (70–99%) or with mild (0–29%) carotid stenosis. European Carotid Surgery Trialists' Collaborative Group, *Lancet* **337**:1235–1243 (1991).

3. Beneficial effect of carotid endarterectomy in symptomatic patients with high-grade carotid stenosis. North American Symptomatic Carotid Endarterectomy Trial Collaborators, *N Engl J Med* **325**:445–453 (1991).

4. Halliday A, Mansfield A, Marro J, Peto C, Peto R, Potter J, Thomas D: Prevention of disabling and fatal strokes by successful carotid endarterectomy in patients without recent neurological symptoms: Randomised controlled trial, *Lancet* **363**:1491–1502 (2004).

5. Pasterkamp G, Smits PC: Imaging of atherosclerosis. Remodelling of coronary arteries, *J Cardiovasc Risk* **9**:229–235 (2002).

6. Glagov S, Zarins C, Giddens DP, Ku DN: Hemodynamics and atherosclerosis. Insights and perspectives gained from studies of human arteries, *Arch Pathol Lab Med* **112**:1018–1031 (1988).

7. Stary HC, Chandler AB, Dinsmore RE, Fuster V, Glagov S, Insull W Jr, Rosenfeld ME, Schwartz CJ, Wagner WD, Wissler RW: A definition of advanced types of atherosclerotic lesions and a histological classification of atherosclerosis. A report from the Committee on Vascular Lesions of the Council on Arteriosclerosis, American Heart Association, *Arterioscler Thromb Vasc Biol* **15**:1512–1531 (1995).

8. Virmani R, Burke AP, Kolodgie FD, Farb A: Vulnerable plaque: The pathology of unstable coronary lesions, *J Interv Cardiol* **15**:439–446 (2002).

9. Virmani R, Burke AP, Kolodgie FD, Farb A: Pathology of the thin-cap fibroatheroma: A type of vulnerable plaque, *J Interv Cardiol* **16**:267–272 (2003).

10. Loree HM, Kamm RD, Stringfellow RG, Lee RT: Effects of fibrous cap thickness on peak circumferential stress in model atherosclerotic vessels, *Circ Res* **71**:850–858 (1992).

11. Davies MJ: Stability and instability: Two faces of coronary atherosclerosis. The Paul Dudley White Lecture 1995, *Circulation* **94**:2013–2020 (1996).

12. Lee RT: Atherosclerotic lesion mechanics versus biology, *Z Kardiol* **89**(Suppl 2):80–84 (2000).

13. Richardson PD: Biomechanics of plaque rupture: Progress, problems, and new frontiers, *Ann Biomed Eng* **30**:524–536 (2002).

14. Barger AC, Beeuwkes R 3rd, Lainey LL, Silverman KJ: Hypothesis: Vasa vasorum and neovascularization of human coronary arteries. A possible role in the pathophysiology of atherosclerosis, *N Engl J Med* **310**:175–177 (1984).

15. Loree HM, Kamm RD, Atkinson CM, Lee RT: Turbulent pressure fluctuations on surface of model vascular stenoses, *Am J Physiol* **261**:H644–H650 (1991).

16. Richardson PD, Davies MJ, Born GV: Influence of plaque configuration and stress distribution on fissuring of coronary atherosclerotic plaques, *Lancet* **2**:941–944 (1989).

17. Huang H, Virmani R, Younis H, Burke AP, Kamm RD, Lee RT: The impact of calcification on the biomechanical stability of atherosclerotic plaques, *Circulation* **103**:1051–1056 (2001).

18. Tang D, Yang C, Zheng J, Woodard PK, Sicard GA, Saffitz JE, Yuan C: 3D MRI-based multicomponent FSI models for atherosclerotic plaques, *Ann Biomed Eng* **32**:947–960 (2004).

19. Cheng GC, Loree HM, Kamm RD, Fishbein MC, Lee RT: Distribution of circumferential stress in ruptured and stable atherosclerotic lesions. A structural analysis with histopathological correlation, *Circulation* **87**:1179–1187 (1993).

20. Stary HC, Chandler AB, Dinsmore RE, Fuster V, Glagov S, Insull W Jr, Rosenfeld ME, Schwartz CJ, Wagner WD, Wissler RW: A definition of advanced types of atherosclerotic lesions and a histological classification of atherosclerosis. A report from the Committee on Vascular Lesions of the Council on Arteriosclerosis, American Heart Association, *Circulation* **92**:1355–1374 (1995).

21. Bennett MR, Boyle JJ: Apoptosis of vascular smooth muscle cells in atherosclerosis, *Atherosclerosis* **138**:3–9 (1998).

22. Littlewood TD, Bennett MR: Apoptotic cell death in atherosclerosis, *Curr Opin Lipidol* **14**:469–475 (2003).

23. Stoneman VE, Bennett MR: Role of apoptosis in atherosclerosis and its therapeutic implications, *Clin Sci* (Lond) **107**:343–354 (2004).

24. Zhang QJ, Goddard M, Shanahan C, Shapiro L, Bennett M: Differential gene expression in vascular smooth muscle cells in primary atherosclerosis and in stent stenosis in humans, *Arterioscler Thromb Vasc Biol* **22**:2030–2036 (2002).

25. Baldewsing RA, de Korte CL, Schaar JA, Mastik F, van der Steen AF: Finite element modeling and intravascular ultrasound elastography of vulnerable plaques: Parameter variation, *Ultrasonics* **42**:723–729 (2004).

26. Lee KW, Wood NB, Xu XY: Ultrasound image-based computer model of a common carotid artery with a plaque, *Med Eng Phys* **26**:823–840 (2004).

27. Lee RT, Schoen FJ, Loree HM, Lark MW, Libby P: Circumferential stress and matrix metalloproteinase 1 in human coronary atherosclerosis. Implications for plaque rupture, *Arterioscler Thromb Vasc Biol* **16**:1070–1073 (1996).

28. Bank AJ, Versluis A, Dodge SM, Douglas WH: Atherosclerotic plaque rupture: A fatigue process? *Med Hypoth* **55**:480–484 (2000).

29. Imoto K, Hiro T, Fujii T, Murashige A, Fukumoto Y, Hashimoto G, Okamura T, Yamada J, Mori K, Matsuzaki M: Longitudinal structural determinants of atherosclerotic plaque vulnerability: A computational analysis of stress distribution using vessel models and three-dimensional intravascular ultrasound imaging, *J Am Coll Cardiol* **46**:1507–1515 (2005).

30. Li ZY, Howarth S, Trivedi RA, U-King-Im JM, Graves MJ, Brown A, Wang L, Gillard JH: Stress analysis of carotid plaque rupture based on in vivo high resolution MRI, *J Biomech* **39**:2611–2622 (2006).

31. Li ZY, Howarth SP, Tang T, Gillard JH: How critical is fibrous cap thickness to carotid plaque stability? A flow-plaque interaction model, *Stroke* **37**:1195–1199 (2006).

32. Haskell WL: Cardiovascular complications during exercise training of cardiac patients, *Circulation* **57**:920–924 (1978).

33. Rochmis P, Blackburn H: Exercise tests. A survey of procedures, safety, and litigation experience in approximately 170,000 tests, *JAMA* **217**:1061–1066 (1971).

34. Chenu P, Zakhia R, Marchandise B, Jamart J, Michel X, Schroeder E: Resistance of the atherosclerotic plaque during coronary angioplasty: A multivariate analysis of clinical and angiographic variables, *Cath Cardiovasc Diagn* **29**:203–209 (1993).

35. Lee RT, Loree HM, Cheng GC, Lieberman EH, Jaramillo N, Schoen FJ: Computational structural analysis based on intravascular ultrasound imaging before in vitro angioplasty: Prediction of plaque fracture locations, *J Am Coll Cardiol* **21**:777–782 (1993).

36. Rekhter MD, Hicks GW, Brammer DW, Work CW, Kim JS, Gordon D, Keiser JA, Ryan MJ: Animal model that mimics atherosclerotic plaque rupture, *Circ Res* **83**:705–713 (1998).

37. McCord BN, Ku DN: Mechanical rupture of the atherosclerotic plaque fibrous cap, *Trans ASME Bioeng Conf* **24**:324–326 (1993).

38. Versluis A, Bank AJ, Douglas WH: Fatigue and plaque rupture in myocardial infarction, *J Biomech* **39**:339–347 (2006).

39. Binns RL, Ku DN: Effect of stenosis on wall motion. A possible mechanism of stroke and transient ischemic attack, *Arteriosclerosis* **9**:842–847 (1989).

40. Mann JM, Davies MJ: Vulnerable plaque. Relation of characteristics to degree of stenosis in human coronary arteries, *Circulation* **94**:928–931 (1996).

41. Falk E, Shah PK, Fuster V: Coronary plaque disruption, *Circulation* **92**:657–671 (1995).

42. Ambrose JA, Tannenbaum MA, Alexopoulos D, Hjemdahl-Monsen CE, Leavy J, Weiss M, Borrico S, Gorlin R, Fuster V: Angiographic progression of coronary artery disease and the development of myocardial infarction, *J Am Coll Cardiol* **12**:56–62 (1988).

43. Little WC, Constantinescu M, Applegate RJ, Kutcher MA, Burrows MT, Kahl FR, Santamore WP: Can coronary angiography predict the site of a subsequent myocardial infarction in patients with mild-to-moderate coronary artery disease? *Circulation* **78**:1157–1166 (1988).

44. Lendon CL, Davies MJ, Richardson PD, Born GV: Testing of small connective tissue specimens for the determination of the mechanical behaviour of atherosclerotic plaques, *J Biomed Eng* **15**:27–33 (1993).

45. Lendon CL, Davies MJ, Born GV, Richardson PD: Atherosclerotic plaque caps are locally weakened when macrophages density is increased, *Atherosclerosis* **87**:87–90 (1991).

46. Lee RT, Grodzinsky AJ, Frank EH, Kamm RD, Schoen FJ: Structure-dependent dynamic mechanical behavior of fibrous caps from human atherosclerotic plaques, *Circulation* **83**:1764–1770 (1991).

47. Lee RT, Richardson SG, Loree HM, Grodzinsky AJ, Gharib SA, Schoen FJ, Pandian N: Prediction of mechanical properties of human atherosclerotic tissue by high-frequency intravascular ultrasound imaging. An in vitro study, *Arterioscler Thromb* **12**:1–5 (1992).

48. Loree HM, Tobias BJ, Gibson LJ, Kamm RD, Small DM, Lee RT: Mechanical properties of model atherosclerotic lesion lipid pools, *Arterioscler Thromb* **14**:230–234 (1994).

49. Topoleski LD, Salunke NV, Humphrey JD, Mergner WJ: Composition- and history-dependent radial compressive behavior of human atherosclerotic plaque, *J Biomed Mater Res* **35**:117–127 (1997).

50. Topoleski LD, Salunke NV: Mechanical behavior of calcified plaques: A summary of compression and stress-relaxation experiments, *Z Kardiol* **89**(Suppl 2):85–91 (2000).

51. Holzapfel GA, Sommer G, Regitnig P: Anisotropic mechanical properties of tissue components in human atherosclerotic plaques, *J Biomech Eng* **126**:657–665 (2004).

52. Holzapfel GA, Gasser TC, Ogden RW: A new constitutive framework for arterial wall mechanics and a comparative study of material models, *J Elast* **61**:1–48 (2000).

53. Zulliger MA, Fridez P, Hayashi K, Stergiopulos N: A strain energy function for arteries accounting for wall composition and structure, *J Biomech* **37**:989–1000 (2004).

54. U-King-Im JM, U. K.-I., Trivedi RA, Sala E, Graves MJ, Gaskarth M, Higgins NJ, Cross JC, Hollingworth W, Coulden RA, Kirkpatrick PJ, Antoun NM, Gillard JH: Evaluation of carotid stenosis with axial high-resolution black-blood MR imaging, *Eur Radiol* **14**:1154–1161 (2004).

55. Trivedi RA, U-King-Im JM, Graves MJ, Horsley J, Goddard M, Kirkpatrick PJ, Gillard JH: Multi-sequence in vivo MRI can quantify fibrous cap and lipid core components in human carotid atherosclerotic plaques, *Eur J Vasc Endovasc Surg* **28**:207–213 (2004).

56. Trivedi RA, U-King-Im JM, Graves MJ, Horsley J, Goddard M, Kirkpatrick PJ, Gillard JH: MRI-derived measurements of fibrous-cap and lipid-core thickness:

The potential for identifying vulnerable carotid plaques in vivo, *Neuroradiology* **46**:738–743 (2004).

57. Hatsukami TS, Ross R, Polissar NL, Yuan C: Visualization of fibrous cap thickness and rupture in human atherosclerotic carotid plaque in vivo with high-resolution magnetic resonance imaging, *Circulation* **102**:959–964 (2000).

58. Yuan C, Beach KW, Smith LH Jr, Hatsukami TS: Measurement of atherosclerotic carotid plaque size in vivo using high resolution magnetic resonance imaging, *Circulation* **98**:2666–2671 (1998).

59. Yuan C, Kerwin WS, Ferguson MS, Polissar N, Zhang S, Cai J, Hatsukami TS: Contrast-enhanced high resolution MRI for atherosclerotic carotid artery tissue characterization, *J Magn Reson Imag* **15**:62–67 (2002).

60. Yuan C, Mitsumori LM, Beach KW, Maravilla KR: Carotid atherosclerotic plaque: Noninvasive MR characterization and identification of vulnerable lesions, *Radiology* **221**:285–299 (2001).

61. Yuan C, Mitsumori LM, Ferguson MS, Polissar NL, Echelard D, Ortiz G, Small R, Davies JW, Kerwin WS, Hatsukami TS: In Vivo accuracy of multispectral magnetic resonance imaging for identifying lipid-rich necrotic cores and intraplaque hemorrhage in advanced human carotid plaques, *Circulation* **104**:2051–2056 (2001).

62. Tang D, Yang J, Yang C, Ku DN: A nonlinear axisymmetric model with fluid-wall interactions for steady viscous flow in stenotic elastic tubes, *J Biomech Eng* **121**:494–501 (1999).

63. Ogden RW: Large deformation isotropic elasticity—on the correlation of theory and experiment for incompressible rubberlike solids, *Proc Roy Soc Lond A* **326**:565–584 (1972).

64. Bank AJ, Wilson RF, Kubo SH, Holte JE, Dresing TJ, Wang H: Direct effects of smooth muscle relaxation and contraction on in vivo human brachial artery elastic properties, *Circ Res* **77**:1008–1016 (1995).

65. Zhao SZ, Ariff B, Long Q, Hughes AD, Thom SA, Stanton AV, Xu XY: Inter-individual variations in wall shear stress and mechanical stress distributions at the carotid artery bifurcation of healthy humans, *J Biomech* **35**:1367–1377 (2002).

66. Chuong CJ, Fung YC: On residual-stresses in arteries, *J Biomech Eng Trans ASME* **108**:189–192 (1986).

67. Han HC, Fung YC: Residual strains in porcine and canine trachea, *J Biomech* **24**:307–315 (1991).

68. Lu X, Gregersen H: Regional distribution of axial strain and circumferential residual strain in the layered rabbit oesophagus, *J Biomech* **34**:225–233 (2001).

69. Fung YC: Stress, strain, growth, and remodeling of living organisms, *Z Angew Math Phys* **46**:S469–S482 (1995).

70. Morrisett J, Vick W, Sharma R, Lawrie G, Reardon M, Ezell E, Schwartz J, Hunter G, Gorenstein D: Discrimination of components in atherosclerotic plaques from human carotid endarterectomy specimens by magnetic resonance imaging ex vivo, *Magn Reson Imag* **21**:465–474 (2003).

71. Alderman EL, Corley SD, Fisher LD, Chaitman BR, Faxon DP, Foster ED, Killip T, Sosa JA, Bourassa MG: Five-year angiographic follow-up of factors associated with progression of coronary artery disease in the Coronary Artery Surgery Study (CASS). CASS Participating Investigators and Staff, *J Am Coll Cardiol* **22**:1141–1154 (1993).

72. Stary HC: Natural history of calcium deposits in atherosclerosis progression and regression, *Z Kardiol* **89**(Suppl 2):28–35 (2000).

73. Mintz GS, Pichard AD, Popma JJ, Kent KM, Satler LF, Bucher TA, Leon MB: Determinants and correlates of target lesion calcium in coronary artery disease: A clinical, angiographic and intravascular ultrasound study, *J Am Coll Cardiol* **29**:268–274 (1997).

74. Raggi P, Callister TQ, Cooil B, He ZX, Lippolis NJ, Russo DJ, Zelinger A, Mahmarian JJ: Identification of patients at increased risk of first unheralded acute myocardial infarction by electron-beam computed tomography, *Circulation* **101**:850–855 (2000).

75. Taylor AJ, Burke AP, O'Malley PG, Farb A, Malcom GT, Smialek J, Virmani R: A comparison of the Framingham risk index, coronary artery calcification, and culprit plaque morphology in sudden cardiac death, *Circulation* **101**:1243–1248 (2000).

76. Schmermund A, Erbel R: Unstable coronary plaque and its relation to coronary calcium, *Circulation* **104**:1682–1687 (2001).

77. Naghavi M, Libby P, Falk E, Casscells SW, Litovsky S, Rumberger J, Badimon JJ, Stefanadis C, Moreno P, Pasterkamp G, Fayad Z, Stone PH, Waxman S, Raggi P, Madjid M, Zarrabi A, Burke A, Yuan C, Fitzgerald PJ, Siscovick DS, de Korte CL, Aikawa M, Juhani Airaksinen KE, Assmann G, Becker CR, Chesebro JH, Farb A, Galis ZS, Jackson C, Jang IK, Koenig W, Lodder RA, March K, Demirovic J, Navab M, Priori SG, Rekhter MD, Bahr R, Grundy SM, Mehran R, Colombo A, Boerwinkle E, Ballantyne C, Insull W Jr, Schwartz RS, Vogel R, Serruys PW, Hansson GK, Faxon DP, Kaul S, Drexler H, Greenland P, Muller JE, Virmani R, Ridker PM, Zipes DP, Shah PK, Willerson JT: From vulnerable plaque to vulnerable patient: A call for new definitions and risk assessment strategies: Part I, *Circulation* **108**:1664–1672 (2003).

78. Stary HC, Chandler AB, Dinsmore RE, Fuster V, Glagov S, Insull W, Rosenfeld ME, Schwartz CJ, Wagner WD, Wissler RW: A definition of advanced types of atherosclerotic lesions and a histological classification of atherosclerosis—a report from the Committee on Vascular-Lesions of the Council on Arteriosclerosis, American Heart Association, *Circulation* **92**:1355–1374 (1995).

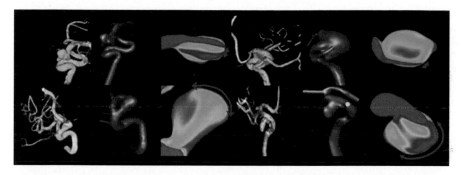

Figure 3.1 Examples of cerebral aneurysms with small (top row) and large (bottom row) flow impaction regions.

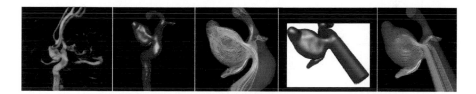

Figure 3.2 Effect of parent artery geometry on intraaneurysmal hemodynamics.

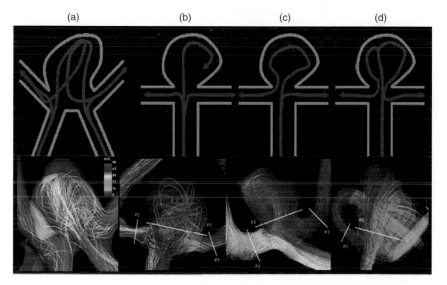

Figure 3.4 Classification of blood flow patterns in anterior communicating artery aneurysms.

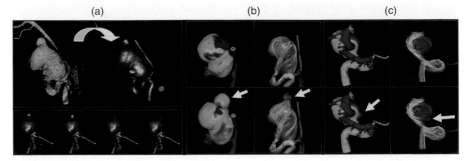

Figure 3.6 (a) Construction of patient-specific models of cerebral aneurysms before and after bleb formation; (b) bleb formation at flow impaction zone; (c) bleb formation at outflow zone.

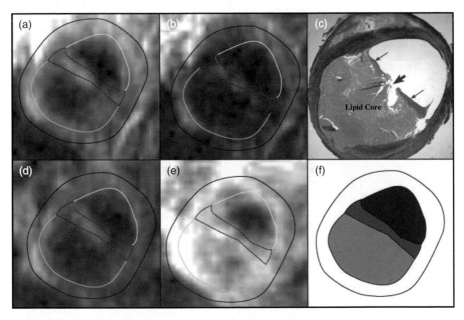

Figure 7.2 Image analysis and plaque segmentation based on multisequence in vivo MR images: (a,b) intermediate T_2-weighted imaging with short and long TEs, respectively; (d) intermediate T_2-weighted with saturated fat; (e) T_1-weighted black blood imaging; (c) H&E histology showing localized hemorrhage and a region of rupture (large, red arrow) in fibrous cap (small red arrows); (f) reconstructed geometry showing fibrous cap (red), lipid core (blue), and lumen (black).

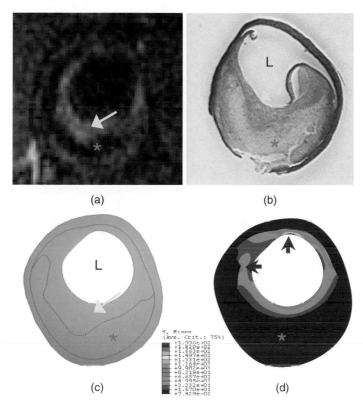

Figure 7.3 Computed Von Mises stress contour of a carotid plaque in a patient with a 60% degree of stenosis based on in vivo MRI plaque geometry: (a) registration of plaque components from in vivo carotid MRI [L—lumen; fibrous cap—yellow arrow; lipid pool—green star (∗)]; (b) histology for coregistration of plaque characterization; (c) plaque geometry for FEA; (d) Von Mises stress contour shows the peak stress concentration on the shoulder of the plaque.

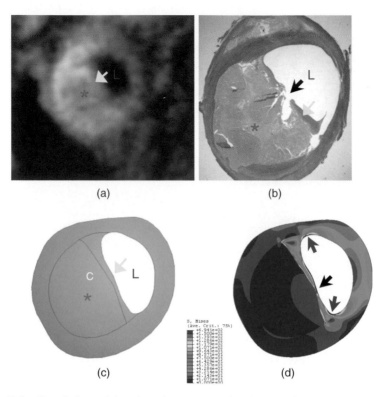

(a)   (b)

(c)   (d)

S, Mises
(Ave. Crit.: 75%)
+6.941e+02
+1.500e+02
+1.393e+02
+1.286e+02
+1.179e+02
+1.071e+02
+9.643e+01
+8.571e+01
+7.500e+01
+6.429e+01
+5.357e+01
+4.286e+01
+3.214e+01
+2.143e+01
+1.071e+01
+0.000e+00

Figure 7.4 Correlation of locations between maximal Von Mises stress concentration and plaque rupture: (a) corresponding T_1-weighted MRI [L—lumen; fibrous cap—yellow arrow; lipid pool—green star (∗)]; (b) EVG and H&E stains demonstrating a complex type IV plaque with rupture of fibrous cap at shoulder region (black arrow), associated with a small area of focal hemorrhage; (c) plaque geometry for FEA; (d) computed stress contour showing high stress in plaque rupture region (black arrow) and shoulder regions (thick red arrow).

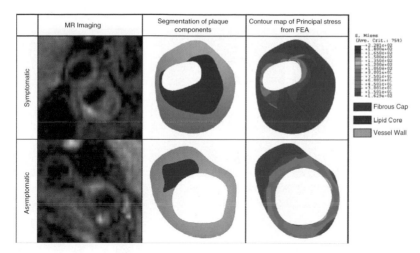

Figure 7.5 A comparison of symptomatic and asymptomatic subjects showing MR, subsequently derived plaque geometry used for FEA and stress maps for each case.

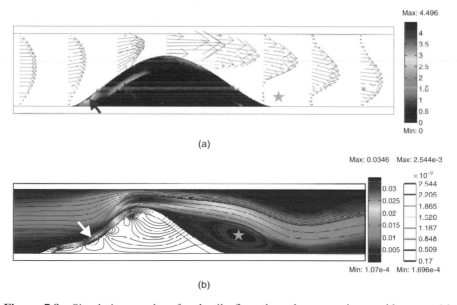

Figure 7.8 Simulation results of pulsatile flow through a stenotic carotid artery. (a) Arrow plot of flow velocity and surface plot of plaque stress (in color) showing the stress distribution within the plaque. The color scale shows the magnitude of plaque stress. In this figure carotid stenosis was 70% and the fibrous cap thickness was 1 mm. Red arrows show the stress concentrations and the star indicates the flow recirculation zone. (b) Surface plot showing the pressure distribution within the artery and streamline flow. The contour plot within the plaque shows the stress distribution. The left scale shows flow velocity, and the right scale shows plaque stress. In this figure, carotid stenosis was 80% and the fibrous cap thickness was 0.5 mm. White arrow shows the maximal plaque deformation, and star indicates the large flow recirculation zone.

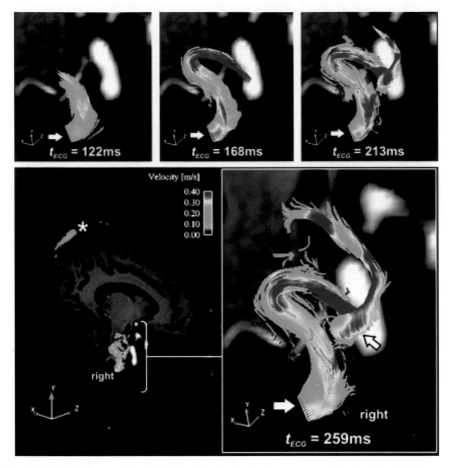

Figure 9.15 Time-resolved 3D particle traces in four consecutive systolic timeframes illustrate the filling of the right carotid siphon.

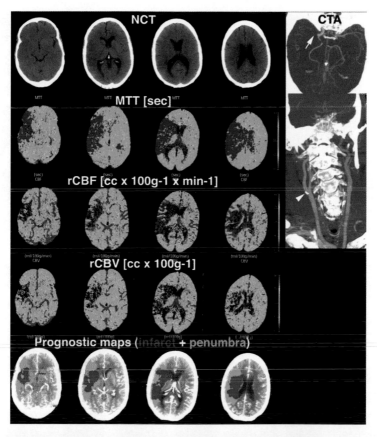

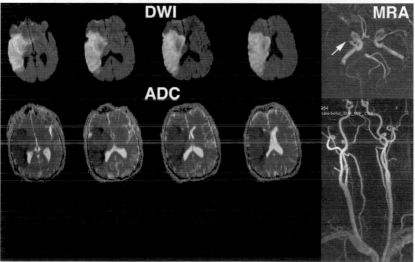

Figure 11.1 Modern CT survey in a 57-year-old male patient admitted in our emergency room with a left hemisyndrome. (See text for complete legend.)

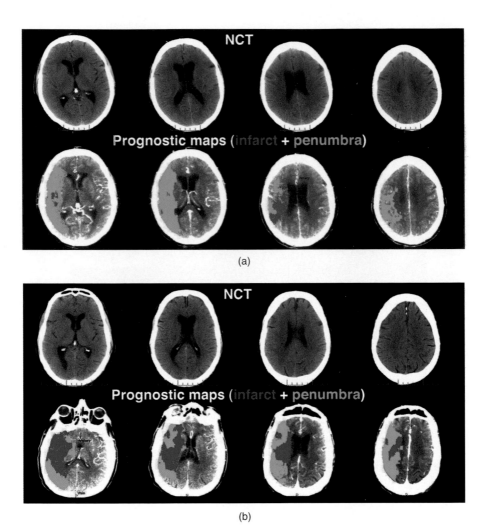

Figure 11.2 These two sets of images feature two cases of acute stroke patients admitted within the first 6 h of symptomatology onset [5 h for patient represented in (a) and 4.5 h for patient represented in (b)]. In both cases, the noncontrast CT is normal. The perfusion CT prognostic map obtained on admission in the patient represented in (a) displays an extensive penumbra (green) and a very limited infarct (red). This first patient would be eligible for intravenous thrombolysis, according to the new criteria developed in our institution, despite a time interval of 5 h since onset. On the other hand, despite identical clinical and conventional noncontrast CT characteristics, the patient represented in (b) shows an extensive infarct extending to more than one-third of the MCA territory. This second patient would not be an adequate candidate for delayed therapy.

CHAPTER 8

The Pressure Gradient at Arterial Stenoses: Towards a Noninvasive Measurement

PETER J. YIM

Department of Radiology, UMDNJ — Robert Wood Johnson Medical School, New Brunswick, New Jersey

Abstract. The hemodynamic significance of, or pressure loss at, arterial stenosis has been found to have considerable prognostic value, beyond that obtained from angiographic measurement of the degree of stenosis. Currently, however, the measurement of transtenotic pressure loss is obtained using primarily invasive techniques. This chapter reviews the burgeoning field of noninvasive imaging for estimation of pressure loss at arterial stenosis. The chapter reviews of clinical studies of transstenotic pressure loss, the fluid dynamics of arterial stenosis, and the various imaging and modeling approaches to estimation of pressure loss. The proposed imaging strategies that are reviewed are wide ranging with modeling based on Bernoulli's law or variations thereof, the Navier-Stokes equation, and turbulence phenomena.

8.1. INTRODUCTION

The obstructive effect of an atherosclerotic lesion on blood flow is a primary consideration in evaluation of the disease. The degree of obstruction or reduction in blood flow that is caused by a given lesion is closely related to the degree of stenosis or percent narrowing of the artery but is not synonymous with it. A variety of other factors also play a role in determining the pressure loss at a stenosis that is closely related to the hypothetical reduction in blood flow. These include the geometry of the stenotic region of the artery, the blood flow rate, and the material properties of the blood.

An appreciation for the importance of assessing the pressure loss at stenoses is growing with a number of studies indicating the diagnostic value of measurement of pressure loss, particularly in the coronary arteries but with implications for the renal and carotid arteries. This first sections of the chapter review clinical findings related to pressure loss at atherosclerotic lesions as measured invasively. The remainder of the chapter presents studies of fluid mechanics related to pressure loss at stenoses and of the development of imaging methodology for noninvasive estimation of pressure loss.

8.2. PRESSURE LOSS MEASUREMENT AND CLINICAL PRACTICE

Coronary Artery Disease

Development of the methodology for measurement of transstenotic pressure loss or gradients and the related quantity, the fractional flow reserve, has been pursued to the greatest extent in the coronary arteries. Studies have demonstrated a strong correlation between the fractional flow reserve measurement and functional cardiac tests. *Fractional flow reserve* is defined as the ratio of the pressure distal to the stenosis to the aortic pressure. Measurements of fractional flow reserve are typically made in intraarterially using an ultraminiature pressure transducer [1].

De Bruyne et al. compared the fractional flow reserve with the magnitude of ST depression during the exercise ECG [2]. They found the fractional flow reserve under both *Re*sting and hyperemic conditions was correlated with ST depression, but the correlation was stronger for fractional flow reserve obtained under hyperemia. Tron et al. compared the fractional flow reserve and coronary flow reserve with myocardial perfusion on SPECT with exercise or pharmacologic stress that detects the presence of reversible myocardial defects [3]. *Coronary flow reserve* is defined as the ratio of the hyperemic mean flow velocity to the baseline mean flow velocity in the stenotic artery. They found a strong association between both the fractional flow reserve and the coronary flow reserve and myocardial perfusion, although the association with coronary flow reserve was strongest. They also found no association between the minimum lumen diameter or the degree of stenosis and myocardial perfusion.

Pijls et al. compared the fractional flow reserve obtained under hyperemia with tests of myocardial ischemia including exercise ECG, exercise thallium scintigraphy, and dobutamine stress echocardiography [4]. They found that a positive fractional flow reserve result, defined as less than or equal to 0.75, coincided with at least one positive result from other tests of myocardial ischemia. The sensitivity of the fractional flow reserve in the identification of reversible ischemia was 88%, and the specificity was 100%. Samady et al. found that fractional flow reserve was effective for the detection of reversible myocardial ischemia with a sensitivity and specificity of 90% and 100% in comparison with dipyridimole myocardial contrast echocardiography obtained after myocardial infarction and at 11 weeks' follow-up to the percutaneous coronary intervention [5].

Bech et al. investigated the use of the fractional flow reserve in deciding whether to perform coronary artery bypass graft surgery in patients with equivocal left main coronary artery disease [6]. They obtained good outcomes in a group of 54 patients, including 100% survival at 3 years in the group that was not originally referred for surgery and 83% in the surgery group. Kern et al. performed a similar study in which patients were selected for immediate coronary angioplasty based on either a positive coronary flow–velocity study, defined as a proximal/distal ratio of less than 1.7, or a positive transstenotic pressure gradient, defined as greater than 25 mmHg [7]. In 88 patients in which angioplasty was deferred, only six procedures were subsequently necessary for the target arteries.

The role of fractional flow reserve in patients with mild stenoses is likely to be less important. Rodes-Cabau et al. found that fractional flow reserve was not associated with myocardial perfusion abnormalities on exercise dipyridmole SPECT in patients with less than 50% coronary artery stenosis [8]. In contrast, plaque burden as assessed by intravascular ultrasound was strongly associated with perfusion abnormalities. Fractional flow reserve was also compared with IVUS in patients with equivocal left main coronary artery stenosis by Jasti et al. [9]. They found that IVUS measurements of lesion severity, including minimum luminal diameter, minimum luminal area, and cross-sectional narrowing, were highly correlated with the fractional flow reserve. In contrast, neither the percent stenosis nor the minimum luminal diameter on quantitative coronary angiography had a significant association with the fractional flow reserve.

Findings related to the use of fractional flow reserve for the diagnosis of coronary artery disease were summarized in a scientific statement of the American Heart Association. In the statement, several indications are recommended for the use of fractional flow reserve, including those for patients with anginal symptoms and moderate coronary artery stenosis, for patients where a functional study is equivocal or unavailable, for evaluating the risk of restenosis after coronary stent implantation and for patients with anginal symptoms without a focal stenosis of a coronary artery [10]. The statement also indicates a variety of other potential indications for the use of fractional flow reserve that are under investigation.

Renal Artery Disease

Although the use of the fractional flow reserve and other indices based on intra-arterial pressure measurements has become relatively well defined for interventional cardiology, the usefulness of such measurements in noncoronary artery disease has not been clearly demonstrated. However, hemodynamic characteristics of renal artery disease have begun to be defined by more recent studies using intraarterial pressure measurement. The aim of these studies is to develop better methodology for selection of patients for renal angioplasty and stenting.

Nahman et al. documented the systolic transstenotic pressure gradients in the renal artery in 138 patients at angioplasty and found the preangioplasty gradient to be 109 ± 50 mmHg [11]. Gross et al. compared angiographic measurements of the degree of stenosis of the renal artery with transstenotic pressure gradients [12]. They found that, as expected, the resting pressure gradient was correlated with the degree of stenosis ($r = 0.6$). Also, they derived a third-order polynomial relation between the resting transstenotic pressure gradient and the degree of stenosis. On the basis of that relation, they determined that a 50% stenosis corresponds to a pressure gradient of 22 mmHg. They also found a very strong correlation ($r = 0.9$), described by a second-order polynomial, between the resting pressure gradient and the pressure gradient obtained following vasodilation by intraarterial administration of nitroglycerine. In another study, Colyer et al. found the correlation between the transstenotic pressure gradient and the percent stenosis to be relatively weak ($r = 0.48$), whereas a somewhat stronger correlation was found with the minimum lumenal diameter ($r = 0.9$) [13].

Renal flow reserve is a related measurement obtained at renal artery angiography that is the ratio of flow at hyperemia to baseline flow. Relative flow rates can be measured based on Doppler ultrasound peak velocity measurements. Manoharan et al. characterized renal flow reserve in patients without renal artery stenosis and found that the renal flow reserve is normally approximately 2.0 and also that an optimal hyperemic response could be obtained with an intrarenal injection of dopamine at 50 μg/kg [14].

The threshold level at which a renal artery stenosis can be considered to be hemodynamically significant is not well defined. A primary adverse effect of renal artery stenosis is a systemic hypertension that is induced by activation of the renin–angiotensin system that occurs when there is inadequate perfusion of a kidney. De Bruyne et al. investigated the relationship between the transstenotic pressure gradient of the renal artery and the plasma renin concentration [15]. In their study, they artificially created stenoses of the renal artery following renal artery stenting and monitored the level of renin concentration in the plasma. They found that a 10% decrease in the distal renal artery pressure relative to the aortic pressure, corresponding to a 0.9 resting fractional flow reserve, was enough to induce an increase in the renin concentration in the stenotic kidney.

The hemodynamics of the renal artery have also been studied extensively with Doppler ultrasound of the intrarenal arteries. The intrarenal Doppler ultrasound provides a measurement of the artery peak velocity waveform within the intrarenal arterial vasculature that has been quantified with the resistive index, RI:

$$RI = \frac{V_{\max} - V_{\mathrm{ed}}}{V_{\max}} \tag{8.1}$$

where $V_{\max}$ is the peak velocity and V_{ed} is the end-diastolic velocity. Also, the waveform has been quantified with the related pulsatility index

$$PI = \frac{V_{\max} - V_{\mathrm{ed}}}{V_{\mathrm{mean}}} \tag{8.2}$$

where V_{mean} is the mean velocity. The RI and PI essentially quantify the relative distribution of flow between systole and diastole. In an experimental canine model, RI was found to strongly correlate with resistance obtained by pressure and flow measurements with variation in vascular resistance obtained by arterial embolization [16]. However, in an experimental study with a rabbit model, systemic factors were shown to have a major effect on RI, particularly the pulse pressure [17]. This association has also been found in clinical studies [18].

Clinical studies have also demonstrated an association between RI and systemic increases in arterial compliance as measured by pulsed-wave velocity [19].

Presumably renal vasculature has both a resistive and a compacitive component and that changes in RI are due, at least in part, to the relative contribution of the resistive and compacitive components in determining flow, and not simply to variations in a resistive component alone. This has been demonstrated in an in vitro model of the renal vasculature in which changes in the renal artery segment compliance produce changes in the RI [20]. The effects of changes in vascular compliance on other aspects of the intrarenal Doppler ultrasound waveform have also been investigated in an in vitro model [21]. This is consistent with the conceptualization of the renal vasculature in a network model in which the vasculature is represented as a capacitor and a resistance in parallel [22].

Both RI and PI may play a role in the detection of renal artery stenosis as well as the selection of patients who should undergo renal artery stenting. Renal artery stenosis can be detected with relatively high accuracy by consideration of left–right differences in RI (ΔRI) with renal artery stenosis producing a reduction in RI [23,24]. The accuracy ΔRI in the detection of renal artery stenosis was found to be improved in patients 50 years old or younger in whom the prevalence of intrarenal atherosclerotic changes or renal insufficiency may be greater and may obscure changes that are purely related to the proximal renal artery stenosis [23]. Confounding effects of variability of the distal vasculature on the PI in have been demonstrated in a canine model of renal artery stenosis [25]. In practice, the accuracy of ΔRI for detection of severe renal artery stenosis is also compromised by the presence of bilateral renal artery stenosis. The tendency of renal artery stenosis to reduce RI is consistent with a network model [22]. In a computational simulation of Doppler ultrasound waveforms, renal artery stenosis produced a progressively decreasing PI with increases in the severity of the renal artery stenosis.

On the other hand, diseases affecting the renal microvasculature have been found to be associated with increases in RI. In a study of patients without renal artery stenosis, increases in RI were found to occur with diabetic nephropathy and with chronic glomerulonephritis even after adjusting for age, sex, systolic blood pressure, and other factors associated with atherosclerotic disease, diabetes, renal insufficiency, and hemodynamic state [19].

Selection of patients to undergo angioplasty and stenting for renal artery stenosis is currently a challenging clinical problem [26,27]. The RI has shown promise with regard to the selection of patient for renal artery revascularization as first reported by Radermacher et al. [28], who found that patients with RI ≥ 0.8 of either kidney were unlikely to benefit from revascularization. This finding was supported by the study of Soulez et al., who found that RI both with and without captopril administration was predictive of the response to renal angioplasty [29]. The value of RI for selecting patients who benefit from revascularization was not supported in the study of Zeller et al. [30]. Differences with respect to the surgical technique may explain the differences in the findings since patients in the study by Radermacher's group underwent angioplasty alone whereas the

Zeller group's patients underwent angioplasty and stenting that is believed to produce a greater rate of technical success. However, another important difference between the two studies was that patients selected for the Zeller group study were only those with a relatively high-grade stenosis of $\geq 70\%$ as determined angiographically.

It is worth noting, apart from the hemodynamic characteristics of the renal vasculature that have been determined from studies of RI, that RI bears certain similarities to a measurement of transstenotic pressure loss. The similarity is that both the transstenotic pressure loss and RI are determined by the opposing influences of the microvascular resistance and the resistance or obstructive effect of the stenosis of the proximal renal artery. RI decreases with increased severity of the proximal renal artery and increases in the presence of disease of the renal microcirculation. Likewise, but with the directionality inverted, the transstenotic pressure gradient increases with increased severity of the proximal renal artery and presumably decreases in the presence of disease of the microcirculation since increases in the overall resistance of the renal vasculature reduce blood flow through the stenosis. Also, the blood flow rate is known to be a major determinant of the pressure gradient across a stenosis and, as discussed above, is likely to be a determinant of RI and PI. Although there are reasons to expect a relationship between these two measurements, the relationship has not been established or even examined experimentally, to date. If such a relationship is found to exist in vivo, RI might serve as at least a foundation for the development of a noninvasive methodology for estimation of the transstenotic pressure gradient.

Other modalities have been developed for measurement of renal blood flow or the related measurement of perfusion. *Perfusion* is defined as the blood flow per volume of tissue. The rate of perfusion of the kidney has been found to be a valid predictor of the response to angioplasty for control of renovascular hypertension. In the study by Gruenewald et al., quantitative perfusion of the kidneys was obtained with single photon emission computed tomography (SPECT) with [^{99m}Tc] DTPA using a dynamic scanning technique [31]. The mean transit time was found to be predictive of those patients in whom an improvement in blood pressure was achieved following angioplasty. More recently, techniques have been developed for assessment of renal perfusion with magnetic resonance imaging and with computed tomography. Michealy et al. found that cine phase contrast magnetic resonance (PC-MR) imaging, which depicts velocities within a cross-section of the artery and can quantify arterial flow, was able to detect the presence of renal artery stenosis or parenchymal disease with a high degree of accuracy [32]. In the study by Binkert et al., presurgical measurements of flow, obtained by PC-MR and measurements of kidney size, were compared with outcomes from renal angioplasty [33]. They found that the combination of renal arterial flow and renal volume could predict the positive outcome with a sensitivity of 91% and a specificity of 67%. One motivation for the use of MR for functional evaluation is that patients with suspicion of renal artery stenosis often undergo a magnetic resonance angiogram for direct detection of the stenosis.

An alternative technique for the assessment of perfusion is based on dynamic imaging of the uptake of contrast media by the kidney parenchyma. Michaely et al. found that differences in renal perfusion by magnetic resonance (MR) perfusion imaging were associated in a statistically significant manner with the presence of hemodynamically significant renal artery stenosis and also with the level of renal function as measured by serum creatinine levels [32]. Measurement of perfusion with this technique can potentially allow for assessment of perfusion defects within the kidney and not merely an overall reduction in flow a given kidney. A similar perfusion imaging technique has been developed using computed tomography [33]. Paul et al. found an asymmetry in the rate of uptake of contrast between the left and right kidneys in patients with unilateral renal artery stenosis [34].

Carotid Artery Disease

Carotid artery disease is a major cause of stroke. The primary mechanism is believed to be through thromboemboli that form at the carotid artery plaque and then dislodge and occlude smaller distal arteries [35]. The flow-limiting effect of carotid artery disease has been considered less important than in coronary and renal artery stenoses, for example, because of the normally high degree of collateralization through the circle of Willis. However, there is growing evidence that carotid artery disease may produce hemispheric cerebral hypoperfusion and that the flow-limiting effect of carotid artery disease may be associated with a higher risk of stroke.

The role of carotid artery stenosis in obstructing cerebral blood flow has been shown by more recent studies in which increases in cerebral blood flow are seen following carotid endarterectomy using phase contrast magnetic resonance imaging [36], transcranial Doppler ultrasound [37–39], and SPECT [40].

In the study by Aleksic et al., flow was measured by transit-time ultrasound and the fractional flow reserve was measured by direct arterial puncture in the internal carotid artery (ICA) [41]. They found a significant increase in blood flow following carotid endarterectomy and noted that this increase was inversely correlated with the fractional flow reserve of the ICA.

Since revascularization of the internal carotid artery may improve cerebral blood flow, various studies have sought to show whether there is an improvement in cognitive function following carotid endarterectomy with both positive and negative results having been reported [42–44]. Subtle preoperative hemodynamic impairment has been found to be associated with improvement in cognitive function following endarterectomy. Kishikawa et al. [45] and Fearn et al. [39] both demonstrated that patients with a diminished preoperative cerebrovascular reserve ipsilateral to the carotid artery stenosis were the most likely to show improvement in cognitive function following carotid endarterectomy. *Cerebrovascular reserve* or *reactivity* is defined as the increase in blood flow to a given region of the brain in response to vasodilation.

The relationship between cerebrovascular reserve and the pressure loss at carotid artery stenosis has not been clearly elucidated. However, a likely mechanism for the decrease in cerebrovascular reserve or reactivity is that vasodilation occurs distal to carotid artery stenoses to compensate for reduced cerebral perfusion pressure. Thus, a reduction in cerebrovascular reserve is expected to occur, perhaps even in a proportional way, with increases in the pressure loss at carotid artery stenosis.

Conversely, preoperative hemodynamic impairment caused by carotid artery stenosis is associated with hyperperfusion syndrome, a major adverse complication of carotid endarterectomy. Nielsen et al. found that patients with a compromised cerebral perfusion pressure index (CPPI) that is associated with large increases in cerebral perfusion following carotid endarterectomy are at a relatively high risk of neurological events at carotid endarterectomy [38]. Ogasawara et al. found that cognitive decline was associated with the incidence of hyperperfusion following endarterectomy [46]. In that same study hyperperfusion was defined as a postoperative ≥ 100% increase in the cerebral blood flow. The patients who were found to have cognitive decline that persisted at 3-month and 6-month follow-ups were primarily those who experienced symptoms of hyperperfusion syndrome.

8.3. FLUID MECHANICS OF ARTERIAL STENOSES

Ordinarily, minimal pressure differences exist within straight segments of large arteries [47]. Pressure differences that do occur are the result of shear stress at the boundary between the blood and the arterial wall. The shear stress is directly proportional to the strain or nonuniformity in the velocity profile in the vicinity of the arterial wall. In an idealistic cylindrical tube, the shear stress at the wall of the artery τ_w is slope of the velocity profile with respect to radius at the wall, multiplied by the viscosity μ

$$\tau_w = \mu \left. \frac{du}{dr} \right|_{r=R} \tag{8.3}$$

where R is the radius of the tube and u is the blood velocity.

The velocity profile in a tube is described by a paraboloid provided that the flow rate is within the laminar domain, or for which the Reynolds number, Re, is less than $\sim$2300. The Reynolds number is defined as

$$\mathrm{Re} = \frac{\rho V D}{\mu} \tag{8.4}$$

where ρ is the density of the fluid, D is the diameter of the tube, and V is the mean velocity in the tube.

In the case of laminar flow, the shear stress at the wall of the tube is given by

$$\tau_w = 4\mu\frac{V}{R} \tag{8.5}$$

where R is the radius of the tube.

The Hagen–Poiseuille relation for pressure loss ΔP along a given length of the tube L can be derived directly from equation (8.5) by integration of the shear stress over the area of the tube, divided by the cross-sectional area of the tube [48]:

$$\Delta P_{HP} = \frac{8\mu L V}{R^2} \tag{8.6}$$

Pressure loss related to wall shear stress, similar to that described by the Hagen–Poiseuille relation, contributes to the total pressure loss at a stenosis. This component of the pressure loss predominates for lower Reynolds numbers and in that domain, the pressure loss is linearly related to the mean velocity. For higher Reynolds numbers, however, the major component of the pressure loss at arterial stenoses is due to a so-called pressure drag that is particularly significant when flow separation occurs downstream from the stenosis.

The pressure loss at arterial stenoses due to flow separation can be modeled with idealistic geometries including the sudden expansion and the orifice obstruction. The sudden-expansion geometry is that of a pipe whose diameter abruptly increases in diameter in the direction of the flow. The idealistic orifice obstruction is a washer-shaped obstruction that has a negligible thickness. At a relatively low Reynolds number, flow separation occurs distal to both the sudden expansion and the orifice geometry.

The pressure–flow relation has been extensively characterized for the orifice obstructions, in part since orifice obstructions are widely used in flow measurement instrumentation. Figure 8.1 shows streamlines of flow at a 6-mm orifice in a 10 mm tube with a Reynolds number of 2000 using a Navier–Stokes axisymmetric finite-element model. The finite-element modeling was performed in Flowlab (Fluent Inc., Lebanon, NH) with the $\kappa-\varepsilon$ turbulence model. The corresponding profile of pressure along the axis of the tube is shown in Figure 8.2. The permanent pressure loss measured between points 1 cm upstream and 6 cm downstream of the orifice is within 12% of those obtained by flowmeter design [49].

The axial pressure profile has a characteristic sharp drop immediately at the stenosis that may extend beyond the stenosis followed by a moderate increase in pressure further downstream known as *pressure recovery*. The minima in pressure along the axis of the tube is relatively accurately predicted by Bernoulli's law. Bernoulli's law is based on the conservation of energy for flow of an inviscid fluid or fluid with no viscosity. Ignoring gravitational effects, we obtain

$$P + \tfrac{1}{2}\rho V^2 = \text{constant} \tag{8.7}$$

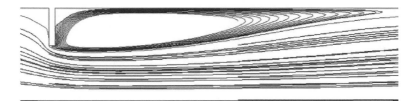

Figure 8.1. Streamlines at 40% orifice obstruction from axisymmetric finite-element model at Reynolds number of 2000. Flow is from left to right. A recirculation region is evident immediately distal to the orifice.

where P is the so-called static pressure that, in practice, is measured from a port that is flush with the wall of a flow system.

By conservation of mass, the flow rate must be the same at each point along a tube, and therefore, at stenoses, where the cross-sectional area is decreased, the mean velocity is proportionately increased and the pressure is decreased. However, the increase in velocity at an orifice is not strictly predicted by the minimum cross-sectional area. Indeed, the flow stream has been found to undergo additional compression distal to the orifice in which the velocity is correspondingly higher. This exaggeration of the compression of the flow channel is seen at stenoses of the aortic valve, for example [50].

The fluid dynamics of stenoses have been characterized extensively in idealistic geometries. As mention above, the flow separation phenomena plays a major role in pressure loss at arterial stenoses. This phenomenon has been characterized for idealistic models of arterial stenoses. By tracking opaque dye released into the flow stream, Golia and Evans studied the conditions of onset of flow separation and the size of the flow separation region in steady flow [51]. Highly linear relations were found between the length of the flow separation, as a fraction of

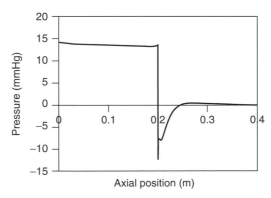

Figure 8.2. Profile of static pressure along central axis of tube with orifice obstruction as shown in Figure 8.1. The location of the orifice is at $x = 0.2$. Calculation obtained by finite-element modeling.

the normal tube radius, and the Reynolds number. The length of the flow separation region was also found to depend on the degree of stenosis and the radius of curvature of the annular obstruction. The separation or critical Reynolds number representing the lowest Reynolds number for which flow separation occurs was found to be described by

$$\mathrm{Re}^* = \frac{4.8}{\bar{\delta}^{1.70}} \tag{8.8}$$

where $\bar{\delta}$ is a geometric factor describing the annular obstruction

$$\bar{\delta} = \frac{\delta}{R} \left(\frac{R}{Z} \right)^{0.138} \tag{8.9}$$

and δ is the radius reduction, R is the normal radius, and Z is the radius of curvature of the annular obstruction. That study included a limited range of flow conditions for which the separation length-to-radius ratio was less than 7.0. As a result, measurements were made only for Reynolds numbers ranging within ≤ 100 for all severe stenoses ($>50\%$ diameter reduction).

Solzbach et al. obtained a similar finding for the relationship between the critical Reynolds number and the degree of stenosis [52]. The study was based on photoelastic imaging of the flow of a birefringent solution that allowed for detection of turbulence and of the reattachment point, or the downstream endpoint of the flow separation region. This technique was used for studying flow in geometries representing varying degrees of stenosis, short versus long stenosis length, concentric versus eccentric location of the stenosis, and perpendicular versus tapered exit angle from the stenosis. The length of the separation region was found to increase with increasing Reynolds number for flow at lower Reynolds numbers, but as the flow rate or Reynolds number increased further, the length of the flow separation region decreased with increasing Reynolds number.

The envelope that includes flow separation, turbulence, and flow instability was also found to increase with increases in the Reynolds number for low-range Re numbers and then decrease gradually with increase in Reynolds number for higher-range Re numbers. Other observations from this study are that onset of flow instabilities at higher Reynolds number occurred for stenoses with longer lengths, stenoses with a tapered exit angle produce shorter separation regions than did those with a perpendicular exit angle, and that instabilities in flow occur at higher Reynolds numbers for eccentric stenoses than do those for concentric stenoses. The inverse relationship between Reynolds number and the flow separation length was also observed using magnetic resonance imaging by Gach et al. [53].

Flow separation has also been investigated in a two-dimensional model representing a channel with an indentation. Experimentation demonstrated that the separation point, or the furthest upstream location of the separation region, was found to move progressively upstream toward the neck of the stenosis with increasing Reynolds number for Reynolds numbers between 1000 and 2000 [54]. A finite-element model based on the one-dimensional form of the Navier–Stokes equations accurately reproduced the experimental finding of the behavior of the separation point [55]. Young and Tsai observed a similar relationship between the flow separation point and Reynolds number for axisymetric models with varying stenosis severity and stenosis length. The axial cross-sectional shape of the constriction region is a partial cosine function [56].

A biphasic behavior of the separation region length was observed for a blunt-plug obstruction in which the separation region length first increases and then decreases with increasing Reynolds number [57]. In the range of Reynolds numbers where the separation region decreases with increases in the Reynolds number, the separation region length could be described by the following equation that is applicable to axisymmetric models with varying decreases of stenosis severity

$$\frac{2L_{\max}}{D_0 - D_1} = \frac{9.52 \times 10^4}{\mathrm{Re}} \left(\frac{D_1^2}{D_0^2} \right) - 1.51 \tag{8.10}$$

where $L_{\max}$ is the length of the separation region downstream from the stenosis, D_0 is the normal tube diameter, and D_1 is the diameter of the opening at the stenosis.

The shape of a constriction in a tube strongly affects the pressure loss–flow relation independent of the maximum degree of reduction in the tube diameter or area. A gradual transition from the point of maximal constriction to the normal tube diameter reduces the pressure loss across the constriction relative to the pressure loss where there is an abrupt transition. The symmetry or asymmetry of a stenosis also affects the pressure loss–flow relation, which Young and Tsai compared for an axisymmetric stenosis with a stenosis formed by a cylindrical indentation in the tube [56]. For equivalent Reynolds number of 1000 and maximal area reduction of 89%, they found an approximately 35% difference between the pressure loss produced by the symmetric and the asymmetric stenoses. Less variability in the pressure loss–flow relation of approximately 5% was observed for a blunt-plug obstruction by Seeley and Young for stenosis with maximal area reduction of 93.8% at a Reynolds number of 1000 [57]. The openings of the blunt-plug obstructions all had a circular cross section but had a variable offset from the centerline of the tube up to an eccentricity of 0.625, where the eccentricity defined the ratio of the off-center distance of the circular opening to the tube radius.

Pressure loss, expressed in nondimensional form as the Euler number, is related to the Reynolds number as follows

$$\frac{\Delta P}{\rho V^2} = \frac{K_v}{\mathrm{Re}} + \frac{K_t}{2} \left[\frac{A_0}{A_1} - 1 \right]^2 \tag{8.11}$$

where K_v and K_t are constants that are dependent on the geometry of the stenosis and A_0 and A_1 are the normal cross-sectional area and the cross-sectional area at the constriction, respectively. This relation has been found to be valid for a variety of geometries, including variation in the degree of stenosis severity, in symmetry of the stenosis, and in the longitudinal profile of the stenosis [56,57].

Fundamentally, the behavior of blood flow is governed by the Navier–Stokes equation for incompressible fluids and the equation for conservation of mass

$$\rho \left(\frac{\partial \mathbf{v}}{\partial t} + \mathbf{v} \cdot \nabla \mathbf{v} \right) = -\nabla p + \mu \nabla^2 \mathbf{v} \tag{8.12}$$

$$\nabla \cdot \mathbf{v} = 0 \tag{8.13}$$

where $\mathbf{v}$ is the velocity vector field and p is the pressure field. In principle, given a complete description of the stenosis geometry and the flow rate, the fluid dynamic conditions within the stenosis can be reconstructed using finite-element modeling. Three-dimensional finite-element models have been constructed, including one based on the specifications of an asymmetric model of Young and Tsai [56]. The finite-element models incorporated the no-slip condition at the arterial walls, such that all components of the fluid velocity are zero at the wall, and also that the fluid had a paraboloid velocity profile at the inlet. The finite-element modeling was based on a discretization of the computational domain by a volumetric mesh of 11,000 nonuniform cells that ranged from 10 radii upstream of the stenosis to 40 radii downstream. Cells of the volumetric mesh were hexahedra with quadrilateral faces. The pressure loss determined from the finite-element modeling was nearly equal to the experimentally measured pressure loss at the stenosis for stenosis severity of 89% area reduction and for Reynolds numbers from 100 to 1000 under steady flow conditions.

Finite-element modeling was also shown to accurately determine pressure loss across a stenosis with a high degree of irregularity in the longitudinal profile [59]. Johnston and Kilpatrick constructed an axisymmetric finite-element model based on measurements of the cross-sectional area made at 50-μm intervals along a cast of a moderately stenotic left circumflex coronary artery. The computational domain extended 8 radii upstream from the stenosis and 80 radii downstream. The finite-element grid was composed of 3629 nonuniform linear quadrilateral elements. The element size was increased in regions with higher velocity gradients, including near the wall of the artery and near the stenosis. The solution to the flow equations was obtained using the Galerkin finite-element method. The pressure losses determined from the finite-element model are very close to the measured pressure losses in the range of Reynolds numbers from 70 to 1000. Some divergence of the finite-element solution from the measured pressure losses was observed for the higher Reynolds numbers with 10–20% difference for Reynolds numbers near 1000.

Our group performed an experimental and numerical study of a model representing the renal artery stenosis (Figure 8.3) [60]. A glass model was constructed with realistic dimensions including the aorta and the renal artery with a 48% stenosis by diameter reduction in a tube whose normal diameter is 5.7 mm. Steady and pulsatile flow conditions were simulated with a glycerol–water solution with

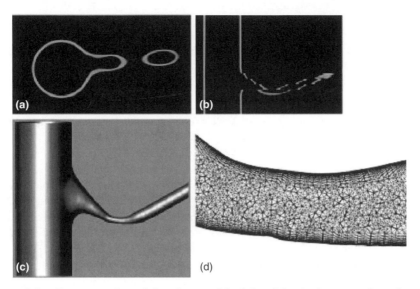

Figure 8.3. Reconstruction of the glass model of the abdominal aorta and renal artery from CT. Axial and coronal cross-sections of the CT image are shown in (a) and (b), respectively. The lumenal surface of the glass model was reconstructed from the CT images using the IDM algorithm. The surface is shown in a shaded surface display in (c). A cut of the finite element mesh in the region of the stenosis showing increased mesh resolution near the vessel walls is presented in (d).

physiologically realistic viscosity of 3.5 cP. The flow rates in the infrarenal aortic segment and the renal segment of the model were measured using transit-time ultrasound, and pressures were measured with a differential pressure transducer. The glass model was imaged with computed tomography (CT) at a resolution of $0.24 \times 0.24 \times 0.63$ mm. The surface of the glass model was reconstructed from the CT image with the *isosurface deformable model* [61], which reconstructs the surface of the model. An unstructured volumetric finite-element mesh, composed of tetrahedral elements, was then constructed with GEN3D (in-house software, George Mason University). The maximal element size was 0.5 mm. The resolution of the volumetric mesh was increased in the vicinity of the wall. Flow solutions were obtained with using FEFLO (in-house software, George Mason University). The numerical technique of Soto et al. was used to obtain the flow solution that can be regarded as incorporating large-eddy simulation of turbulence [62].

For steady flow conditions, the mean error in the measurement of the transstenotic pressure gradient was 21.4 mmHg for all flow conditions through 33 cm^3/s (Re = 2100) but was only 5.5 mmHg for flow conditions less than 22 cm^3/s (Re = 1400). Experimental and numerical measurements of the transstenotic pressure gradient are compared in Figure 8.4. In the study of pulsatile flow conditions, the transstenotic pressure gradient determined numerically

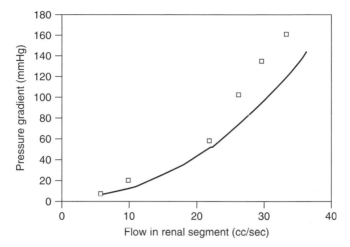

Figure 8.4. Accuracy of CFD estimation of differential pressure under steady flow conditions. Differential pressures estimated with CFD (box) and measured by transducer (solid line) are plotted against renal artery flow.

was 5.7% and 9.9% greater than the pressure determined experimentally in its peak and mean values, respectively.

8.4. IMAGE-BASED MODELS

The prospect of noninvasive measurement, or imaging, of pressure loss at arterial stenoses is intriguing and has been the subject of numerous investigations. Progress in this area of research is discussed below.

Bernoulli Models

Technology has matured in the related area of measurement of transvalvular pressure gradients. In this area Doppler ultrasound measurements of peak velocity are considered to be almost interchangeable with pressure gradients obtained at catheterization [63,64]. The Doppler peak velocity has been found to be related to the transvalvular pressure gradient by the simplified or modified Bernoulli equation [65]

$$\Delta P = 4V^2 \qquad (8.14)$$

where the velocity is implicitly in units of m/s and the pressure is implicitly in units of mmHg. The simplified Bernoulli equation is based on the assumption that pressure loss across the valve or other obstruction is equal to the maximal pressure drop from a proximal position to the valve or obstruction to the *vena contracta* or the point of maximal constriction of the flow stream. Also, the simplied Bernoulli equation is based on the assumption that mean blood velocity proximal to the valve or obstruction is negligible relative to the peak velocity.

Comparable measurements of peak velocity at stenotic valves have been obtained by the technique of phase contrast magnetic resonance (PC-MR) imaging to those obtained by Doppler ultrasound [66]. Velocity–time integrals that represent the mean systolic velocity in both the left ventricular outflow tracts and at the stenosis of the aortic valve were found to be highly correlated between PC-MR and Doppler ultrasound blood. However, velocities at the highest range were consistently underestimated by PC-MR with respect to Doppler ultrasound. The origin of the discrepancy between PC-MR and Doppler ultrasound is unknown. In any case, the presumed inaccuracy of PC-MR in this range is not expected to have a negative effect on its diagnostic accuracy since it occurs beyond the threshold for defining critical stenoses.

Kawarada et al. compared trans-stenotic renal artery pressure gradients measured at catheterization in a series of 60 patients with 75 stenoses [67]. Both the peak systolic velocity and the degree of stenosis were found to be correlated with the transstenotic pressure gradient. The correlation coefficients between peak systolic velocity and degree of stenosis with the pressure gradient were 0.743 and 0.701, respectively. An optimal threshold for detection of a hemodynamically significant stenosis was found to be 219 cm/s, which gave both a sensitivity and a specificity of 89%. The relationship between imaging variables and transstenotic pressure loss in the renal artery is shown in Figure 8.5.

Sudden-Expansion Models

The major limitation of the simplified Bernoulli equation for estimation of transvalvular pressure loss is that pressure recovery occurs distal to the *vena contracta* and that the magnitude of that pressure recovery is variable. The degree of pressure recovery has been found to be related to the ratio of distal aortic cross-sectional area and the stenotic cross-sectional area of the valve. Combined with the simplified Bernoulli equation, the total transvalvular pressure loss is [68]

$$\Delta P = 4V^2 - 8V^2 \frac{A_1}{A_0} \left(1 - \frac{A_1}{A_0} \right) \tag{8.15}$$

where A_0 and A_1 are the cross-sectional areas of the normal and constricted segments of the vessel, respectively.

In a study of 14 pediatric patients with aortic valve stenosis, Villavicencio et al. found that the limits of agreement between Doppler pressure loss measurements and pressure loss measurements obtained at catheterization were reduced using the pressure recovery correction to the simplified Bernoulli equation [68]. The limits of agreement ranged from -9 to 19 and from 2 to 83 mmHg for pressure loss corrected by pressure recovery and by using only the simplified Bernoulli equation, respectively. However, the correlations with pressure loss at

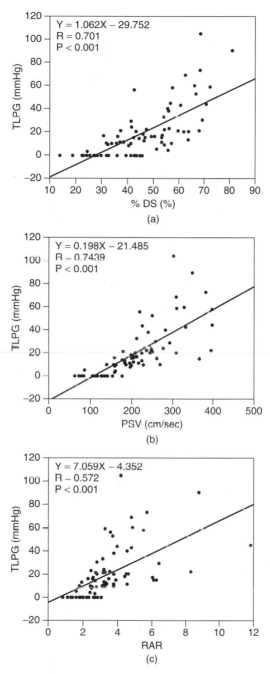

Figure 8.5. A: Correlation between %DS and TLPG. (b) Correlation between PSV and TLPG. (c) Correlation between RAR and TLPG. [DS, percent diameter stenosis; TLPG, translesional pressure gradient;. PSV, peak systolic velocity; RAR, renal artery to aorta ratio.] (Reprinted with permission from *Catheterization and Cardiovascular Interventions*.)

catheterization of both the pressure recovery model and the simplified Bernoulli equation model were identical ($r = 0.92$).

Variability in the peak velocity in the *vena contracta* was found to be produced by variability in valve geometry by Gilon et al. [69]. In this study, realistic models of aortic valves were constructed using stereolithography based on 3D echocardiography. Valves with more gradual tapering proximal to the orifice were found to have a relatively wider *vena contracta* in comparison to valves with more abrupt tapering to the orifice. Asymmetry of the flow at a stenotic valve may cause additional inaccuracy of the simplified Bernoulli equation as shown by VanAuker et al. [70].

The simplified Bernoulli equation has been found to be less accurate for determination of the pressure gradient from peak velocity for aortic coartation. Oshinski et al. studied the peak velocity–pressure relation in a series of in vitro models of aortic coarctation with varying degrees of stenosis severity [71]. They found that for each coarctation model, the pressure loss was proportional to the square of the peak velocity but the proportionality constant, or the loss coefficient, differed among the models with the loss coefficient increasing for increased stenosis severity. In a series of 6 patients, pressure gradients from PC-MR peak velocity using severity-based loss coefficients were more accurate than were pressure gradients from Doppler ultrasound using the simplified Bernoulli equation in comparison with gold-standard pressure gradient measurements at catheterization.

The effect of variations in stenosis geometry on the pressure loss determination from the simplified Bernoulli equation were also investigated in in vitro models by Baumgartner et al. [72]. Axisymmetric models were constructed in which the normal segment had a diameter of 2.4 cm. Physiological pulsatile flow conditions were imposed. The models had varying degrees of stenosis between 90% and 98% area reduction and with varying rates of taper proximal and distal to the neck of the stenosis. The measurement of the maximal pressure gradient by catheter in which the distal pressure measurement was obtained where the pressure was at a minimum correlated strongly with the pressure gradient from the simplified Bernoulli equation independent of the stenosis model. However, pressure gradient measurements obtained by catheter with the distal position 10 cm distal to the stenosis, representing the true pressure loss, depended significantly on the stenosis geometry. This suggests that variation in pressure loss across the stenoses in the models studied was due primarily to variability in pressure recovery.

Lien et al. compared the accuracy of the simplified Bernoulli equation and the Young–Tsai equation for determining transstenotic pressure gradients [73]. In their study, four stenosis models were constructed from silicone tubing with varying degrees of stenosis severity and length. The models were contructed from silicone, and sonographic contrast material was added to the circulating fluid to allow for ultrasonic imaging. Dimensional imaging of cross-sectional areas by B-mode ultrasound were found to be within 3% of measurements made by high-resolution X-ray images. The peak velocity used for determining the pressure gradient from the simplified Bernoulli equation was derived from the mean velocity in a normal segment of the model on the basis of the continuity equation. Thus, the results of the study may not be strictly interpreted with respect to pressure gradients obtained from direct measurements of peak velocity, which are usually the basis for pressure gradient estimates. Pressures measured by the Young–Tsai method were highly correlated with the gold-standard pressure measurements with a correlation coefficient of >0.988 for each stenosis model. The slope of the best-fit equations for each model ranged from 0.924 to 1.07 among the four models. Determination of the pressure gradient from the Young–Tsai equation was found to be generally better than that obtained by the simplified Bernoulli equation.

Navier–Stokes Models

As discussed previously, the mechanics of fluids is fundamentally governed by the Navier–Stokes equation and, in the case of incompressible fluids, the divergence-free condition as given in equations (8.12) and (8.13).

The gradient of the pressure can be expressed as a function of the velocity field and thus is uniquely determined by the velocity field. Given an adequate measurement of the velocity field in the vicinity of an arterial stenosis, the (mathematical) gradient of the pressure can be calculated. Given the pressure gradient field, the transstenotic pressure gradient can be calculated by a line integral of the pressure gradient

$$\Delta P = \oint_{\lambda} \left(\frac{\partial p}{\partial x} \, dx + \frac{\partial p}{\partial y} \, dy + \frac{\partial p}{\partial z} \, dz \right) \tag{8.16}$$

where λ is a path between the two points for which the pressure gradient is to be determined.

This approach for estimation of transstenotic pressure gradients was proposed by Yang et al., who determined the velocity field using phase contrast magnetic resonance (PC-MR) imaging [74]. The velocity field obtained by PC-MR has imperfections, of course, and those imperfections tend to be amplified by Navier–Stokes operations needed to calculate the pressure gradient field. Thus, considerable attention has been given to deriving the pressure gradient field from the velocity field in an optimal manner. An approach was proposed by Song et al. in the context of analysis of intraventricular fluid dynamics conditions from 4D computed tomography [75]. They showed that the optimal pressure gradient field, based on the least-squares criterion, could be obtained by solving the pressure Poisson equation that is derived from the Navier–Stokes equation subject within the blood pool

$$\nabla^2 p = \nabla \cdot \mathbf{b}_F \tag{8.17}$$

where $\mathbf{b}_F$ is a quantity calculated directly from the measured velocity field as

$$\mathbf{b}_F = \mu \nabla^2 \mathbf{v_F} - \rho \left(\frac{\partial \mathbf{v_F}}{\partial t} + \mathbf{v_F} \cdot \nabla \mathbf{v_F} \right) \tag{8.18}$$

$\mathbf{v}_F$ is the measured velocity vector field. The solution is subject to the Neumann boundary condition on the boundary of the blood pool

$$\nabla p \cdot \hat{n} = \mathbf{b}_F \cdot \hat{n} \tag{8.19}$$

where $\hat{n}$ is an outward normal vector to the boundary. An iterative approach to solving this set of equations was proposed by Yang et al. [74].

A similar approach has been taken for estimation of transvalvular gradients by Thompson and McVeigh [76]. In their study, only the blood was considered to be inviscid. In a canine model, measurements of pressure gradients derived from cine 2D PC-MR were very highly correlated with direct measurement of transvalvular pressures, although the magnitude of the pressure gradients was less than 4 mmHg throughout the cardiac cycle. Transvalvular pressure gradients were calculated using the iterative method of Yang et al. and also in terms of the pressure gradients calculated directly from the velocity fields. Differences in their study between transvalvular pressure gradients determined using the iterative approach and the direct approach were found to be minimal. The methodology was extended for use with cine 3D PC-MR for measurement of intracardiac relative pressure distribution [77,78].

The solution of the pressure–Poisson equation provides an optimal pressure gradient field by the least-squares criterion, but pressure differences calculated from the estimated pressure field are still dependent on the path chosen for performing the line integral. An alternative approach for determining the pressure gradient field is to constrain, a priori, the solution to the pressure gradient field functions within an integrable subspace or to functions for which line integrals between any pair of points are independent of the choice of the path of integration [79]. This is a concept that was previously proposed in the field of computer vision for reconstruction of shape from shading [80].

This methodology was evaluated with an axisymmetric in vitro model with varying flow rates and degrees of stenosis severity. Transstenotic pressure gradients were derived from PC-MR using pressure gradient fields based on the least-squares optimization and based on projection into an integrable subspace. The estimates of axial pressure profiles were compared with calculations made with finite-element modeling in FLUENT with a laminar flow model. Differences between pressure fields determined from PC-MR and by FLUENT were similar for the projection method and the least-squares method. However, the projection method was found to have greater accuracy than the least-squares optimization when various degrees of Gaussian noise were added to the PC-MR. The results of the comparison between the projection method and the least-squares method should not be considered definitive, however, even for this in vitro model since gold-standard measurements of pressure gradients were not obtained.

Acquisition of the velocity field within an artery at sufficient resolution and within a practical period of time is a significant challenge. The technique of phase contrast with vastly undersampled isotropic projection reconstruction (PC-VIPR) has been developed that allows for high-speed image acquisition that is potentially within clinically acceptable limits for acquisition time and at relatively high 3D resolution [81]. In cine PC MR, a sequence of images is acquired representing each timepoint throughout the cardiac cycle. In PC-VIPR, the acquisition speed is accelerated by acquiring only the low spatial frequencies for each image in the sequence during the corresponding limited time window. The higher spatial frequencies in the images are assumed to remain relatively constant throughout the cardiac cycle and are thus acquired with a broad time window. Using this technique, the 4D image of the blood's 3D velocity vector can be acquired in about 10 min.

Navier–Stokes analysis was applied to the velocity field obtained by PC-VIPR in the canine model, and transstenotic pressure gradients were compared with measurements at catheterization [82]. A strong correlation was found between the pressure determined by PC-VIPR and by catheterization ($r = 0.91$), whereas there was virtually no correlation between the degree of stenosis and the pressure measured at catheterization (correlation coefficient not reported). The linear fit of the relationship between PC-VIPR pressure and catherization pressure was found to be weakest in the range of pressures above ∼17 mmHg (Figure 8.6).

Finite-element modeling of arterial hemodynamics, as was described previously, has been widely used to study hemodynamic phenomena and their relation to vascular disease [83–85]. With advances in medical imaging methodology that allow for both highly detailed structural imaging of the arterial lumen and measurements of blood flow, finite-element models have become increasingly realistic. My colleagues and I and other groups have begun to explore the potential

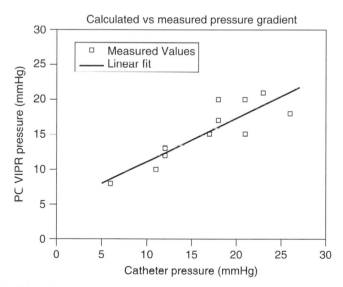

Figure 8.6. Plot showing correlation of actual measured microcatheter values versus calculated pressure gradients from PC-VIPR across the stenosis. (Reprinted with permission from AJNR.)

use of such finite-element modeling for diagnostic purposes. Technology for performing finite-element modeling on a patient-specific basis requires a relatively automated process for construction of the finite-element models from the imaging, as well as for reconstruction of the arterial surface from the angiography and for construction of a volumetric finite-element mesh from the surface geometry.

Work in these areas by my colleagues and I and others is reviewed elsewhere [86,87]. The methodology for construction of the finite-element models includes geometrically deformable models for reconstruction of the arterial geometry from contrast-enhanced magnetic resonance angiography [61,88]. In these models, geometries, that is, triangulated surfaces that are initialized with relatively minimal user interaction, are deformed subject to various forces, as if the vertices of the triangulated mesh were point masses that are joined to the neighboring vertices by spring and other forces. Also, in the mechanical analogy, the additive inverse of the magnitude of the gradient of the image is considered to be the gravitational potential energy. A mechanical deformation is then simulated to let the geometry reach an equilibrium state. In the equilibrium state, the geometry is both relatively smooth as a result of the forces between neighboring vertices and is aligned with the boundaries of the lumen because of the influence of the gravitational potential energy derived from the image.

In principle, this methodology can be applied for estimation of translesional pressure gradients as we have previously proposed [60]. This approach to estimation of the transstenotic pressure gradient has the advantage over the methods for direct calculation of the pressure gradient field from the velocity field on the basis of the Navier–Stokes relation, in that velocity measurements do not need to be made in a three-dimensional manner and can, in fact, be made in regions with less complex flow patterns where the technique of PC-MR imaging or other techniques for flow measurement are likely to be more reliable. Also, in this approach the governing equations of flow can be solved in a more rigorous manner at arbitrarily high resolution.

Feasibility of the finite-element modeling approach was established in an in vitro study, as discussed previously, in which the transstenotic pressure gradient was determined only on the basis of CT imaging of the lumen of the glass model and measurements of flow in the aortic and renal segments of the model using the transit-time ultrasound technique. The applicability of this technique to in vivo measurements, however, has not yet been established. Measurements of the transstenotic pressure gradient using this technique are likely to have considerable dependence on the accuracy of the reconstructed arterial geometry, particularly in the area of maximal stenosis.

Turbulence Models

Nonlaminar, or turbulent, flow conditions are a hallmark of arterial stenosis. In such flow conditions, by definition, flow does not occur along strictly parallel streamlines. Rather, turbulent flow is characterized by intersecting streamlines caused by eddies. The velocity in the turbulent flow field is subject to random fluctuations.

The potential relationship between turbulence and the transstenotic pressure gradient was first suggested by Mustert et al. [89]. That study was based on the phenomena of poststenotic signal attenuation, which was a prominent artifact in magnetic resonance angiography with earlier-generation MR systems. This phenomena is believed to be associated with turbulence on the basis of both experimental and numerical simulations [90,91]. Mustert et al. demonstrated in in vitro models that the transstenotic pressure gradient is directly related to the volume of fluid in the poststenotic region that undergoes signal attenuation. The in vitro models in that study encompassed a wide range of severity of stenosis and two steady-flow rates.

The hypothesis of poststenotic signal attenuation in magnetic resonance angiography is supported by the study of Iseda et al. [92]. In a series of 44 patients with carotid artery disease, they found that poststenotic attenuation in phase contrast magnetic resonance angiography of the carotid artery was associated with a significant decrease in regional blood flow to the brain. Also, notably, in all patients with poststenotic attenuation, collateral flow through the anterior or posterior communicating arteries was absent. Flow through those arteries typically compensates for disruption of flow due to carotid artery stenosis.

Improvements in detection or quantification of turbulence in the poststenotic flow field may be derived from improved phase contrast magnetic resonance (PC-MR) imaging techniques. More recent studies have demonstrated the potential of PC MR for assessing the velocity spectrum at each point within the flow stream. Methodology for estimating the standard deviation of the velocities have been proposed by Pipe [93] and by Dyverfeldt et al. assuming a normal velocity distribution [94]. (See Figure 8.7 for example images of intravoxel velocity variation.) Methodology has also been developed that potentially allows for direct quantification of the velocity spectra in an efficient manner from PC MR [95]. Alternatively, the use of pulsed-wave Doppler ultrasound has been proposed for characterization of turbulence at arterial stenoses [96]. In this study, turbulence in the Doppler frequency spectrum was modeled as a random fluctuation in the mean frequency of the spectrum. The potential accuracy of pulsed-wave Doppler ultrasound was demonstrated for characterization of both the turbulent intensity and of the bandwidth of the Kolmogorov spectrum associated with turbulence.

8.5. CONCLUSIONS

Measurement of transstenotic pressure loss by imaging is a tantalizingly simple problem. However, the potential solutions to this problem are just beginning to emerge, and these solutions draw on the upper limits of existing imaging and computational methodologies. In this chapter, a broad framework to this problem has been developed. The potential clinical value of such methodology

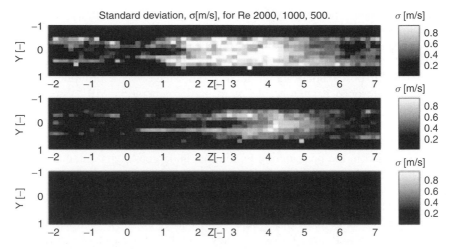

Figure 8.7. Maps of standard deviation of velocity at stenosis for Re 2000 (upper panel), 1000 (middle panel), and 500 (lower panel), velocity encoded in the Z-direction. Z and Y show the normalized distance from the center of the stenosis (Z, $Y = 1 = 14.6\,\text{mm}$). The direction of flow is the positive Z-direction. (Reprinted with permission from MRM.)

has been assessed in the context of coronary artery disease, renal artery disease, and carotid artery disease. The evidence suggests that there is very significant potential value of this methodology in all of those vascular territories. Although studies from other vascular territories were not included in this review, there is no inference that the technology would exclusively, or even primarily, apply to the vascular territories discussed. A second broad field that has a bearing on the measurement of transstenotic pressure loss is, of course, that of fluid mechanics. The problem of characterization of the fluid dynamics at arterial stenoses and analogous conditions in pipes is a classical one, and highly relevant findings are drawn from the literature in that field. Finally, a number of approaches to imaging of transstenotic pressure loss are reviewed. These approaches can be classified as being derived from the Bernoulli model, the sudden-expansion model, the Navier–Stokes model, or a turbulence model. While imaging of transstenotic pressure loss is at a relatively preliminary stage, there is clearly a powerful array of theory and technology available for further advancement of this field.

REFERENCES

1. Abildgaard A, Klow NE: A pressure-recording guidewire for measuring arterial transstenotic gradients: In vivo validation, *Acad Radiol* **2**(1):53–60 (1995).
2. De Bruyne B, Bartunek J, Sys SU, Heyndrickx GR: Relation between myocardial fractional flow reserve calculated from coronary pressure measurements and exercise-induced myocardial ischemia, *Circulation* **92**(1):39–46 (1995).

3. Tron C, Donohue TJ, Bach RG, Aguirre FV, Caracciolo EA, Wolford TL, Miller DD, Kern MJ: Comparison of pressure-derived fractional flow reserve with poststenotic coronary flow velocity reserve for prediction of stress myocardial perfusion imaging results, *Am Heart J* **130**(4):723–733 (1995).

4. Pijls NH, De Bruyne B, Peels K, Van Der Voort PH, Bonnier HJ, Bartunek J, Koolen JJ, Koolen JJ: Measurement of fractional flow reserve to assess the functional severity of coronary-artery stenoses, *N Engl J Med* **334**(26):1703–1708 (1996).

5. Samady H, Lepper W, Powers ER, Wei K, Ragosta M, Bishop GG, Sarembock IJ, Gimple L, Watson DD, Beller GA, Barringhaus KG: Fractional flow reserve of infarct-related arteries identifies reversible defects on noninvasive myocardial perfusion imaging early after myocardial infarction, *J Am Coll Cardiol* **47**(11):2187–2193 (2006).

6. Bech GJ, Droste H, Pijls NH, De Bruyne B, Bonnier JJ, Michels HR, Peels KH, Koolen JJ: Value of fractional flow reserve in making decisions about bypass surgery for equivocal left main coronary artery disease, *Heart* **86**(5):547–552 (2001).

7. Kern MJ, Donohue TJ, Aguirre FV, Bach RG, Caracciolo EA, Wolford T, Mechem CJ, Flynn MS, Chaitman B: Clinical outcome of deferring angioplasty in patients with normal translesional pressure-flow velocity measurements, *J Am Coll Cardiol* **25**(1):178–187 (1995).

8. Rodes-Cabau J, Candell-Riera J, Angel J, de Leon G, Pereztol O, Castell-Conesa J, Soto A, Anivarro I, Aguade S, Vazquez M, Domingo E, Tardif JC, Soler-Soler J: Relation of myocardial perfusion defects and nonsignificant coronary lesions by angiography with insights from intravascular ultrasound and coronary pressure measurements, *Am J Cardiol* **96**(12):1621–1626 (2005).

9. Jasti V, Ivan E, Yalamanchili V, Wongpraparut N, Leesar MA: Correlations between fractional flow reserve and intravascular ultrasound in patients with an ambiguous left main coronary artery stenosis, *Circulation* **110**(18):2831–2836 (2004).

10. Kern MJ, Lerman A, Bech JW, De Bruyne B, Eeckhout E, Fearon WF, Higano ST, Lim MJ, Meuwissen M, Piek JJ, Pijls NH, Siebes M, Spaan JA; American Heart Association Committee on Diagnostic and Interventional Cardiac Catheterization, Council on Clinical Cardiology: Physiological assessment of coronary artery disease in the cardiac catheterization laboratory: A scientific statement from the American Heart Association Committee on Diagnostic and Interventional Cardiac Catheterization, Council on Clinical Cardiology, *Circulation* **14**(12):1321–1341 (2006).

11. Nahman NS Jr, Maniam P, Hernandez RA Jr, Falkenhain M, Hebert LA, Kantor BS, Stockum AE, VanAman ME, Spigos DG: Renal artery pressure gradients in patients with angiographic evidence of atherosclerotic renal artery stenosis, *Am J Kidney Dis* **24**(4):695–699 (1994).

12. Gross CM, Kramer J, Weingartner O, Uhlich F, Luft FC, Waigand J, Dietz R: Determination of renal arterial stenosis severity: Comparison of pressure gradient and vessel diameter, *Radiology* **220**(3):751–756 (2001).

13. Colyer WR Jr, Cooper CJ, Burket MW, Thomas WJ: Utility of a 0.014″ pressure-sensing guidewire to assess renal artery translesional systolic pressure gradients, *Cath Cardiovasc Interv* **59**(3):372–377 (2003).

14. Manoharan G, Pijls NH, Lameire N, Verhamme K, Heyndrickx GR, Barbato E, Wijns W, Madaric J, Tielbeele X, Bartunek J, De Bruyne B: Assessment of renal flow and flow reserve in humans, *J Am Coll Cardiol* **47**(3):620–625 (2006).

15. De Bruyne B, Manoharan G, Pijls NH, Verhamme K, Madaric J, Bartunek J, Vander-heyden M, Heyndrickx GR: Assessment of renal artery stenosis severity by pressure gradient measurements, *J Am Coll Cardiol* **48**(9):1851–1855 (2006).

16. Norris CS, Barnes RW: Renal artery flow velocity analysis: A sensitive measure of experimental and clinical renovascular resistance, *J Surg Res* **36**(3):230–236 (1984).

17. Tublin ME, Tessler FN, Murphy ME: Correlation between renal vascular resistance, pulse pressure, and the resistive index in isolated perfused rabbit kidneys, *Radiology* **213**(1):258–264 (1999).

18. Heine GH, Reichart B, Ulrich C, Kohler H, Girndt M: Do ultrasound renal resistance indices reflect systemic rather than renal vascular damage in chronic kidney disease? *Nephrol Dial Transplant* **22**(1):163–170 (2007).

19. Ohta Y, Fujii K, Arima H, Matsumura K, Tsuchihashi T, Tokumoto M, Tsuruya K, Kanai H, Iwase M, Hirakata H, Iida M: Increased renal resistive index in atherosclerosis and diabetic nephropathy assessed by Doppler sonography, *J Hypertens* **23**(10):1905–1911 (2005).

20. Bude RO, Rubin JM: Relationship between the resistive index and vascular compliance and resistance, *Radiology* **211**(2):411–417 (1999).

21. Halpern EJ, Deane CR, Needleman L, Merton DA, East SA: Normal renal artery spectral Doppler waveform: A closer look, *Radiology* **196**(3):667–673 (1995).

22. John LR: Forward electrical transmission line model of the human arterial system, *Med Biol Eng Comput* **42**(3):312–321 (2004).

23. Ripolles T, Aliaga R, Morote V, Lonjedo E, Delgado F, Martinez MJ, Vilar J: Utility of intrarenal Doppler ultrasound in the diagnosis of renal artery stenosis, *Eur J Radiol* **40**(1):54–63 (2001).

24. Schwerk WB, Restrepo IK, Stellwaag M, Klose KJ, Schade-Brittinger C: Renal artery stenosis: Grading with image-directed Doppler US evaluation of renal resistive index, *Radiology* **190**(3):785–790 (1994).

25. Evans DH, Barrie WW, Asher MJ, Bentley S, Bell PR: The relationship between ultrasonic pulsatility index and proximal arterial stenosis in a canine model, *Circ Res* **46**(4):470–475 (1980).

26. van Jaarsveld B, Krijnen P, Bartelink A, Dees A, Derkx F, Man in't Veld A, Schalekamp M, The Dutch Renal Artery Stenosis Intervention Cooperative (DRASTIC) Study: Rationale, design and inclusion data, *J Hypertens Suppl* **16**(6):S21–S27 (1998).

27. Ives NJ, Wheatley K, Stowe RL, Krijnen P, Plouin PF, van Jaarsveld BC, Gray R: Continuing uncertainty about the value of percutaneous revascularization in atherosclerotic renovascular disease: A meta-analysis of randomized trials, *Nephrol Dial Transplant* **18**(2):298–304 (2003).

28. Radermacher J, Chavan A, Bleck J, Vitzthum A, Stoess B, Gebel MJ, Galanski M, Koch KM, Haller H: Use of Doppler ultrasonography to predict the outcome of therapy for renal-artery stenosis, *N Engl J Med* **344**(6):410–417 (2001).

29. Soulez G, Therasse E, Qanadli SD, Froment D, Leveille M, Nicolet V, Turpin S, Giroux MF, Guertin MC, Oliva VL: Prediction of clinical response after renal angioplasty: Respective value of renal Doppler sonography and scintigraphy, *Am J Roentgenol* **181**(4):1029–1035 (2003).

30. Zeller T, Frank U, Muller C, Burgelin K, Sinn L, Bestehorn HP, Cook-Bruns N, Neumann FJ: Predictors of improved renal function after percutaneous stent-supported angioplasty of severe atherosclerotic ostial renal artery stenosis, *Circulation* **108**(18):2244–2249 (2003).

31. Gruenewald SM, Collins LT, Antico VF, Farlow DC, Fawdry RM: Can quantitative renography predict the outcome of treatment of atherosclerotic renal artery stenosis? *J Nucl Med* **30**(12):1946–1954 (1989).

32. Michaely HJ, Schoenberg SO, Ittrich C, Dikow R, Bock M, Guenther M: Renal disease: Value of functional magnetic resonance imaging with flow and perfusion measurements, *Invest Radiol* **39**(11):698–705 (2004).

33. Binkert CA, Debatin JF, Schneider E, Hodler J, Ruehm SG, Schmidt M, Hoffmann U: Can MR measurement of renal artery flow and renal volume predict the outcome of percutaneous transluminal renal angioplasty? *Cardiovasc Interv Radiol* **24**(4):233–239 (2001).

34. Paul JF, Ugolini P, Sapoval M, Mousseaux E, Gaux JC: Unilateral renal artery stenosis: Perfusion patterns with electron-beam dynamic CT—preliminary experience, *Radiology* **221**(1):261–265 (2001).

35. Hennerici MG: The unstable plaque, *Cerebrovasc Dis* **17**(Suppl 3):17–22 (2004).

36. Vanninen R, Koivisto K, Tulla H, Manninen H, Partanen K: Hemodynamic effects of carotid endarterectomy by magnetic resonance flow quantification, *Stroke* **26**(1):84–89 (1995).

37. Zachrisson H, Blomstrand C, Holm J, Mattsson E, Volkmann R: Changes in middle cerebral artery blood flow after carotid endarterectomy as monitored by transcranial Doppler, *J Vasc Surg* **36**(2):285–290 (2002).

38. Nielsen MY, Sillesen HH, Jorgensen LG, Schroeder TV: The haemodynamic effect of carotid endarterectomy, *Eur J Vasc Endovasc Surg* **24**(1):53–58 (2002).

39. Fearn SJ, Hutchinson S, Riding G, Hill-Wilson G, Wesnes K, McCollum CN: Carotid endarterectomy improves cognitive function in patients with exhausted cerebrovascular reserve, *Eur J Vasc Endovasc Surg* **26**(5):529–536 (2003).

40. Lishmanov Y, Shvera I, Ussov W, Shipulin V: The effect of carotid endarterectomy on cerebral blood flow and cerebral blood volume studied by SPECT, *J Neuroradiol* **24**(2):155–162 (1997).

41. Aleksic M, Matoussevitch V, Heckenkamp J, Brunkwall J: Changes in internal carotid blood flow after CEA evaluated by transit-time flowmeter, *Eur J Vasc Endovasc Surg* 2006 Jan; **31**(1):14–7.

42. Lunn S, Crawley F, Harrison MJ, Brown MM, Newman SP: Impact of carotid endarterectomy upon cognitive functioning. A systematic review of the literature, *Cerebrovasc Dis* **9**(2):74–81 (1999).

43. Grunwald IQ, Supprian T, Politi M, Struffert T, Falkai P, Krick C, Backens M, Reith W: Cognitive changes after carotid artery stenting, *Neuroradiology* **48**(5):319–323 (2006).

44. Xu G, Liu X, Meyer JS, Yin Q, Zhang R: Cognitive performance after carotid angioplasty and stenting with brain protection devices, *Neurol Res* **29**(3):251–255 (2007).

45. Kishikawa K, Kamouchi M, Okada Y, Inoue T, Ibayashi S, Iida M: Effects of carotid endarterectomy on cerebral blood flow and neuropsychological test performance in patients with high-grade carotid stenosis, *J Neurol Sci* **213**(1–2):19–24 (2003).

46. Ogasawara K, Yamadate K, Kobayashi M, Endo H, Fukuda T, Yoshida K, Terasaki K, Inoue T, Ogawa A: Postoperative cerebral hyperperfusion associated with impaired cognitive function in patients undergoing carotid endarterectomy, *J Neurosurg* **102**(1):38–44 (2005).

47. Pijls NH, Van Gelder B, Van der Voort P, Peels K, Bracke FA, Bonnier HJ, el Gamal MI: Fractional flow reserve. A useful index to evaluate the influence of an epicardial coronary stenosis on myocardial blood flow, *Circulation* **92**(11):3183–3193 (1995).

48. White FM: *Fluid Mechanics*, 2nd ed, McGraw-Hill, 1986.

49. http://www.lmnoeng.com/Flow/SmallOrificeLiq.htm.

50. Garcia D, Pibarot P, Landry C, Allard A, Chayer B, Dumesnil JG, Durand LG: Estimation of aortic valve effective orifice area by Doppler echocardiography: Effects of valve inflow shape and flow rate, *J Am Soc Echocardiogr* **17**(7):756–765 (2004).

51. Golia C, Evans NA: Flow separation through annular constrictions in tubes, *Exp Mech* **13**(4):157–162 (1973).

52. Solzbach U, Wollschlager H, Zeiher A, Just H: Effect of stenotic geometry on flow behavior across stenotic models, *Med Biol Eng Comput* **25**(5):543–550 (1987).

53. Gach HM, Lowe IJ: Measuring flow reattachment lengths downstream of a stenosis using MRI, *J Magn Reson Imag* **12**(6):939–948 (2000).

54. Matsuzaki Y, Ikeda T, Matsumoto T, Kitagawa T: Experiments on steady and oscillatory flows at moderate Reynolds numbers in a quasi-two-dimensional channel with a throat, *J Biomech Eng* **120**(5):594–601 (1998).

55. Kalse SGC, Bijl H, VAN Oudheusden BW: A one-dimensional viscous-inviscid strong interaction model for flow in indented channels with separation and reattachment, *J Biomech Eng* **125**(3):355–362 (2003).

56. Young DF, Tsai FY: Flow characteristics in models of arterial stenoses. I. Steady flow, *J Biomech* **6**(4):395–410 (1973).

57. Seeley BD, Young DF: Effect of geometry on pressure losses across models of arterial stenoses, *J Biomech* **9**(7):439–448 (1976).

58. Ang KC and Mazumdar JN: Mathematical modeling of three-dimensional flow through an asymmetric arterial stenosis, *Math Comput Model* **25**(1):19–29 (1997).

59. Johnston PR, Kilpatrick D: Mathematical modelling of flow through an irregular arterial stenosis, *J Biomech* **24**(11):1069–1077 (1991).

60. Yim PJ, Cebral JR, Weaver A, Lutz RJ, Soto O, Vasbinder GB, Ho VB, Choyke PL: Estimation of the differential pressure at renal artery stenoses, *Magn Reson Med* **51**(5):969–977 (2004).

61. Yim PJ, Vasbinder GB, Ho VB, Choyke PL: Isosurfaces as deformable models for magnetic resonance angiography, *IEEE Trans Med Imag* **22**(7):875–881 (2003).

62. Soto O, Loehner R, Cebral J: An implicit monolithic time accurate finite element scheme for incompressible flow problems, AIAA-2001-2616, 15th AIAA Computational Fluid Dynamics Conf. Anaheim, CA, June 11– 14, 2001.

63. Khalid O, Luxenberg DM, Sable C, Benavidez O, Geva T, Hanna B, Abdulla R: Aortic stenosis: The spectrum of practice, *Pediatr Cardiol* **27**(6):661–669 (2006).

64. Nitter-Hauge S: Does mitral stenosis need invasive investigation? *Eur Heart J* **12**(Suppl B):81–83 (1991).

65. Popp RL, Teplitsky I: Lessons from in vitro models of small, irregular, multiple and tunnel-like stenoses relevant to clinical stenoses of valves and small vessels, *J Am Coll Cardiol* **13**(3):716–722 (1989).

66. Caruthers SD, Lin SJ, Brown P, Watkins MP, Williams TA, Lehr KA, Wickline SA: Practical value of cardiac magnetic resonance imaging for clinical quantification of aortic valve stenosis: Comparison with echocardiography, *Circulation* **108**(18):2236–2243 (2003).

67. Kawarada O, Yokoi Y, Takemoto K, Morioka N, Nakata S, Shiotani S: The performance of renal duplex ultrasonography for the detection of hemodynamically significant renal artery stenosis, *Cath Cardiovasc Interv* **68**(2):311–318 (2006).

68. Villavicencio RE, Forbes TJ, Thomas RL, Humes RA: Pressure recovery in pediatric aortic valve stenosis, *Pediatr Cardiol* **24**(5):457–462 (2003).

69. Gilon D, Cape EG, Handschumacher MD, Song JK, Solheim J, VanAuker M, King ME, Levine RA: Effect of three-dimensional valve shape on the hemodynamics of aortic stenosis: Three-dimensional echocardiographic stereolithography and patient studies, *J Am Coll Cardiol* **40**(8):1479–1486 (2002).

70. VanAuker MD, Chandra M, Shirani J, Strom JA: Jet eccentricity: A misleading source of agreement between Doppler/catheter pressure gradients in aortic stenosis, *J Am Soc Echocardiogr* **14**(9):853–862 (2001).

71. Oshinski JN, Parks WJ, Markou CP, Bergman HL, Larson BE, Ku DN, Mukundan S Jr, Pettigrew RI: Improved measurement of pressure gradients in aortic coarctation by magnetic resonance imaging, *J Am Coll Cardiol* **28**(7):1818–1826 (1996).

72. Baumgartner H, Schima H, Tulzer G, Kuhn P: Effect of stenosis geometry on the Doppler-catheter gradient relation in vitro: A manifestation of pressure recovery, *J Am Coll Cardiol* **21**(4):1018–1025 (1993).

73. Lien WW, Lee AH, Kono Y, Steinbach GC, Mattrey RF: Noninvasive estimation of the pressure gradient across stenoses using sonographic contrast: In vitro validation, *J Ultrasound Med* **23**(5):683–691 (2004).

74. Yang GZ, Kilner PJ, Wood NB, Underwood SR, Firmin DN: Computation of flow pressure fields from magnetic resonance velocity mapping, *Magn Reson Med* **36**(4):520–526 (1996).

75. Song SM, Leahy RM, Boyd DP, Brundage BH, Napel S: Determining cardiac velocity fields and intraventricular pressuredistribution from a sequence of ultrafast CT cardiac images, *IEEE Trans Med Imag* **13**(2):386–397 (1994).

76. Thompson RB, McVeigh ER: Fast measurement of intracardiac pressure differences with 2D breath-hold phase-contrast MRI, *Magn Reson Med* **49**(6):1056–1066 (2003).

77. Ebbers T, Wigstrom L, Bolger AF, Engvall J, Karlsson M: Estimation of relative cardiovascular pressures using time-resolved three-dimensional phase contrast MRI, *Magn Reson Med* **45**(5):872–879 (2001).

78. Tyszka JM, Laidlaw DH, Asa JW, Silverman JM: Three-dimensional, time-resolved (4D) relative pressure mapping using magnetic resonance imaging, *J Magn Reson Imag* **12**(2):321–329 (2000).

79. Wang Y, Moghaddam AN, Behrens G, Fatouraee N, Cebral J, Choi E, Amini AA: Pulsatile pressure measurements via harmonics-based orthogonal projection of noisy pressure gradients, *Proc SPIE* **6143**:95–110 (2006).

80. Frankot R, Chellappa R: A method for enforcing integrability in shape from shading algorithms, *IEEE Trans Pattern Anal Machine Intell* **10**(4):439–451 (1988).

81. Gu T, Korosec FR, Block WF, Fain SB, Turk Q, Lum D, Zhou Y, Grist TM, Haughton V, Mistretta CA: PC VIPR: A high-speed 3D phase-contrast method for flow quantification and high-resolution angiography, *Am J Neuroradiol* **26**(4):743–749 (2005).

82. Turk AS, Johnson KM, Lum D, Niemann D, Aagaard-Kienitz B, Consigny D, Grinde J, Turski P, Haughton V, Mistretta C: Physiologic and anatomic assessment of a canine carotid artery stenosis model utilizing phase contrast with vastly undersampled isotropic projection imaging, *Am J Neuroradiol* **28**(1):111–115 (2007).

83. Perktold K, Hilbert D: Numerical simulation of pulsatile flow in a carotid bifurcation model, *J Biomed Eng* **8**(3):193–199 (1986).

84. Perktold K, Kenner T, Hilbert D, Spork B, Florian H: Related articles, links numerical blood flow analysis: Arterial bifurcation with a saccular aneurysm, *Basic Res Cardiol* **83**(1):24–31 (1988).

85. Stroud JS, Berger SA, Saloner D: Numerical analysis of flow through a severely stenotic carotid artery bifurcation, *J Biomech Eng* **124**(1):9–20 (2002).

86. Yim PJ, Demarco JK, Castro MA, Cebral J: Characterization of shear stress on the wall of the carotid artery using magnetic resonance imaging and computational fluid dynamics, *Stud Health Technol Inform* **113**:412–442 (2005).

87. Yim PJ, DeMarco JK: Measurement of carotid artery stenosis from magnetic resonance angiography, in Leondes CT, ed, *Medical Imaging Systems Technology*, World Scientific, Singapore, 2005.

88. Yim PJ, Cebral JJ, Mullick R, Marcos HB, Choyke PL: Vessel surface reconstruction with a tubular deformable model, *IEEE Trans Med Imag* **20**(12):1411–1421 (2001).

89. Mustert BR, Williams DM, Prince MR: In vitro model of arterial stenosis: Correlation of MR signal dephasing and trans-stenotic pressure gradients, *Magn Reson Imag* **16**(3):301–310 (1998).

90. Oshinski JN, Ku DN, Pettigrew RI: Turbulent fluctuation velocity: The most significant determinant of signal loss in stenotic vessels, *Magn Reson Med* **33**(2):193–199 (1995).

91. Siegel JM Jr, Oshinski JN, Pettigrew RI, Ku DN: Computational simulation of turbulent signal loss in 2D time-of-flight magnetic resonance angiograms, *Magn Reson Med* **37**(4):609–614 (1997).

92. Iseda T, Nakano S, Miyahara D, Uchinokura S, Goya T, Wakisaka S: Poststenotic signal attenuation on 3D phase-contrast MR angiography: A useful finding in haemodynamically significant carotid artery stenosis, *Neuroradiology* **42**(12):868–873 (2000).

93. Pipe JG: A simple measure of flow disorder and wall shear stress in phase contrast MRI, *Magn Reson Med* **49**(3):543–550 (2003).

94. Dyverfeldt P, Sigfridsson A, Kvitting JP, Ebbers T: Quantification of intravoxel velocity standard deviation and turbulence intensity by generalizing phase-contrast MRI, *Magn Reson Med* **56**(4):850–858 (2006).

95. Hansen MS, Baltes C, Tsao J, Kozerke S, Pruessmann KP, Boesiger P, Pedersen EM: Accelerated dynamic Fourier velocity encoding by exploiting velocity-spatio-temporal correlations, *MAGMA* **17**(2):86–94 (2004).

96. Cloutier G, Chen D, Durand LG: Performance of time-frequency representation techniques to measure blood flow turbulence with pulsed-wave Doppler ultrasound, *Ultrasound Med Biol* **27**(4):535–550 (2001).

CHAPTER 9

Measurement of Blood Flow with Phase Contrast Magnetic Resonance Imaging

REZA NEZAFAT

Department of Medicine, Division of Cardiology, Beth Israel Deaconess Medical Center and Harvard Medical School, Boston, Massachusetts

RICHARD B. THOMPSON

Department of Biomedical Engineering, University of Alberta, Canada

Abstract. Magnetic resonance imaging (MRI) is a noninvasive imaging modality that can be used to measured anatomical, functional, metabolic, and chemical characteristics of lliving tissues. MR imaging can be used to measure motion using a phase contrast imaging sequence. In this sequence, the motion information is encoded in the phase of an image. This imaging technique can be used for in vivo imaging of the blood flow within the cardiovascular system, myocardial motion through cardiac cycle, or flow of cerebral spinal fluid, to name a few applications, In this chapter, we will review the fundamentals of phase contrast MR and provide an overview of clinical and basic physiologic science applications of this technique in cardiovascular imaging, limiting our consideration to the imaging of blood flow.

9.1. INTRODUCTION

Magnetic resonance imaging is based on the NMR phenomena initially observed by two Nobel Prize winners, Felix Block and Edward Purcell. When nuclei with a net magnetic dipole moment were placed in a magnetic field, they absorbed energy in the radiofrequency range of the electromagnetic spectrum, and reemitted this energy when the nuclei transferred to their original state. The strength of

Vascular Hemodynamics: Bioengineering and Clinical Perspectives, Edited by Peter J. Yim
Copyright © 2008 John Wiley & Sons, Inc.

the magnetic field and the frequency of the absorption and emission of energy matched each other. The ability of NMR to generate images using the signal radiated by nuclei was pioneered by two other Nobel Prize winners, Paul Lauterbur and Sir Peter Mansfield, who created two-dimensional images by introducing spatial gradients in the magnetic fields. The motion sensitivity of nuclear MR was initially observed by Carr and Purcell in 1954, followed by a study by Hahn in 1960 measuring the motion of seawater. The first formal description of phase velocity magnetic resonance imaging was introduced in 1982 by Moran [1]. In the presence of specially designed patterns of magnetic field gradients (a pair of balanced or "bipolar" gradients), the moving nuclei will create a phase shift that is proportional to the velocity of spins. Therefore, in a phase contrast imaging study, the motion information is encoded in the phase of an image. This imaging technique can be used for in vivo imaging of blood flow within the cardiovascular system, myocardial motion through cardiac cycle, or flow of cerebral spinal fluid.

9.2. IMAGING PRINCIPLES AND TECHNIQUES

Physical Basis of Phase Contrast MRI

The source of the signal in MRI is the precessing magnetic dipole moments from the nuclei of interest (predominantly hydrogen atoms in water, ^{1}H), which, acting in unison, are termed *magnetization*. The signal that is acquired in magnetic resonance experiments has a magnitude component and a phase component, reflecting the vector nature of the magnetization, so is most conveniently expressed in the complex domain. The MRI signals are acquired in the time domain, but it is convenient to use an alternate domain termed *k space*, which accounts for the effects of the magnetic field gradients that are used to spatially localize the source of the MRI signals. The complex MR signal $s(k_x, k_y)$ from a moving magnetization $m(x, y)$ with velocity vector $v = (v_x, v_y, v_z)$ acquired along the k-space trajectory $k(t) = (k_x(t), k_y(t))$ can be expressed as

$$s(k_x, k_y) = \iint\limits_{x,y} m(x, y) e^{-i2\pi(k_x x + k_y y) + \gamma(M_{1x} v_x + M_{1y} v_y + M_{1z} v_z)} \qquad (9.1)$$

The same magnetic field gradients that are used to encode the spatial location of the magnetization are also used to encode the velocity of the magnetization to image phase. In equation (9.1), $M_1 = (M_{1x}, M_{1y}, M_{1z})$ is the first moment of the gradient shape in the imaging sequence, which is a scaling term for velocity encoding, that relates the magnetization velocity in the presence of given gradient field to the image phase that is induced. Recall that the raw MR signal $s(k_x, k_y)$ contains two components: a magnitude and a phase. The magnitude contains anatomic information, while the phase contains velocity information, in addition to various background sources of image phase. The signal phase induced by motion is proportional to the velocity of spins as follows

$$\varphi = \gamma M_1 v = \gamma (M_{1x} v_x + M_{1y} v_y + M_{1z} v_z) \qquad (9.2)$$

in which M_1 is the first moment of the applied gradient waveform G and γ is the gyromagnetic ratio, which is a constant (42.58 MHz/T for ^{1}H). The first moment M_1 of applied gradient G is to be calculated as follows:

$$M_1 = \int G(t) t \, dt \qquad (9.3)$$

Figure 9.1 shows a bipolar gradient that is applied before the signal acquisition to create a nonzero first moment M_1. Note that because the net area under this bipolar gradient (the zero moment) is null, it does not affect the stationary tissues. The phase of the magnetization in a given image voxel will exhibit a change proportional to the velocity of the spins. In the presence of this bipolar gradient, the accumulated phase of static tissue (solid line) in the first lobe will be compensated in the second phase; however, for the moving spins there will be a residual phase (dashed line) that is proportional to the velocity of the moving spins in the direction of the magnetic field gradient.

In addition to the motion-induced phase in each voxel, there exist additional background phases due to the radiofrequency (RF) coils (antenna) used to receive the signal, off-resonance effects, and unavoidable imperfections in the experimental design and hardware such as pulse sequence timing errors, eddy currents, Maxwell term effects, and RF saturations. To resolve the motion-induced phase from these background image phases, a second image is acquired with a different gradient first moment, so that a difference in the first moments (ΔM_1) will exist

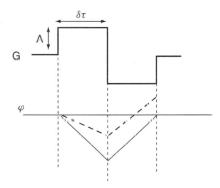

Figure 9.1. Bipolar flow encoding gradient G and phase f accumulation for a static spin (solid line) and dynamic (dashed line) spins; in a phase contrast MRI a bipolar gradient is added to induce motion sensitivity in the phase. The accumulated phase of the static spins in the first half will be compensated in the second half, while the dynamic spins will accumulate an extra phase that is proportional to the velocity of the spins.

between the two acquisitions. The unwanted phase difference, which is assumed to be consistent in the two images, will be removed by subtracting the image phases. Phase contrast imaging experiments thus typically require two or more flow-encoding steps, with different first moments, to uniquely identify the image phase that is proportional to the magnetization velocity. Figure 9.2 shows how the phase contrast MR images are acquired using a reference scan to measure the background phase image followed by a velocity-encoded image. Velocity maps are then reconstructed using the phase difference between the two acquisitions.

Velocity Encoding and Aliasing

The difference in the first-moment gradients ΔM_1 determines the strength of velocity encoding, commonly termed the v_{enc} (cm/s). The v_{enc} is an imaging parameter, specified by the user that will determine the velocity that will produce a π phase shift in the image signal. The velocities between $-v_{\mathrm{enc}}$ and v_{enc} will be distributed linearly between $-\pi$ to π. In order to design the magnetic field

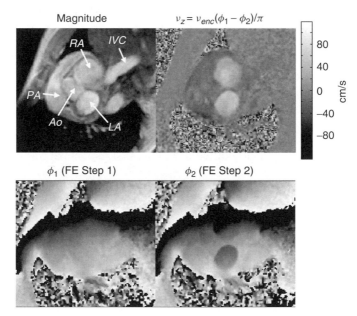

Figure 9.2. Sample phase contrast images of blood flow in the heart: A magnitude image, which shows the relevant anatomy, is shown in the top left. The corresponding phase contrast image is in the top right, in this case sensitive to the velocity in the through-plane direction. A single frame during diastole (ventricular filling) is shown. The individual raw phase images, from the two flow encoding steps are shown in the bottom row, with the left frame flow-compensated (no velocity information in the phase). The background phase is present in both phase images, and is subtracted out in the phase difference image. (RA = right atrium, IVC = inferior vena cava, PA = pulmonary artery, LA, left atrium, Ao = aorta.)

gradients to generate a target v_{enc}, the first moment ΔM_1 is determined by the prescribed v_{enc} as follows:

$$\Delta M_1 = \frac{\pi}{\gamma v_{enc}} \tag{9.4}$$

The v_{enc} can also be described as the maximum velocity that can be measured in a phase contrast image without any phase wrapping, also termed *aliasing*. An image phase that exceeds $180°$ ($\pi + \Delta\phi$) cannot be distinguished from the negative phase ($-\pi + \Delta\phi$), so that large positive and negative velocities can become ambiguous. To avoid velocity aliasing, the v_{enc} should be prescribed to a value higher than the maximum expected velocity in the field of view. However, because the signal-to-noise ratio in the ultimate velocity image is inversely proportional to v_{enc}, excessively large values are undesirable owing to the loss in sensitivity. Figure 9.3 shows a sample magnitude and phase contrast image frame from a normal heart, showing the velocity of the blood in the left ventricle and ascending aorta during systole (ejection of blood from the heart). The v_{enc} was set to 90 cm/s, but the peak velocity in the ejecting blood in this subject reached 110 cm/s, so velocity aliasing resulted, clearly visible in the figure.

Flow-Encoding Methods

In a phase contrast experiment, bipolar velocity-encoding gradients are used to encode a first-moment difference of ΔM_1 between two acquisitions, by

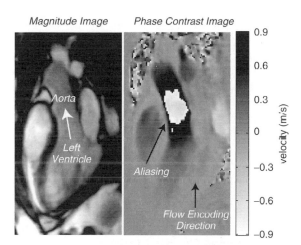

Figure 9.3. A sample magnitude and phase contrast image frame from a normal heart, showing the velocity of the blood in the left ventricle and ascending aorta during systole (ejection of blood from the heart). The v_{enc} was set to 90 cm/s, but the peak velocity in the ejecting blood in this subject reached 110 cm/s, so velocity aliasing resulted, clearly visible in the figure.

controlling the M_1 values in each acquisition. This encoding can be achieved via different schemes. In the "one-sided technique," the first image is acquired using a flow-compensated gradient ($M_1 = 0$), followed by the second image with the first moment of $M_1 = \Delta M_1$. Figure 9.2 shows an example phase contrast image acquired using the one-sided technique for a slice prescribed at the base of the heart, which would be used for measurement of the blood flow into the filling ventricles. The figure shows the magnitude and phase contrast velocity image in the top row, and the two raw phase images used to reconstruct the velocity image. Note that the left phase image has no phase information regarding velocity while the right image clearly shows the velocity phase in addition to the background phases, the through-plane velocity in this example.

In the "two-sided" strategy, the first moment of the bipolar flow-encoding gradients are symmetrically placed around zero in two acquisitions (i.e., $M_1 = \pm \Delta M_1 / 2$). In a method optimized for efficiency, the predetermined first-moment gradient value in each acquisition is relaxed to yield two different bipolar gradients with a ΔM_1 difference [2]. In other words, the first-moment difference between two flow-encoding steps (i.e., two acquisitions) is used as the bipolar gradient design constraint without regard to individual first-moment values. This strategy results in the shortest possible total duration of the velocity-encoding gradients (a shorter echo time).

In order to add sensitivity to motion in a specified direction, the bipolar flow encoding will be added to the physical axis of the corresponding gradient. Through-plane and in-plane blood flow is measured by addition of the bipolar gradient to the slice-selective or phase-encoding (or frequency-encoding) gradients, or equivalently, the z, y, or x gradient directions, as shown in Figure 9.4. Various methods exist for encoding all three directions of the flow in a single phase contrast study. Table 9.1 summarizes two schemes commonly used for imaging all three directions of the flow: the four-point and balanced four-point. Four acquisitions are required for measurement of all three directions of flow. In the four-point method, a reference image will be acquired with a flow-compensated gradient. Three additional images, each with a bipolar gradient in a target direction, are acquired. The velocity in each direction is calculated by combining the motion-sensitized acquisition in the target direction with the reference image. In the balanced four-point method, four symmetric acquisitions are performed in which each acquisition carries the phase from all three directions but with different weights. The velocity information in each direction is calculated from the four acquisitions outlined in Table 9.1.

Pulse Sequences for Phase Contrast MR

Figure 9.4 outlines the basic structure of the phase contrast pulse sequence. A bipolar gradient is added to an imaging pulse sequence to add sensitivity to motion as discussed previously. A minimum of two images are acquired with two different bipolar gradients, and the subtraction of the phases from the two

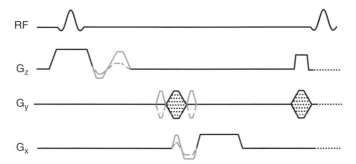

Figure 9.4. A typical phase contrast MR pulse sequence used for imaging the blood flow velocity. A bipolar gradient (light grayline) is added to an MR pulse sequence to enhance sensitivity to motion. Two images acquired with two different bipolar gradients (solid and dashed graylines) are acquired to compensate for the background phase information using phase subtraction of the acquired phase contrast MR images. The direction of motion sensitivity is determined by the gradient axis where the bipolar gradient is applied.

TABLE 9.1. Balanced and Simple Four-Point Velocity-Encoding Schemes in Phase Contrast MR^a

Phase Contrast	Balanced Four-Point Encoding			Simple Four-Point Encoding		
MR Experiment	Readout	Phase	Slice	Readout	Phase	Slice
1	$-M_1$	$-M_1$	$-M_1$	0	0	0
2	$+M_1$	$+M_1$	$-M_1$	M_1	0	0
3	$+M_1$	$-M_1$	$+M_1$	0	M_1	0
4	$-M_1$	$+M_1$	$+M_1$	0	0	M_1
	$v_x = (-f_4 + f_3 + f_2 - f_1)/(4\gamma M_1)$			$v_x = (f_2 - f_1)/(\gamma M_1)$		
	$v_x = (+f_4 - f_3 + f_2 - f_1)/(4\gamma M_1)$			$v_x = (f_3 - f_1)/(\gamma M_1)$		
	$v_z = (+f_4 + f_3 - f_2 - f_1)/(4\gamma M_1)$			$v_z = (f_4 - f_1)/(\gamma M_1)$		

^{a}All three velocity directions (v_x, v_y, v_z) are included here; M_1 is the first moment amplitude used to encode velocity to phase; f_1, f_2, f_3, and f_4 are the phase images generated from experiments 1, 2, 3, and 4, respectively; and γ is the gyromagnetic ratio (42.58 MHz/T for ^{1}H)

images removes the background phase. While all phase contrast experiments have in common the use of bipolar gradients for velocity encoding, there are several choices of k-space sampling, which determines how the image data themselves are acquired. These different sampling trajectories can directly influence the imaging contrast, noise, artifacts, and reconstruction. Figure 9.5 shows three k-space sampling techniques that are commonly used in phase contrast MR. Figure 9.5a illustrates a Cartesian k-space sampling scheme that is the predominant imaging sequence in MRI. All sampling lines are on a linear path, parallel to each other with the same distance. A simple 2D Fourier transform

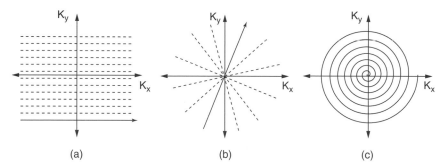

Figure 9.5. Different sampling trajectories in k space can be used for phase contrast MR: (a) Cartesian sampling, (b) radial (projection reconstruction), and (c) spiral sampling are three commonly used sampling sequences.

is used to reconstruct images acquired with Cartesian imaging. The acquisition efficiency can be improved using an echo–planar imaging (EPI) readout in which multiple lines of k space are acquired in a single repetition time (i.e., excitation). However, this improvement in efficiency increases sensitivity to imaging artifacts such as ghosting and image distortions. Radial (projection reconstruction) sampling is shown in Figure 9.5b, where the raw data are sampled using a set of radial spokes. Each radial acquisition is equivalent to a projection of the object at a different angle. Although this sampling trajectory has good motion artifact reduction properties, it is seldom used in phase contrast MR because of the presence of streaking artifacts and reduced signal-to-noise ratios. A more common sampling technique in phase contrast MR is spiral imaging (Figure 9.5c) [3,4]. A spiral sampling trajectory starts at the center of k space and *spirals* out radially, most commonly at either a constant angular velocity or a constant linear velocity. This sampling is more efficient than the Cartesian or radial trajectory; however, it is prone to blurring owing to the effects of off-resonances (inhomogeneities in the main static magnetic field) [5]. This sampling has been used widely for real-time phase contrast MR, which we will discuss in the following sections. A full description of the k-space formalism, and several other aspects of magnetic resonance imaging physics are beyond the scope of this work.

Phase Contrast MR Reconstruction

The radiofrequency signals emitted by resonating nuclei in an MR experiment are received with one, or more commonly, multiple, antennas (radiofrequency receiver coils) placed near the target anatomy. The optimal method of combining the signals from multiple coils to generate an image is by weighting the contributions by the sensitivities of coils. To reconstruct phase contrast images a good approximation of this weighting strategy is given by

$$\Delta\varphi = \text{angle}(\Sigma I_1 \times I_2^*) \tag{9.5}$$

where I_1 and I_2 are the complex representation of the two differentially flow-encoded images ($I_1 = I_1^{\text{real}} + iI_1^{\text{imag}}$) and I_2^* is the conjugate of complex image I_2 ($I_2^{\text{real}} - iI_2^{\text{imag}}$). The phase image is then converted to velocity according to

$$v = \frac{v_{\text{enc}}\Delta\varphi}{\pi} \tag{9.6}$$

As shown in Figure 9.3, the raw phase images for each flow-encoding step have contributions from nonvelocity sources that are assumed to be identical in the two steps, so that they can be completely subtracted when equation (9.5) is applied. In practice, there some phase difference will always result from magnetic field gradient imperfections and physical limitations of the magnetic field gradients, but fortunately these residual phases are of very low spatial frequency in nature, and are constant over time.

Figure 9.6 shows a simple and robust user-independent method for removing this contaminant background phase. The ability to measure this residual background phase is made possible by the fact that most phase contrast experiments are time-resolved, with multiple images acquired over a cardiac cycle. A mask

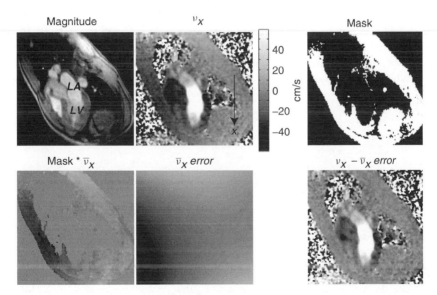

Figure 9.6. Phase contrast background phase corrections. The phase contrast image v_x shows the velocities in the heart (LV—left ventricle, LA—left atrium) in the up/down direction. Nonzero velocities in the chest wall to the left of the heart from unwanted background nonvelocity phases are clearly visible. A mask is generated from the phase contrast images by selecting only those pixels whose phase does not vary significantly over the cardiac cycle. The phase in the masked image is fit with a low-spatial-frequency function, and subsequently subtracted from the entire time series of phase contrast images, to generate a background-free velocity image.

can then be generated from the phase contrast images by selecting only those pixels whose standard deviation over the cardiac cycle are below a threshold. This mask will thus select pixels that have sufficient signal-to-noise ratio and are not within the blood pool or tissue that has significant phase variations (i.e., significant velocity variations) over the cardiac cycle. In other words, the mask selects static tissue that can be used to estimate the background phases. The phase in the masked image is fit with a low-spatial-frequency function, and subsequently subtracted from the entire time series of phase contrast images. This process is shown in Figure 9.6.

Complex-difference reconstruction is an alternative to the phase difference reconstruction [6–8]. In this technique, the reconstruction is performed by subtracting the complex data. This technique was originally proposed for MR angiography to image the vessels [8]. The flow information can be extracted from the complex-difference images using postprocessing [8–10]. This subtraction can be performed in the image or k-space domain. A significant advantage of complex-difference reconstruction over the phase difference reconstruction is the superiority of the complex difference if a voxel contains both stationary and flowing spins [11]. Figure 9.7 shows a simple diagram illustrating how the presence of static spins in a voxel results in inaccuracy in phase difference reconstruction. However, in the complex difference reconstruction, the signals associated with the stationary spins will not change between the two bipolar imaging steps; therefore, this signal will be subtracted out in the complex-difference subtraction [9,10]. This property can be exploited further to reduce the image acquisition time, to acquire flow images in real time [9,10]. A drawback of the complex-difference approach is that the resulting images

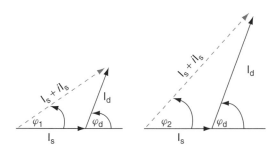

Figure 9.7. Vector diagram illustrating the partial voluming effect in a phase contrast MR study. If a voxel contains both stationary spins ($\mathbf{I}_s$) and dynamic spins ($\mathbf{I}_d$), the complex sum of the two vectors, stationary spins with $0°$ and dynamic spins with ϕ_d, will result in a complex vector ($\mathbf{I}_s + i\mathbf{I}_d$) that estimates the velocity in a voxel, which contains partial voluming errors due to the presence of the stationary spins. The true phase due to the moving spins should be calculated as f_d in the diagram. This calculated phase velocity will be affected as the proportion of the static and dynamic spins in the voxel changes as shown by the length of the arrows in the two diagrams. As the length of $\mathbf{I}_d$ increases, the phase velocity measurement changes from φ_1 to φ_2 both different from true velocity phase of f_d.

are now dependent on several factors in addition to the actual spin velocity, so quantitative velocity imaging is challenging.

Cardiac Phase Contrast Imaging

Cardiac motion and function and blood flow are best evaluated by acquisition of a time series of images that span the cardiac cycle [12 14]. One imaging approach is to acquire consecutive images through the cardiac cycle, which is referred to as *real-time imaging* [15,16]. All the k-space lines for each frame are sampled sequentially in 70–150 ms before moving to the next phase or the next image in the time series. While the image acquisition and reconstruction are straightforward, MRI is intrinsically a low-bandwidth modality and the acquired images usually suffer from low spatial and temporal resolution. As an alternative, the required k-space data for acquisition of a complete image are often segmented into different portions or *segments*, each taking 20–40 ms to acquire. Each segment can be repeated several times in each cardiac cycle to allow many images to be reconstructed for a cine or movie acquisition. A different portion (segment) of each image is acquired in sequential heartbeats. Figure 9.8 shows the schematic of the segmented k space cine acquisition for a single slice acquiring multiple cardiac phases. Breath holding is generally necessary to reduce motion artifacts due to respiration-induced cardiac motion. As shown in Figure 9.8, each cardiac cycle, identified by the R–R interval, is divided into n different cardiac phases, and a portion (segment) of k-space data for each of cardiac phase is acquired. The k-space matrix is filled by acquiring all the required k-space data through m heartbeats. The total number of heartbeats is determined by the total required lines of k space and how many lines are acquired in each segment of k space (i.e., in each heartbeat).

In cardiac imaging, an electrocardiogram or ECG signal, which is a representative of the electrical activity of the heart muscle, is used to synchronize a pulse sequence to the cardiac cycle. There are two schemes for using the ECG for image acquisition and reconstruction: prospective triggering and retrospective gating. For *retrospective* acquisitions the ECG signal is recorded and used only at the time of image reconstruction to align the data into cardiac phases. *Prospective* experiments are actually triggered to the measured ECG signal in real time, telling the scanner to start acquiring the next segment of k space. With this approach there is typically a trigger window in which no data will be acquired at the end of each cardiac cycle, while the scanner is searching for the ECG signal. The trigger window is commonly set to 5–20% of the duration of the cardiac cycle.

Phase contrast images can also be acquired with both cine and real-time approaches [3,4,17–21]. We will discuss the real-time approach in more detail in the following sections. In the segmented cine acquisition, two flow-encoded images can be acquired in an interleaved order in the same cardiac cycle, which will maintain the breath-hold duration, although with a lower temporal resolution. The flow-encoded images can be acquired in consecutive heartbeats to increase

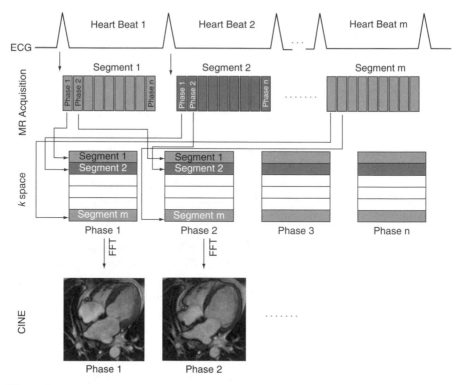

Figure 9.8. Cardiac cine imaging. The cardiac cycle and k-space data matrix is divided into n segments and m phases, respectively. After each ECG trigger, a segment of the k space is acquired repeatedly throughout the cardiac cycle and the acquired data are assigned to difference phases, which corresponds to different cardiac phases through the cardiac cycle. The total m-segment data are acquired during m consecutive heartbeats.

the temporal resolution, although at the price of longer scan durations. Images acquired using the latter method could also suffer from misregistration due to variability in the heart rate and inconsistencies due to respiratory motion. In general, respiratory motion is a source of artifact in all forms of cardiac imaging, which can cause significant aliasing and blurring. Three methods have been used to reduce the effect of respiratory motion in cardiac imaging (including phase contrast imaging): breath-hold, respiratory navigators, and averaging. The simplest method to suppress the artifacts associated with respiratory motion is a breath-hold image acquisition, in which the patient stops breathing at end expiration. The images are limited in both spatial and temporal resolution due to limited breath-hold duration, especially in patients. A second method is to measure and compensate for respiratory motion using respiratory bellows physically placed around the abdomen or MR navigators [22–24]. In navigator gating, the respiratory motion is monitored using a cylindrical pencil beam usually placed in the at the lung–liver intersection. The k-space data are used for a final image reconstruction only if the respiratory motion falls in a predefined window set in an initial training phase. This method can be used for acquiring images with high spatial and temporal resolution [25]; however, the total image acquisition will be longer compared to the breath-hold acquisition. While non-breath-hold acquisition using respiratory gating or navigator compensation yields accurate flow measurement, it is not commonly used in clinical practice owing to lengthy acquisition times. The third approach for suppressing motion artifacts in phase contrast imaging is to average over multiple acquisitions. This technique is commonly used in clinical practice to measure volumetric blood flow in great vessels (where respiratory blurring is less serious) because of its ease of use and robustness.

Rapid Phase Contrast MR

Phase contrast imaging is intrinsically less efficient than conventional magnitude cine MRI because of the requirement for multiple flow-encoding steps, and the overhead associated with the bipolar flow-encoding gradients. Several efficient acquisition methods have been used to improve temporal and spatial resolution in phase contrast imaging. Echo–planar imaging, in which multiple lines of k-space are sampled within a single excitation, has been used to improve the temporal resolution of flow imaging. This concept was one of the earliest in magnetic resonance imaging, proposed and developed by Sir Peter Mansfield [26]. Figure 9.9 shows how the data acquisition efficiency can be improved

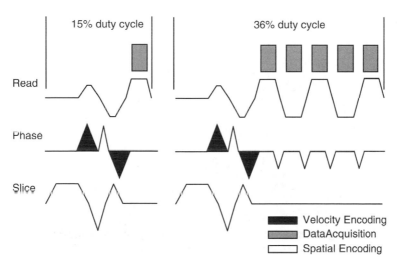

Figure 9.9. The collection of a single line of k space in a phase contrast experiment with a conventional acquisition scheme is compared to an echo–planar acquisition. The conventional experiment has a low acquisition duty cycle, owing in large part to the time required for velocity encoding, which is improved by acquiring multiple lines of k space per excitation.

using an echo–planar readout acquisition. The concept of maximizing acquired data per excitation has been further expanded using alternate k-space trajectories, most commonly the spiral readout [3,4]. A sample spiral trajectory is shown in Figure 9.5c. Images can be acquired a single spiral interleave (real-time imaging) or multiple interleaves, which are then defined as segmented imaging as described above for conventional cine imaging. Nayak et al. developed a real-time color flow phase contrast MR system that can be used in an interactive framework to image and display blood flow using rapid spiral readout [4,21]. Ungated spiral phase contrast has also the potential for rapid measurement of time-averaged blood flowrates in the presence of pulsatility [27–29]. Another k-space trajectory that has been exploited for fast imaging is the radial pattern, shown in Figure 9.5b, which has been combined with a bipolar flow encoding to image the blood flow with high efficiency [30]. Figure 9.10 shows a real-time flow image measuring the blood flow through the aortic valve, using a spiral k-space trajectory for data acquisition.

Since the mid-1990s, a new approach for fast MR imaging commonly termed *parallel imaging* has seen massive growth and now mainstream clinical use. Parallel imaging exploits the unique spatial sensitivity maps of arrays of radiofrequency coils (antennas used to receive the MRI signal) to allow a significant reduction in the coverage of k space necessary to reconstruct an image, at the cost of signal-to-noise ratio [31,32]. The accuracy and reproducibility of blood flow velocity measurements using parallel image reconstruction with Cartesian sampling at different acceleration factors shows an accurate estimate of flow measurement [33]. Temporal resolution of the flow images can be accelerated

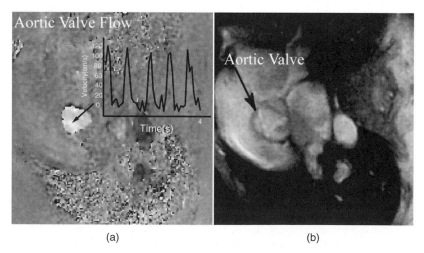

(a)   (b)

Figure 9.10. Real-time through-plane blood flow in the aortic valve acquired with a temporal resolution of 91.2 ms and an in-plane resolution of 1:8 × 1:8 mm². The trace on the phase contrast image shows the calculated through-plane velocity through an ROI placed in the middle of the valve.

by a factor of ≥ 3 while preserving spatial resolution and acceptable image quality.

Complex-difference processing can be used to further reduce the required k-space data in phase contrast MR by removing the signal from stationary tissue. This approach reduced the field of view that must be imaged by retaining signal only from flowing blood. A real-time volumetric flow measurement using complex-difference processing can provide an integral of volumetric blood flow in a single projection [9]. Figure 9.11 shows a sample real-time flow image acquired from the popliteal artery, which passes through the knee to feed the lower leg. A partial field of view (pFOV) spiral motion-encoded technique for rapid flow imaging is another approach to increase the efficiency of acquisition [10]. This approach again takes advantage of the reduced imaging field of view

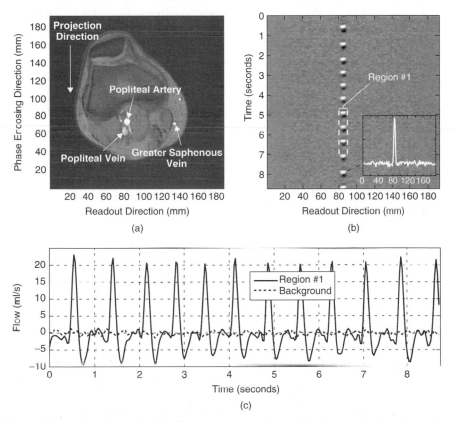

(a)

(b)

(c)

Figure 9.11. The image in (a) shows a cross section of the knee, showing the major arteries and veins. The image is (b) is a series of real-time flow projections through this knee. Complex-difference subtraction is used to remove the signal from the stationary tissue, which allows the entire image to be collapsed into a single line without interference from the nonflowing spins. The time curve in (c) shows the real-time measurement of flow in the popliteal artery using the single-projection complex-difference approach.

required when the stationary tissue in the chest and back and other tissues are removed with a complex-difference subtraction.

Flow Visualization

While the visualization of anatomy and even cardiovascular function via cine imaging is straightforward in most cases, the visualization of blood flow can be significantly more challenging because of vector nature of blood velocity and potentially complex spatiotemporal patterns. Vector field maps and particle paths are thus useful tools for representing the flow of blood. Figure 9.12 shows a still-frame image of a heart (standard three-chamber view) with three velocity images that correspond to the three component directions for a single timeframe during the filling of the left ventricle (diastole). The vector image on the right displays the magnitude and direction of the blood velocity within the left ventricle calculated using the in-plane velocity components v_x and v_y. Figure 9.13 shows a time series of vector field maps around the anterior mitral valve leaflet, again during the filling phase of the left ventricle. The vector field shows the complex patterns of blood flow associated with the leaflets in a normal filling heart, and how they rapidly evolve during the cardiac cycle. Figure 9.14 shows another example of blood flow patterns around a valve leaflet, for visualization of the flow vortex that forms in a sinus of Valsalva, which is the anatomic

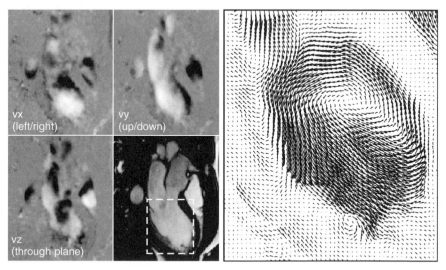

Figure 9.12. Phase contrast velocity images for the three component directions are shown from a three-chamber image view of the heart at a single cardiac phase, late in the filling phase (diastole). The corresponding magnitude image shows the anatomy; most important here is the left ventricle, which is seen in the center of the dashed box. The vector image on the right shows the velocity (magnitude and direction) using a vector display. This vector field clearly shows the large flow vortex that fills the ventricle, a pattern that is not obvious by examining the raw velocity images.

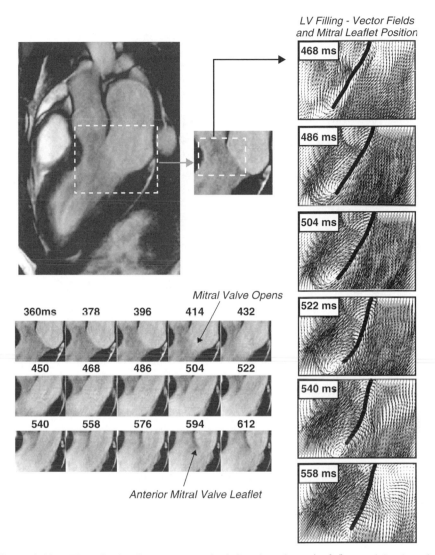

Figure 9.13. The mitral valves separate the left atrium from the left ventricle. A series of MR images show the anterior mitral valve leaflet position as a function of time in the cardiac cycle, since the QRS complex. The series of vector plots on the right shows the complex flow patterns are associated with the leaflet and its motion. The leaflet position is highlighted in these frames.

dilation of the ascending aorta just above the aortic valve. The flow behind the leaflets is thought to play a role in normal valve operation. Another visualization tool that has been used in conjunction with MR velocity data is the particle path display [34]. Figure 9.15 shows the complex three-dimensional paths taken by blood flow in the intracranial arteries [35]. Four consecutive systolic timeframes illustrate the filling of the right carotid siphon. Note the

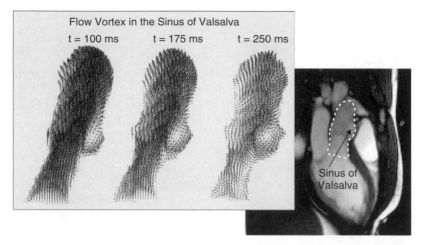

Figure 9.14. Similar to the approach seen in Figure 9.12, a vector display approach is used to clearly visualize a complex flow pattern, in this case the flow vortex that forms in the sinus of Valsalva, just beyond the aortic valve leaflet, in the ascending aorta.

complex and counterclockwise helical flow pattern (if viewed along the flow direction) in the C5 segment (*open arrow*). The emitter plane from which particle traces were released from equidistant grid points is indicated by the solid white arrow. In the superior sagittal sinus (*asterisk*), particle traces demonstrate lower flow velocities and thus reduced tracer length compared with arterial blood flow.

9.3. CLINICAL APPLICATIONS OF PHASE CONTRAST IMAGING

Volumetric Flow Measurements and Applications

The instantaneous volume flowrate through a pixel in a given direction is equal to the product of the velocity in that direction and the pixel area perpendicular to the velocity. The flow through a region of interest, most commonly through a blood vessel or across a valve, is thus the sum of the flowrates of the pixels of interest. Using velocity images alone to identify lumen pixels can be confounded by low flowrates near the boundaries, which reduces the contrast at the lumen edges, so pixels are often identified using the magnitude and velocity images. The cumulative or total flow per cardiac cycle, which is a common clinical parameter of interest, is measured by integrating the flowrate over the cardiac cycle.

Figure 9.16 shows the measurement of flowrate and cumulative flow in the aortic valve through the cardiac cycle. The cumulative flow is measured by integrating the flowrate through the cardiac cycle. A common application for volumetric flow imaging for the diagnosis of valvular disease, in which flow can

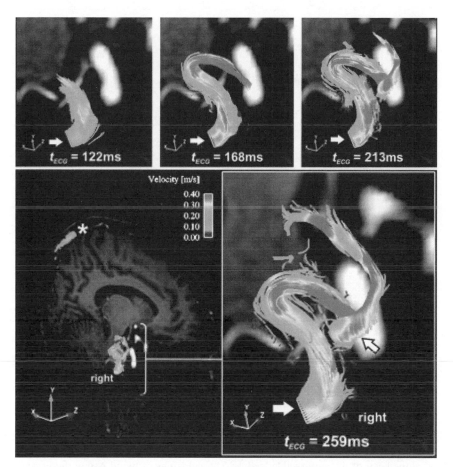

Figure 9.15. Time-resolved 3D particle traces in four consecutive systolic timeframes illustrate the filling of the right carotid siphon. Note the complex and counterclockwise helical flow pattern (if viewed along the flow direction) in the C5 segment (open arrow). The emitter plane from which particle traces were released from equidistant grid points is indicated by the solid white arrow. In the superior sagittal sinus (asterisk), particle traces demonstrate lower flow velocities and thus reduced tracer length compared with arterial blood flow. [Reproduced from Wetzel S et al: In vivo assessment and visualization of intracranial arterial hemodynamics with flow-sensitized 4D MR imaging at 3T, *Am J Neuroradiol* 28:433–438 (March 2007) [35], with permission from the publisher.]

be impeded during the valve's open phase, or blood flow can leak in the valve's closed phase.

Figure 9.17 shows an example image series of the aortic valve in which the valve does not close completely as shown in frames (c) and (d). Flow measurement through this valve shows negative flow during the normally closed phase, which is an indication of backward flow or aortic regurgitation. The severity of

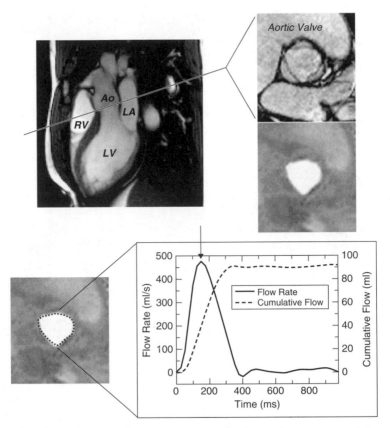

Figure 9.16. The volumetric flowrate of blood ejected from the contracting left ventricle is measured by orienting a phase contrast imaging plane perpendicular to the direction of flow, at the level of the aortic valve leaflets. The velocities of blood within the lumen are summed to calculate the instantaneous flowrate or the total cumulative flow, by integrating the flowrate over time.

valvular regurgitation for the aortic and pulmonic valves can be calculated by quantifying the backward flow during diastole compared with the forward flow ejected from the ventricle during systole.

Quantitative measures of blood flow abnormalities are based on standard measures such as the stroke volume of the heart, which is calculated as the flow across the aortic valve during systole, as shown in Figure 9.16. The stroke volume multiplied by the heart rate yields the cardiac output, another standard clinical measure, typically ~5 L/min. Mitral and tricuspid regurgitation, which is backward flow through these values during systole, which reduces the total effective stroke volume, can be measured using multiple methods. Direct measurement of the regurgitant volume can be difficult because of turbulence in the high-velocity jets. Comparison of the forward stroke volume measured in the aorta (Figure 9.16) and the true volume change measured from anatomic images of the ventricle can

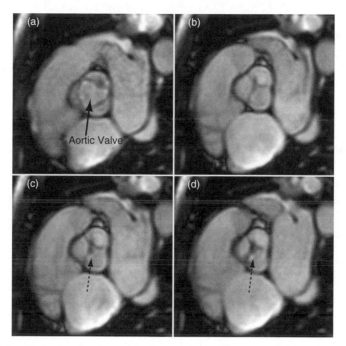

Figure 9.17. Four phases of a cardiac cine acquisition of the aortic valve showing all three leaflets and insufficiency of the valve closure. The retrograde flow can be quantified using a phase contrast image prescribed perpendicular to the aortic 2 3 mm superior to the valve.

yield an indirect measure of the regurgitant volumes. Intercardiac shunts occur when there is abnormal passage of blood from one side of cardiac circulation to the other, such as through atrial septal defects, ventricular septal defects, or anomalous pulmonary veins. If the flow of blood exiting the right ventricle to the main pulmonary artery (pulmonary circulation) is not equal to the flow of blood exiting the left ventricle to the aorta (systemic circulation), the presence of a shunt is implied. The ratio of pulmonary to systemic flow $(Q_p/Q_s) > 1.2$ suggests the presence of abnormal left-to-right shunting. These imaging parameters are commonly extracted from clinical phase contrast MR studies in evaluation of the cardiac function. For the quantification of flow, MRI offers the ability to measure through-plane velocities for planes in arbitrary orientations, so it is not limited by the complex anatomy often associated with cardiovascular disease.

Coronary Flow and Flow Reserve

Coronary artery disease is one of the leading causes of death in cardiovascular disease. Coronary magnetic resonance imaging has shown promise for the assessment of significant coronary artery disease in proximal and mid segments of the coronary arteries [36]. Currently coronary MR imaging cannot reliably predict the physiological significance of stenosis of intermediate severity, and X-ray angiography has a similar limitation [37,38]. Measurement of *coronary flow reserve*, which is defined as the ratio of the maximal hyperemic coronary flow to the baseline coronary flow, can be used for physiological assessment of functional severity of intermediate stenosis [39,40]. In humans, it has been shown that basal myocardial blood flow remains constant regardless of the severity of coronary artery stenosis [41]. However, during hyperemia, flow progressively decreases when the degree of stenosis is about $\geq 40\%$ and does not differ significantly from basal flow when stenosis is $\geq 80\%$ [41]. Therefore, the measurement of flow reserve with phase contrast MR in complement with MR angiography could lead to a diagnostically complete exam assessing both vessel stenosis and its physiological significance [42–44]. Phase contrast MR measurement of flow reserve has been validated in canine and humans against both Doppler flow wire [45,46] and positron emission tomography [47]. Coronary phase contrast MR measurement can be performed either in a free-breathing acquisition using a respiratory navigator [48] or a breath-hold acquisition [49]. However, breath-held acquisition results in lower spatiotemporal resolution compared to a free-breathing acquisition, which affects the accuracy of the measurement [48]. For example, a temporal resolution of less than 25 ms is required to resolve the peak velocity in the right coronary artery and less than 120 ms in the left [50]. Imaging with insufficient temporal resolution results in significant underestimation of the peak velocity and motion, leading to artifactual reduction of the coronary flow reserve. Low spatial resolution will also affect the accuracy of flow quantification by increasing partial-volume error, which reduces the flow values measured due to averaging of neighboring tissue signals [51,52]. The in vitro results suggested that at least 16 voxels must cover the cross section of the vessel lumen to obtain a measurement accuracy to within 10% [52]. The signal-to-noise and velocity-to-noise ratios in a phase contrast study increase by a factor of 2.5 at 3 T compared to 1.5 T [53]. This improvement could be used to measure the blood flow velocity through small vessels such as coronary arteries, allowing for acquisitions with both increased spatial and temporal resolutions. Figure 9.18 shows blood flow through the right coronary artery (RCA) imaged at 3 T (a) magnitude image acquired during the phase contrast scan (b) flow map through the RCA shown at peak systole during the cardiac cycle. An increased number of pixels in the RCA can be visualized, which has the potential to improve the accuracy of flow measurements.

MR Pressure Gradients

Blood flow is driven by gradients in pressure, so the evaluation of these gradients can provide fundamental physiologic information. For example, the drop in

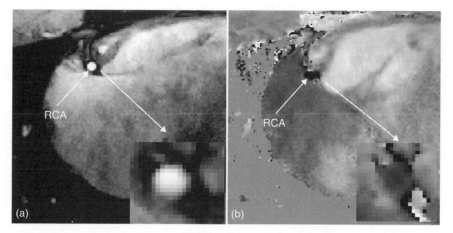

Figure 9.18.   Blood flow through right coronary artery (RCA) imaged at 3 T: (a) magnitude image acquired during the phase contrast scan; (b) flow map through the RCA shown at peak systole during cardiac cycle.

pressure across a stenotic valve or coronary artery provides a direct measure of the severity of the restriction. More subtle changes in intracardiac pressure differences reflect ventricular relaxation and compliance, and atrial filling pressures. Phase contrast MR offers the ability to accurately resolve the pressure gradients in vivo in three dimensions with unrestricted image orientation [54–57]. The Navier–Stokes (NS) equations relate the blood velocity fields to the driving pressure gradients. A simplified form of these equations that has been used in conjunction with MRI-measured velocity fields is shown here:

$$-\frac{\partial P}{\partial x_i} = \rho \frac{\partial v_i}{\partial t} + \rho \left[v_1 \frac{\partial v_i}{\partial x_1} + v_2 \frac{\partial v_i}{\partial x_2} + v_3 \frac{\partial v_i}{\partial x_3} \right] - \mu \left[\frac{\partial^2 v_i}{\partial x_1^2} + \frac{\partial^2 v_i}{\partial x_2^2} + \frac{\partial^2 v_i}{\partial x_3^2} \right]$$
$$-F_i, i = x, y, z \tag{9.7}$$

The x_i are the x, y, and z axes in the image frame and the v_i are the corresponding velocities, μ is the coefficient of viscosity ($\mu_{\text{blood}} = 4$ cP), and ρ is the fluid density ($\rho_{\text{blood}} = 1060$ kg/m^3). From left to right in equation (9.7), the NS equations relate the pressure gradients to the local and convective accelerations as well as the viscosity or frictional effects and finally, the global body force terms, the F_i (gravity). It is commonplace to omit the viscous terms for regions outside of the thin boundary layer that exists at the blood–tissue interface [58]. Figure 9.19 shows sample pressure gradient time series between various locations within the left atrium and left ventricle, measured during filling of the left ventricle. Equation (9.7) was evaluated using blood velocity values measured with phase contrast MRI. Figure 9.20 shows the visualization of pressure gradient waves in a dog aorta. Pressure gradients were calculated over a 1 cm distance at several locations along the ascending and descending aorta, as a function of

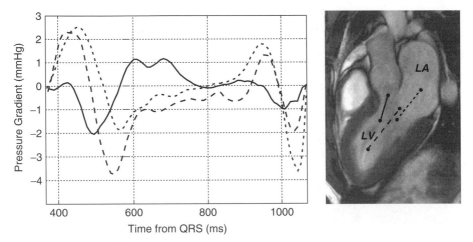

Figure 9.19. Pressure gradients within the left atrium (LA) and left ventricle (LV) between fixed points in space are plotted over the filling interval of the cardiac cycle (diastole). Note the significant variation in patterns as a function of space. The early peaks at 400 ms are associated with the early-filling or E wave and the second set of peaks at ~950 ms are associated with the late-filling or A wave.

time in the cardiac cycle. Forward and backward waves are sufficiently separated to visualize the wave propagation. The wave speed in the aorta can be directly measured as ~4 m/s. The ability of MRI to quantify blood velocities in all three component directions, which cannot be achieved with other imaging modalities, makes this approach particularly appealing for the study of cardiovascular hemodynamics, given the often complex anatomy and flow patterns.

9.4. OTHER APPLICATIONS

In addition to cardiovascular applications, phase contrast imaging has been used to image the blood flow in the peripheral arteries and veins and neurovascular systems [59–70]. The flow of cerebrospinal fluid (CSF) throughout the ventricles and subarachnoid space can be measured using phase contrast MR that can provide sufficient accuracy to enable distinction between normal and hyperdynamic CSF flow [70]. Time-resolved 3D particle tracing is an emerging technique for visualization of the blood flow in the neurovascular and great vessels [71–77]. Figure 9.15 showed four consecutive systolic timeframes that illustrate the filling of the right carotid siphon. Phase contrast and MR angiography have also been used extensively in the field of computational fluid dynamics, as a means to provide both boundary conditions within which numerical calculations will be carried out, and to provide flow boundary conditions and a method to validate calculated flow fields [78–81]. As MRI scanners become more commonplace in the clinical setting and technology continues to improve, the applications of blood velocity imaging with MRI will undoubtedly continue to increase as well.

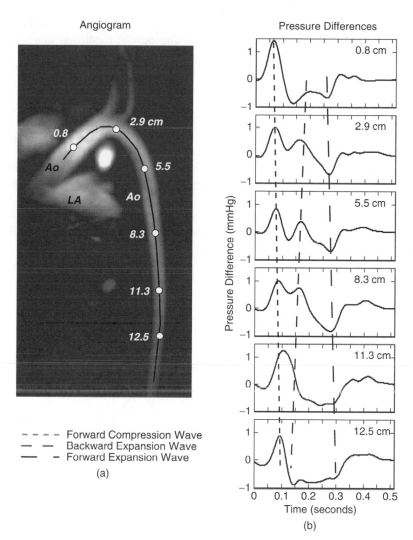

Figure 9.20. Phase contrast MRI was used to measure the blood velocity field in the ascending and descending aorta of a dog. The local pressure gradients (over a 1 cm length) at a series of points along the aorta are plotted as a function of time in the cardiac cycle. The forward and reverse (reflected) pressure waves associated with the contraction and relaxation of the heart are clearly visible, as shown by the dashed lines.

9.5. SUMMARY

Phase contrast MR imaging has the capability to image the blood velocities in vivo. The appeal of MRI for imaging blood velocities is the intrinsically three-dimensional nature of the modality and the sensitivity to all three component velocities, which, when combined with time-resolved imaging, represented the complete blood velocity field. We have outlined a sampling of the applications in which phase contrast MR can be used in the human cardiovascular system. Volumetric flow measurements such as cardiac output and valvular regurtation are commonly used in clinical practice, but other applications will undoubtedly translate in the near future. A rich variety of approaches, ranging from real-time phase contrast to much more extensive 3D time-resolved phase contrast studies are continually undergoing technical development as approaches for accelerated acquisition and imaging hardware continue to improve. Equally important, imaging scientists and clinicians together are also developing visualization and quantitative tools to take advantage of the sometimes overwhelming amount of information in the complex multidimensional velocity fields. Phase contrast and a variation called *displacement-encoded MRI* have also been used extensively to image the motion of the myocardium and the mechanics of other muscles throughout the body, but a full consideration of these works is the beyond the scope of the overview provided here.

REFERENCES

1. Moran PR: A flow velocity zeugmatographic interlace for NMR imaging in humans, *Magn Reson Imag* **1**(4):197–203 (1982).

2. Bernstein MA, Shimakawa A, Pelc NJ: Minimizing TE in moment-nulled or flow-encoded two- and three-dimensional gradient-echo imaging, *J Magn Reson Imag* **2**(5):583–588 (1992).

3. Gatehouse PD, Firmin DN, Collins S, Longmore DB: Real time blood flow imaging by spiral scan phase velocity mapping, *Magn Reson Med* **31**(5):504–512 (1994).

4. Nayak KS, Pauly JM, Kerr AB, Hu BS, Nishimura DG: Real-time color flow MRI, *Magn Reson Med* **43**(2):251–258 (2000).

5. Noll DC, Meyer C, Pauly JM, Nishimura DG, Macovski A: A homogeneity correction method for magnetic resonance imaging with time-varying gradients, *IEEE Trans Med Imag* **10**(4):629–637 (1991).

6. Polzin JA, Alley MT, Korosec FR, Grist TM, Wang Y, Mistretta CA: A complex-difference phase-contrast technique for measurement of volume flow rates, *J Magn Reson Imag* **5**(2):129–137 (1995).

7. Hamilton CA: Effects of intravoxel velocity distributions on the complex difference method of phase-contrast MR angiography, *J Magn Reson Imag* **6**(2):409–410 (1996).

8. Bernstein MA, Ikezaki Y: Comparison of phase-difference and complex-difference processing in phase-contrast MR angiography, *J Magn Reson Imag* **1**(6):725–729 (1991).

9. Thompson RB, McVeigh ER: Real-time volumetric flow measurements with complex-difference MRI, *Magn Reson Med* **50**(6):1248–1255 (2003).

10. Nezafat R, Thompson RB, Derbyshire JA, McVeigh ER: Partial field-of-view spiral phase-contrast imaging using complex difference processing, *Magn Reson Med* **56**(3):676–680 (2006).

11. Hamilton CA: Effects of intravoxel velocity distributions on the complex difference method of phase-contrast MR angiography, *J Magn Reson Imag* **6**(2):409–410 (1996).

12. Semelka RC, Tomei E, Wagner S, Mayo J, Kondo C, Suzuki J, Caputo GR, Higgins CB: Normal left ventricular dimensions and function: Interstudy reproducibility of measurements with cine MR imaging, *Radiology* **174**(3 Pt 1):763–768 (1990).

13. Carr JC, Simonetti O, Bundy J, Li D, Pereles S, Finn JP: Cine MR angiography of the heart with segmented true fast imaging with steady-state precession, *Radiology* **219**(3):828–834 (2001).

14. McVeigh ER: MRI of myocardial function: Motion tracking techniques, *Magn Reson Imag* **14**(2):137–150 (1996).

15. Farzaneh F, Riederer SJ, Lee JN, Tasciyan T, Wright RC, Spritzer CE: MR fluoroscopy: Initial clinical studies, *Radiology* **171**(2):545–549 (1989).

16. Riederer SJ, Tasciyan T, Farzaneh F, Lee JN, Wright RC, Herfkens RJ: MR fluoroscopy: Technical feasibility, *Magn Reson Med* **8**(1):1–15 (1988).

17. Pelc NJ, Herfkens RJ, Shimakawa A, Enzmann DR: Phase contrast cine magnetic resonance imaging, *Magn Reson Q* **7**(4):229–254 (1991).

18. Nayler GL, Firmin DN, Longmore DB: Blood flow imaging by cine magnetic resonance, *J Comput Assist Tomogr* **10**(5):715–722 (1986).

19. Lingamneni A, Hardy PA, Powell KA, Pelc NJ, White RD: Validation of cine phase-contrast MR imaging for motion analysis, *J Magn Reson Imag* **5**(3):331–338 (1995).

20. Keegan J, Gatehouse PD, Mohiaddin RH, Yang GZ, Firmin DN: Comparison of spiral and FLASH phase velocity mapping, with and without breath-holding, for the assessment of left and right coronary artery blood flow velocity, *J Magn Reson Imag* **19**(1):40–49 (2004).

21. Nayak KS, Hu BS, Nishimura DG: Rapid quantitation of high-speed flow jets, *Magn Reson Med* **50**(2):366–372 (2003).

22. McConnell MV, Khasgiwala VC, Savord BJ, Chen MH, Chuang ML, Edelman RR, Manning WJ: Comparison of respiratory suppression methods and navigator locations for MR coronary angiography, *Am J Roentgenol* **168**(5):1369–1375 (1997).

23. Wang Y, Rossman PJ, Grimm RC, Riederer SJ, Ehman RL: Navigator-echo-based real time respiratory gating and triggering for reduction of respiration effects in three-dimensional coronary MR angiography, *Radiology* **198**(1):55–60 (1996).

24. Wang Y, Grimm RC, Rossman PJ, Debbins JP, Riederer SJ, Ehman RL: 3D coronary MR angiography in multiple breath-holds using a respiratory feedback monitor, *Magn Reson Med* **34**(1):11–16 (1995).

25. Stuber M, Botnar RM, Danias PG, Sodickson DK, Kissinger KV, Van CM, De BJ, Manning WJ: Double-oblique free-breathing high resolution three-dimensional coronary magnetic resonance angiography, *J Am Coll Cardiol* **34**(2):524–531 (1999).

26. Ordidge RJ, Mansfield P, Doyle M, Coupland RE: Real time movie images by NMR, *Br J Radiol* **55**(658):729–733 (1982).

27. Park JB, Olcott EW, Nishimura DG: Rapid measurement of time-averaged blood flow using ungated spiral phase-contrast, *Magn Reson Med* **49**(2):322–328 (2003).

28. Park JB, Hu BS, Conolly SM, Nayak KS, Nishimura DG: Rapid cardiac-output measurement with ungated spiral phase contrast, *Magn Reson Med* **56**(2):432–438 (2006).

29. Park JB, Santos JM, Hargreaves BA, Nayak KS, Sommer G, Hu BS, Nishimura DG: Rapid measurement of renal artery blood flow with ungated spiral phase-contrast MRI, *J Magn Reson Imag* **21**(5):590–595 (2005).

30. Barger AV, Peters DC, Block WF, Vigen KK, Korosec FR, Grist TM, Mistretta CA: Phase-contrast with interleaved undersampled projections, *Magn Reson Med* **43**(4):503–509 (2000).

31. Sodickson DK, Manning WJ: Simultaneous acquisition of spatial harmonics (SMASH): Fast imaging with radiofrequency coil arrays, *Magn Reson Med* **38**(4):591–603 (1997).

32. Pruessmann KP, Weiger M, Scheidegger MB, Boesiger P: SENSE: Sensitivity encoding for fast MRI, *Magn Reson Med* **42**(5):952–962 (1999).

33. Thunberg P, Karlsson M, Wigstrom L: Accuracy and reproducibility in phase contrast imaging using SENSE, *Magn Reson Med* **50**(5):1061–1068 (2003).

34. Wigstrom L, Ebbers T, Fyrenius A, Karlsson M, Engvall J, Wranne B, Bolger AF: Particle trace visualization of intracardiac flow using time-resolved 3D phase contrast MRI, *Magn Reson Med* **41**(4):793–799 (1999).

35. Wetzel S, Meckel S, Frydrychowicz A, Bonati L, Radue EW, Scheffler K, Hennig J, Markl M: In vivo assessment and visualization of intracranial arterial hemodynamics with flow-sensitized 4D MR imaging at 3T, *Am J Neuroradiol* **28**(3):433–438 (2007).

36. Kim WY, Danias PG, Stuber M, Flamm SD, Plein S, Nagel E, Langerak SE, Weber OM, Pedersen EM, Schmidt M, Botnar RM, Manning WJ: Coronary magnetic resonance angiography for the detection of coronary stenoses, *N Engl J Med* **345**(26):1863–1869 (2001).

37. Joye JD, Schulman DS, Lasorda D, Farah T, Donohue BC, Reichek N: Intracoronary Doppler guide wire versus stress single-photon emission computed tomographic thallium-201 imaging in assessment of intermediate coronary stenoses, *J Am Coll Cardiol* **24**(4):940–947 (1994).

38. Vogel RA: Assessing stenosis significance by coronary arteriography: Are the best variables good enough ? *J Am Coll Cardiol* **12**(3):692–693 (1988).

39. Gould KL, Lipscomb K: Effects of coronary stenoses on coronary flow reserve and resistance, *Am J Cardiol* **34**(1):48–55 (1974).

40. Miller DD, Donohue TJ, Younis LT, Bach RG, Aguirre FV, Wittry MD, Goodgold HM, Chaitman BR, Kern MJ: Correlation of pharmacological 99mTc-sestamibi myocardial perfusion imaging with poststenotic coronary flow reserve in patients with angiographically intermediate coronary artery stenoses, *Circulation* **89**(5):2150–2160 (1994).

41. Uren NG, Melin JA, De Bruyne B, Wijns W, Baudhuin T, Camici PG: Relation between myocardial blood flow and the severity of coronary-artery stenosis, *N Engl J Med* **330**(25):1782–1788 (1994).

42. Edelman RR, Manning WJ, Gervino E, Li W: Flow velocity quantification in human coronary arteries with fast, breath-hold MR angiography, *J Magn Reson Imag* **3**(5):699–703 (1993).

43. Hundley WG, Lange RA, Clarke GD, Meshack BM, Payne J, Landau C, McColl R, Sayad DE, Willett DL, Willard JE, Hillis LD, Peshock RM: Assessment of coronary arterial flow and flow reserve in humans with magnetic resonance imaging, *Circulation* **93**(8):1502–1508 (1996).

44. Clarke GD, Eckels R, Chaney C, Smith D, Dittrich J, Hundley WG, NessAiver M, Li HF, Parkey RW, Peshock RM: Measurement of absolute epicardial coronary artery flow and flow reserve with breath-hold cine phase-contrast magnetic resonance imaging, *Circulation* **91**(10):2627–2634 (1995).

45. Bedaux WL, Hofman MB, de Cock CC, Stoel MG, Visser CA, van Rossum AC: Magnetic resonance imaging versus Doppler guide wire in the assessment of coronary flow reserve in patients with coronary artery disease, *Coron Artery Dis* **13**(7):365–372 (2002).

46. Shibata M, Sakuma H, Isaka N, Takeda K, Higgins CB, Nakano T: Assessment of coronary flow reserve with fast cine phase contrast magnetic resonance imaging: Comparison with measurement by Doppler guide wire, *J Magn Reson Imag* **10**(4):563–568 (1999).

47. Sakuma H, Koskenvuo JW, Niemi P, Kawada N, Toikka JO, Knuuti J, Laine H, Saraste M, Kormano M, Hartiala JJ: Assessment of coronary flow reserve using fast velocity-encoded cine MR imaging: Validation study using positron emission tomography, *Am J Roentgenol* **175**(4):1029–1033 (2000).

48. Nagel E, Bornstedt A, Hug J, Schnackenburg B, Wellnhofer E, Fleck E: Noninvasive determination of coronary blood flow velocity with magnetic resonance imaging: Comparison of breath-hold and navigator techniques with intravascular ultrasound, *Magn Reson Med* **41**(3):544–549 (1999).

49. Davis CP, Liu PF, Hauser M, Gohde SC, von Schulthess GK, Debatin JF: Coronary flow and coronary flow reserve measurements in humans with breath-held magnetic resonance phase contrast velocity mapping, *Magn Reson Med* **37**(4):537–544 (1997).

50. Hofman MB, Wickline SA, Lorenz CH: Quantification of in-plane motion of the coronary arteries during the cardiac cycle: Implications for acquisition window duration for MR flow quantification, *J Magn Reson Imag* **8**(3):568–576 (1998).

51. Wolf RL, Ehman RL, Riederer SJ, Rossman PJ: Analysis of systematic and random error in MR volumetric flow measurements, *Magn Reson Med* **30**(1):82–91 (1993).

52. Tang C, Blatter DD, Parker DL: Accuracy of phase-contrast flow measurements in the presence of partial-volume effects, *J Magn Reson Imag* **3**(2):377–385 (1993).

53. Lotz J, Doker R, Noeske R, Schuttert M, Felix R, Galanski M, Gutberlet M, Meyer GP: In vitro validation of phase-contrast flow measurements at 3T in comparison to 1.5T: Precision, accuracy, and signal-to-noise ratios, *J Magn Reson Imag* **21**(5):604–610 (2005).

54. Ebbers T, Wigstrom L, Bolger AF, Engvall J, Karlsson M: Estimation of relative cardiovascular pressures using time-resolved three-dimensional phase contrast MRI, *Magn Reson Med* **45**(5):872–879 (2001).

55. Tyszka JM, Laidlaw DH, Asa JW, Silverman JM: Three-dimensional, time-resolved (4D) relative pressure mapping using magnetic resonance imaging, *J Magn Reson Imag* **12**(2):321–329 (2000).

56. Tasu JP, Mousseaux E, Delouche A, Oddou C, Jolivet O, Bittoun J: Estimation of pressure gradients in pulsatile flow from magnetic resonance acceleration measurements, *Magn Reson Med* **44**(1):66–72 (2000).

57. Thompson RB, McVeigh ER: Fast measurement of intracardiac pressure differences with 2D breath-hold phase-contrast MRI, *Magn Reson Med* **49**(6):1056–1066 (2003).

58. Wood NB: Aspects of fluid dynamics applied to the larger arteries, *J Theor Biol* **199**(2):137–161 (1999).

59. Rutgers DR, Blankensteijn JD, van der Grond J: Preoperative MRA flow quantification in CEA patients: Flow differences between patients who develop cerebral ischemia and patients who do not develop cerebral ischemia during cross-clamping of the carotid artery, *Stroke* **31**(12):3021–3028 (2000).

60. van Everdingen KJ, Klijn CJ, Kappelle LJ, Mali WP, van der Grond J: MRA flow quantification in patients with a symptomatic internal carotid artery occlusion. The Dutch EC-IC Bypass Study Group, *Stroke* **28**(8):1595–1600 (1997).

61. Yamashita S, Isoda H, Hirano M, Takeda H, Inagawa S, Takehara Y, Alley MT, Markl M, Pelc NJ, Sakahara H: Visualization of hemodynamics in intracranial arteries using time-resolved three-dimensional phase-contrast MRI, *J Magn Reson Imag* **25**(3):473–478 (2007).

62. Turk AS, Johnson KM, Lum D, Niemann D, agaard-Kienitz B, Consigny D, Grinde J, Turski P, Haughton V, Mistretta C: Physiologic and anatomic assessment of a canine carotid artery stenosis model utilizing phase contrast with vastly undersampled isotropic projection imaging, *Am J Neuroradiol* **28**(1):111–115 (2007).

63. Bagan P, Vidal R, Martinod E, Destable MD, Tremblay B, Dumas JL, Azorin JF: Cerebral ischemia during carotid artery cross-clamping: Predictive value of phase-contrast magnetic resonance imaging, *Ann Vasc Surg* **20**(6):747–752 (2006).

64. Oktar SO, Yucel C, Karaosmanoglu D, Akkan K, Ozdemir H, Tokgoz N, Tali T: Blood-flow volume quantification in internal carotid and vertebral arteries: Comparison of 3 different ultrasound techniques with phase-contrast MR imaging, *Am J Neuroradiol* **27**(2):363–369 (2006).

65. Bagan P, Azorin J, Salama J, Dumas JL: The value of phase-contrast magnetic resonance angiography of the circle of Willis in predicting cerebral ischemia-hypoxia (shunt need) during carotid endarterectomy, *Surg Radiol Anat* **27**(6):544–547 (2005).

66. Cosottini M, Pingitore A, Michelassi MC, Puglioli M, Lazzarotti G, Caniglia M, Parenti G, Bartolozzi C: Redistribution of cerebropetal blood flow in patients with carotid artery stenosis measured non-invasively with fast cine phase contrast MR angiography, *Eur Radiol* **15**(1):34–40 (2005).

67. de Boorder MJ, Hendrikse J, van der Grond J: Phase-contrast magnetic resonance imaging measurements of cerebral autoregulation with a breath-hold challenge: A feasibility study, *Stroke* **35**(6):1350–1354 (2004).

68. Kim DS, Choi JU, Huh R, Yun PH, Kim DI: Quantitative assessment of cerebrospinal fluid hydrodynamics using a phase-contrast cine MR image in hydrocephalus, *Childs Nerv Syst* **15**(9):461–467 (1999).

69. Henry-Feugeas MC, Idy-Peretti I, Blanchet B, Hassine D, Zannoli G, Schouman-Claeys E: Temporal and spatial assessment of normal cerebrospinal fluid dynamics with MR imaging, *Magn Reson Imag* **11**(8):1107–1118 (1993).

70. Nitz WR, Bradley WG, Jr., Watanabe AS, Lee RR, Burgoyne B, O'Sullivan RM, Herbst MD: Flow dynamics of cerebrospinal fluid: Assessment with phase-contrast velocity MR imaging performed with retrospective cardiac gating, *Radiology* **183**(2):395–405 (1992).

71. Frydrychowicz A, Markl M, Harloff A, Stalder AF, Bock J, Bley TA, Berger A, Russe MF, Schlensak C, Hennig J, Langer M: Flow-sensitive in-vivo 4D MR imaging at 3T for the analysis of aortic hemodynamics and derived vessel wall parameters, *Rofo* **179**(5):463–472 (2007).

72. Frydrychowicz A, Winterer JT, Zaitsev M, Jung B, Hennig J, Langer M, Markl M: Visualization of iliac and proximal femoral artery hemodynamics using time-resolved 3D phase contrast MRI at 3T, *J Magn Reson Imag* **25**(5):1085–1092 (2007).

73. Frydrychowicz A, Bley TA, Dittrich S, Hennig J, Langer M, Markl M: Visualization of vascular hemodynamics in a case of a large patent ductus arteriosus using flow sensitive 3D CMR at 3T, *J Cardiovasc Magn Reson* **9**(3):585–587 (2007).

74. Wetzel S, Meckel S, Frydrychowicz A, Bonati L, Radue EW, Scheffler K, Hennig J, Markl M: In vivo assessment and visualization of intracranial arterial hemodynamics with flow-sensitized 4D MR imaging at 3T, *Am J Neuroradiol* **28**(3):433–438 (2007).

75. Markl M, Harloff A, Bley TA, Zaitsev M, Jung B, Weigang E, Langer M, Hennig J, Frydrychowicz A: Time-resolved 3D MR velocity mapping at 3T: Improved navigator-gated assessment of vascular anatomy and blood flow, *J Magn Reson Imag* **25**(4):824–831 (2007).

76. Frydrychowicz A, Harloff A, Jung B, Zaitsev M, Weigang E, Bley TA, Langer M, Hennig J, Markl M: Time-resolved, 3-dimensional magnetic resonance flow analysis at 3T: Visualization of normal and pathological aortic vascular hemodynamics, *J Comput Assist Tomogr* **31**(1):9–15 (2007).

77. Markl M, Draney MT, Hope MD, Levin JM, Chan FP, Alley MT, Pelc NJ, Herfkens RJ: Time-resolved 3-dimensional velocity mapping in the thoracic aorta: Visualization of 3-directional blood flow patterns in healthy volunteers and patients, *J Comput Assist Tomogr* **28**(4):459–468 (2004).

78. Botnar R, Rappitsch G, Scheidegger MB, Liepsch D, Perktold K, Boesiger P: Hemodynamics in the carotid artery bifurcation: A comparison between numerical simulations and in vitro MRI measurements, *J Biomech* **33**(2):137–144 (2000).

79. Steinman DA: Image-based computational fluid dynamics modeling in realistic arterial geometries, *Ann Biomed Eng* **30**(4):483–497 (2002).

80. Wood NB, Weston SJ, Kilner PJ, Gosman AD, Firmin DN: Combined MR imaging and CFD simulation of flow in the human descending aorta, *J Magn Reson Imag* **13**(5):699–713 (2001).

81. Saber NR, Wood NB, Gosman AD, Merrifield RD, Yang GZ, Charrier CL, Gatehouse PD, Firmin DN: Progress towards patient-specific computational flow modeling of the left heart via combination of magnetic resonance imaging with computational fluid dynamics, *Ann Biomed Eng* **31**(1):42–52 (2003).

CHAPTER 10

Measuring Cerebral Perfusion Using Magnetic Resonance Imaging

FERNANDO CALAMANTE

Brain Research Institute, Austin Health, Victoria, Australia

Abstract. Since the first studies in the late 1980s, dynamic susceptibility contrast MRI (DSC-MRI, also known as *bolus tracking*) has become a very powerful technique for the assessment of perfusion and perfusion-related parameters. The lack of ionizing radiation, combined with the good spatial resolution and extra information available within an MR examination, has made DSC-MRI one of the techniques of choice for the in vivo investigation of cerebral perfusion in clinical studies. A significant expansion in the availability of MRI scanners has taken place since the mid-1990s, and DSC-MRI has become an important diagnostic technique. The technical advances achieved since then have transformed DSC-MRI into essential tools in many clinical and basic research investigations. This chapter describes the underlying principles and models to quantify perfusion using DSC-MRI. The main assumptions and steps required for perfusion quantification are described, and the main limitations and artifacts that can affect its accuracy are discussed. Many of the initial technical limitations have now been circumvented, and the remaining issues are currently a very active area of research in the field. In the interim, these issues should be considered whenever DSC-MRI is used to measure perfusion, and the users of these techniques should be aware of the potential problems to avoid misinterpretation of the findings, and make the most of the invaluable information provided by perfusion MRI.

10.1. INTRODUCTION

The term *perfusion* is often used very loosely, and its meaning is interpreted in different ways depending on the particular technique and application concerned. [*Note*: Throughout this chapter the terms *perfusion* and *cerebral blood flow* (CBF) will be used interchangeably.] In the context of modern magnetic resonance imaging (MRI) studies, *cerebral perfusion* is often defined as the volume of

Vascular Hemodynamics: Bioengineering and Clinical Perspectives, Edited by Peter J. Yim
Copyright © 2008 John Wiley & Sons, Inc.

blood [i.e., milliliter (mL) of blood] delivered to the capillary beds of a block of tissue (i.e., per 100 g of tissue) in a given time period (i.e., per minute), and its units are therefore mL $(100 \text{ g})^{-1}$ $\min^{-1}$ or mL g^{-1} s^{-1} (*Note:* The typical cerebral perfusion value in normal gray-matter tissue is 60 mL $(100 \text{ g})^{-1}$ $\min^{-1}$ or 0.01 mL g^{-1} s^{-1} [1]). It can also be interpreted as the rate of blood delivery to brain tissue. However, it is important to distinguish between perfusion and bulk flow; perfusion is concerned with flow at the capillary level, where exchange of nutrients between blood and tissue occurs, whereas bulk flow (as measured, for example, by MR angiography) corresponds to flow through major vessels such as arteries and veins, where no exchange takes place. The survival of the brain is dependent on a continuous and adequate supply of blood, and failure of the cerebral circulation can result in cell death or malfunction. Similarly, some clinical conditions are associated with a hyperperfusion status (such as epilepsy and tumors) because of their increased energy demand. For these reasons, the ability to measure perfusion accurately, noninvasively, and with good spatial resolution would offer the chance to identify and characterize abnormal tissue in many clinical conditions. A further advantage of MRI methods to measure perfusion is that they can be easily combined in the same examination with other MR techniques, which can provide complementary anatomical (using T_1- and T_2-weighted imaging), bioenergetics (using diffusion MRI), vascular anatomy (using MR angiography), and biochemical information (using MR spectroscopy), thus providing a more complete understanding of the developing pathophysiologic mechanism.

Since the mid–late 1980s, two distinct perfusion MRI techniques have been the subject of significant improvements, which have transformed them into essential tools in many clinical and basic research investigations. The two methods differ with regard to their respective use of an exogenous (in the *dynamic susceptibility contrast MRI* (DSC-MRI) and endogenous (in a technique known as *arterial spin labeling* (ASL)) MRI-visible tracer (see the literature [1–4] for review work on these methodologies). Despite the need for an exogenous MR agent, DSC-MRI is currently the most common MR perfusion methodology in clinical studies. A significant expansion in the availability of MRI scanners has taken place since the mid-1990s and DSC-MRI has become an important diagnostic technique. This chapter describes the underlying principles and models applied or used to quantify perfusion using DSC-MRI, as well as the state of the art and limitations of this methodology.

10.2. DYNAMIC SUSCEPTIBILITY CONTRAST MRI

Dynamic susceptibility contrast magnetic resonance imaging (DSC-MRI; also known as *bolus-tracking MRI*) relies on the injection of a bolus of a paramagnetic contrast agent (usually gadolinium-DTPA), which produces a transient decrease in signal intensity on a series of gradient-echo (i.e., T_2^*-weighted) or spin echo (i.e., T_2-weighted) images acquired during its passage through the brain

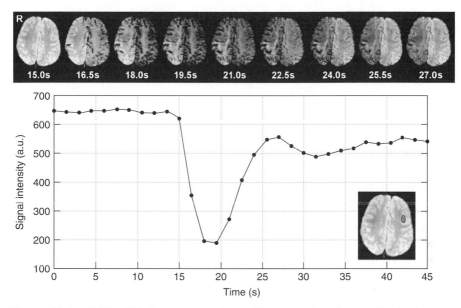

Figure 10.1. DSC-MRI data on a patient with a vascular abnormality in the right anterior, posterior, and middle cerebral arteries. The patient had no infarctions at the time of MR examination. The nine images in the top row are nine time samples of the gradient–echo echo–planar images acquired during passage of the bolus of contrast agent (TR = 1.5 s). These images show the transient decrease in signal intensity induced by the passage of the bolus. Note the asymmetric behavior due to abnormalities on the right major cerebral arteries. The bottom graph shows the signal intensity time course for a region of interest in the contralateral cortical gray matter (see inset). Three different periods can be observed: the baseline (before arrival of the bolus to the region, approximately 0–14 s), the first passage (approximately 14–26 s), and the recirculation (times approximately greater than 26 s).

[5] (see Figure 10.1). The loss in signal intensity is due to the decrease in T_2^* associated with the susceptibility-induced gradients surrounding the paramagnetic contrast agent [6]. (*Note*: For the remainder of this chapter, all the statements referring to T_2^* are also applicable to T_2, unless otherwise stated.) This effect is more significant in areas where the contrast agent is compartmentalized (since this increases the induced gradients) and makes quantification of cerebral perfusion in areas with blood–brain barrier (BBB) leakage more complex. (*Note*: The BBB is a physical barrier that limits the transport of substances from the blood into the central nervous system; in particular, an intact BBB will make the MR contrast agent used in DSC-MRI an effective intravascular contrast agent.)

Since the passage of the bolus through brain tissue is of the order of only a few seconds [1], a very fast MR imaging method is required to fully characterize the induced MR signal changes. The most common imaging technique currently used is echo–planar imaging (EPI) [7], which allows for a good compromise between time resolution (typical imaging repetition time 1–2 s), image coverage (typically 10–15 slices), and spatial resolution (typical imaging voxel size $2 \times 2 \times 5$ mm^3). However, other image acquisitions can be used if full brain coverage is necessary (e.g., 3D-PRESTO [8]), or if reduced (susceptibility-related) image distortions are required for a particular application (e.g., by using the HASTE method [9]) or parallel imaging acquisition [10]).

10.3. QUANTIFICATION AND MEASUREMENT METHODS

Perfusion Quantification: Indicator Dilution Theory

The changes in relaxation rate (ΔR_2^*, where $R_2^* = 1/T_2^*$) are related to the time-dependent concentration of the contrast agent; the greater the concentration, the greater the observed MRI effect. Early work has suggested that, for typical doses used in clinical studies, this relationship can be assumed to be linear [5,6,11]:

$$C(t) = k \cdot \Delta R_2^*(t) \tag{10.1}$$

where $C(t)$ is the time-dependent concentration of the contrast agent and k is a proportionality constant that depends on the tissue type, the contrast agent, the field strength, and the particular MRI pulse sequence used for image acquisition.

For a gradient–echo sequence, the signal intensity during a DSC-MRI study depends on the R_2^* and the longitudinal relaxation rate ($R_1 = 1/T_1$):

$$S(t) = S_0 \cdot \left(1 - e^{-\text{TR} \cdot R_1(t)}\right) \cdot e^{-\text{TE} \cdot R_2^*(t)} \tag{10.2}$$

where S_0 is the signal intensity in the absence of relaxation, TR is the repetition time, and TE is the echo time of the MR sequence. Therefore, by assuming that the contribution from longitudinal relaxation effects during the bolus passage is negligible, one can calculate $C(t)$ from the changes in signal intensity with respect to its baseline value (i.e., preinjection):

$$C(t) = -\frac{k}{TE} \cdot \ln\left(\frac{S(t)}{S(0)}\right) \tag{10.3}$$

where $S(t)$ is the signal intensity at time t and $S(0)$ is its baseline value (see Figure 10.2).

Although early studies assessed perfusion by calculating summary parameters of the concentration–time course profile (e.g., the time to peak, or time to reach maximum concentration) [1], the concentration in the tissue is not only proportional to CBF but is also affected by how the study is done [for example, a slower injection will lead to a wider $C(t)$, even for a stable CBF] [12,13].

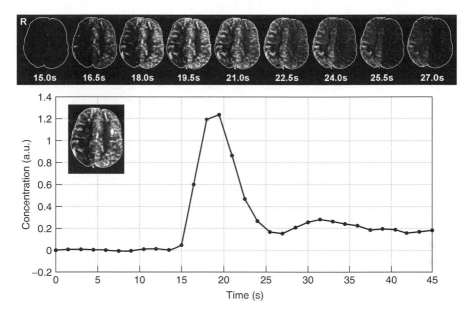

Figure 10.2. Concentration time course on a patient with vascular abnormality in the right major cerebral arteries (same patient as in Figure 10.1). The nine images in the top row are nine time samples of the concentration of the contrast agent during passage of the bolus (TR = 1.5 s); the images show a transient increase in contrast concentration with the bolus. Note the asymmetric behavior due to abnormalities on the right major cerebral arteries. The bottom graph shows the concentration time course for a region of interest in the contralateral cortical gray matter (see inset). As expected, the concentration is zero before arrival of the bolus (during the baseline period).

Using indicator dilution theory, the concentration time course can be shown to be expressed by a convolution equation [14–16]:

$$C(t) = \alpha \cdot \text{CBF}\big(\text{AIF}(t) \otimes R(t)\big) = \alpha \cdot \text{CBF} \int_0^t \text{AIF}(\tau) R(t - \tau) d\tau \qquad (10.4)$$

where AIF is the *arterial input function* (i.e., the function describing the contrast agent input to the tissue of interest) and $R(t\text{-}\tau)$ is the tissue *residue function*, which describes the fraction of contrast agent remaining in the tissue at time t, following the injection of an ideal instantaneous bolus at time τ. [*Note*: By definition, $R(0) = 1$, i.e., no contrasts agent has left the tissue at time $t = \tau$ after an ideal instantaneous bolus injected at time τ, and $R(\infty) = 0$, i.e., after a very long time, no tracer remains in the tissue if the BBB is intact and the contrast is washed out by perfusion.] The proportionality constant α depends on the density of brain tissue, and the difference in hematocrit levels between capillaries and large vessels (to compensate for the fact that only the plasma volume is accessible to the contrast agent) [1]. The convolution accounts for the fact that for a nonideal bolus, part of the spread in the concentration time curve is due to the finite length of the injected bolus. The integral expression in equation (10.4) can be interpreted by considering the AIF as a superposition of consecutive ideal boluses "AIF$(\tau)d\tau$" injected at time τ. For each ideal bolus, according to the definition of the residue function, the concentration still present in the tissue at time t will be proportional to "CBF·AIF$(\tau)R(t\text{-}\tau)d\tau$," and the total concentration $C_t(t)$ will be given by the sum (or integral) of all these contributions. The factor CBF reflects the fact that the concentration in the tissue is proportional to the amount of blood [with concentration AIF(τ)] being delivered to the tissue per unit time (i.e., CBF).

Perfusion Quantification: The Deconvolution Step

Quantification of CBF therefore involves inversion of Equation (10.4), a mathematical process known as *deconvolution* [16]. This requires measurement of the AIF, and calculating the scaled residue function CBF·$R(t)$ (known as the *impulse response function*). Once this function is obtained, perfusion can be calculated from its initial value, since $R(t=0)=1$ by definition (see Figure 10.3) [17]. Although in theory the initial value of the impulse response determines perfusion, the presence of bolus dispersion distorts the shape of the calculated impulse response function such that $R(0)=0$ (see "Measurement of the AIF: Bolus Delay and Dispersion" section below). In practice, it is therefore common to estimate perfusion from the maximum value of the function [16].

The inverse problem involved in Equation (10.4) (i.e., performing the deconvolution) is known mathematically as an "ill-posed problem." This means that even a small amount of noise in the measured concentration curves [i.e., $C(t)$ and the AIF] has a huge effect on the calculated impulse response (and thus on the CBF estimate). To address this issue, special approach is required to make the inversion problem more robust to the presence of noise, an approach known as *regularization* (e.g., see Hansen [18]); it can be seen as a "filter" applied *during* the inversion problem, which aims at reducing the effect of noise while recovering the true impulse response function (see Figure 10.4). The development, implementation, assessment, and comparison of regularization methods have been a very active area of research in the field of perfusion MRI. Many methods have been developed, depending on the characteristics of the "filter"; for any of these methods, a key (and usually very complex) aspect is to determine the right amount of filtering once the filter type is chosen (see Figure 10.4). Some of the algorithm proposed to date include the Fourier transform approach [16,19], truncated singular value decomposition [16,20] and its variants [21,22], Tikhonov regularization [23], maximum-likelihood maximization [24,25], expansion in orthogonal polynomials [26], and Gaussian processes deconvolution [27]. Ideally, an algorithm should produce accurate measurements under a wide a range of practical situations, such as with various tissue characteristics (e.g., perfusion values, residue function models), and imaging

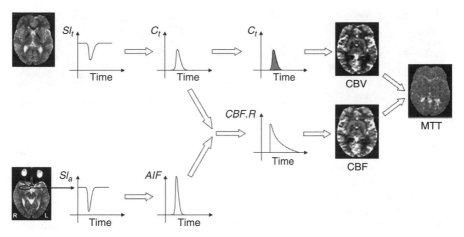

Figure 10.3. Schematic representation of the steps involved in the quantification of DSC-MRI data. From each pixel in the image (spin echo echo–planar image in this example), the signal intensity time course is obtained (SI_t). Using equation (10.3), the SI_t is converted to the tissue concentration time course (C_t). From the area under the peak [see equation (10.5)], a map of CBV can be calculated. From pixels on a major artery (right middle cerebral artery in this example), the arterial signal intensity time course is measured (SI_a). The AIF is obtained by converting SI_a to concentration of contrast agent [see (10.3)]. The AIF information is the used to deconvolve C_t [see (10.4)] to obtain the product of CBF times the residue function R. From the initial value of this resulting curve, a map of CBF can be generated. By using the central volume theorem, the MTT can be calculated as the ratio of CBV to CBF. (Image previously published in Ref. 17, © 2005, Springer-Verlag.)

characteristics (e.g., signal-to-noise levels), sequence parameters (e.g., TR, TE), as well as for other experimental conditions (such as the presence of bolus delay to areas with abnormal vascular supply). Furthermore, the algorithm should be fast and require minimum user interaction so that it can be easily implemented in a clinical environment. Unfortunately, there is currently no single algorithm that fulfills all these requirements; this is the likely reason for the lack of consensus between users of DSC-MRI. It is for this reason that this remains an area of very active research.

DSC-MRI Quantification: Further Information Available

Apart from estimates of cerebral perfusion, DSC-MRI can provide information about other physiological and hemodynamic parameters. It is this wealth of information available, as well as its fast acquisition time (<1 min) and relatively high contrast-to-noise ratio, that have made DSC-MRI the perfusion MRI technique of choice for the rapid assessment of patients in clinical investigations. In particular, owing to the compartmentalization of the contrast agent within the intravascular

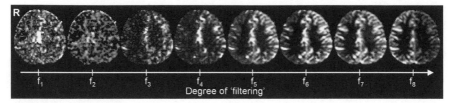

Figure 10.4. Illustration of the regularization step required in CBF quantification by deconvolution analysis. The eight images show the corresponding CBF maps calculated with increasing degree of regularization (i.e., "filtering"), with increasing filtering from left to right. The example shows the results for a patient with right internal carotid artery stenosis and regularization using the truncated singular value decomposition method (increasing regularization corresponding to increasing amount of truncation). As can be seen in the figure, with little regularization (f_1 and f_2 filter levels in the figure), the solution is completely dominated by noise. On the other hand, with overregularization (f_8 filter level) the estimated impulse response function is excessively smoothed, leading (in this case) to the erroneous identification of the abnormal tissue: note that the normal left hemisphere is incorrectly displayed as hypoperfused on the CBF map calculated for this filter level. The optimum degree of regularization in this particular case corresponds to the f_6 filter level.

space (for an intact BBB), the *cerebral blood volume* (CBV) is proportional to the normalized total amount of tracer [1] (see Figure 10.3):

$$\text{CBV} = \alpha^{-1} \frac{\int C(t)dt}{\int \text{AIF}(t)dt} \tag{10.5}$$

where the proportionality factor α^{-1} is the inverse of the factor in Equation (10.4). (NB. The CBV measures the fraction of the tissue volume occupied by the blood, and it is commonly measured in mL/100 g of tissue; the typical value in normal gray-matter tissue is 4 mL/100 g or, given that the density of tissue is approximately 1 g/mL, 4% [1].) The area under the concentration time curve $C(t)$ in equation (10.5) represents the entire amount of contrast agent passing through the voxel, and is therefore an indication of the capability of the region to pass blood through it. The normalization to the integral of AIF accounts for the fact that the more tracer that is injected, the greater concentration will reach the tissue, regardless of the CBV.

A third physiological parameter accessible by DSC-MRI is the *mean transit time* (MTT: the average time for a molecule of contrast agent to pass through the tissue vasculature following an ideal instantaneous bolus injection). The typical value in normal gray-matter tissue is 4 s [1]. These three physiological parameters are not independent, but they are related via the *central volume theorem* [28]: MTT=CBV/CBF (see Figure 10.3). The MTT has been found to be a very useful hemodynamic parameter in the investigation of acute stroke; its value is significantly increased in affected tissue, which, combined with the relatively low

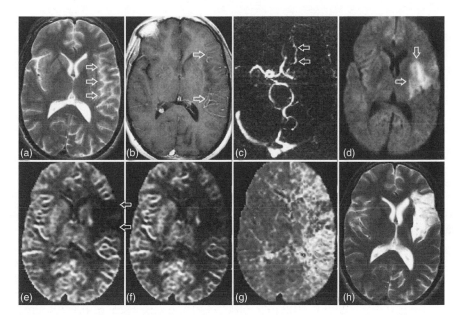

Figure 10.5. DSC-MRI from a patient with acute stroke, scanned 4 h after onset of symptoms (right-sided hemiplegia and mutism). The T_2-weighted image (a) shows sulcal enhancement (arrows). The contrast material-enhanced T_1-weighted image (b) demonstrates contrast in multiple dilated vessels (arrows) in the affected hemisphere, consistent with slow flow. The phase contrast MR angiogram (c) demonstrates absence of flow in the left internal carotid and middle cerebral arteries. Note the prominent ophthalmic artery (arrows), which directional MR angiography (not shown) depicted as having retrograde flow. The diffusion-weighted image (d) demonstrates hyperintensity (arrows) in the left hemisphere consistent with patient's symptoms. Hemodynamic images including CBV (e), CBF (f), and MTT (g) depict a larger area of abnormality, consistent with occlusion of the middle cerebral artery branch but collateral flow. As can be in these maps, the area of hemodynamic abnormality is more easily demarcated as prolonged MTT in (g). The follow-up T_2-weighted image obtained at 7 months (h) depicts the infarction as smaller than the DSC-MRI abnormality but larger than the diffusion abnormality in (d). (Image kindly provided by Dr. A. G. Sorensen, and previously published in Ref. 29, © 1999, RSNA.)

contrast between normal gray- and white-matter MTT values, makes identification of abnormal MTT areas straightforward [29] (see Figure 10.5).

Other summary parameters reflecting different hemodynamic aspects can be calculated *directly* from the profile of the $C(t)$ curve [1], including bolus arrival time (BAT), time to peak (TTP), maximum peak concentration (MPC) [i.e., maximum value of $C(t)$], and full-width at half-maximum (FWHM). These parameters were used in early studies as indirect perfusion measures, but it should be noted that most of these parameters can be influenced not only by CBF but also by CBV, MTT, and the injection conditions (volume injected, injection rate, cannula size, etc.), as well as the vascular structure, and the cardiac output of the patient. Therefore, the interpretation of abnormalities observed in these parameters in terms of perfusion is not straightforward [12,13]. Nevertheless, they are simpler to calculate (they do not require deconvolution or knowledge of the AIF) and can provide useful information. In particular, some of them can provide very important clinical complementary information; for example, the BAT map can be used to identify areas for which the bolus of contrast agent is delayed, which can provide information regarding the presence of collateral blood supply in patients with stroke or vascular abnormalities.

Perfusion Quantification: CBF in Absolute Units

Various methods have been proposed to calculate CBF in absolute units (i.e., in mL $(100 \text{ g})^{-1} \text{ min}^{-1}$). These can be divided in three main approaches:

1. *Measurements Based on an Internal Standard*. Early CBF measurements using position emission tomography (PET) suggested a relatively age-independent and uniform value in white-matter tissue in normal adult subjects (CBF = 22 mL $(100 \text{ g})^{-1} \text{ min}^{-1}$ [30]); on the basis of these findings, a region in normal white matter was proposed as an internal standard to convert the measurement in MR units to absolute units [31].
2. *Measurements Based on Knowledge of the Proportionality Constants*. If the values of the constants appearing in the equations above (e.g., k) were known, the deconvolution method would lead to absolute measurements [19,26,32–34].
3. *Measurements Based on a Scaling Factor Obtained from a Cross-Calibration Study*. The MR CBF values can be converted to absolute units by using an empirical conversion factor calculated (usually from a separate study) by cross-calibration of DSC-MRI to a "gold standard" technique (e.g., PET) [35,36].

Each of these methods has been used to calculate perfusion in absolute units, and the values obtained in normal subjects were consistent with expected CBF values. However, there are still some concerns for all these approaches regarding their accuracy under various physiological conditions [37–40], and the agreement might have been fortuitous. In principle, all the approaches can potentially lead to errors, particularly in the presence of pathology. For example, one study has shown a wide variability in white-matter CBF values measured with PET on the contralateral hemisphere in patients with chronic carotid occlusion [41], which would suggest that method 1 can lead to erroneous measures. Similarly, some studies have shown that the constant k in equations (10.1) and (10.3) may vary between tissue types and subjects, as well as between tissue and arteries [i.e., it would be different for $C(t)$ and AIF(t)] [42,43]. Furthermore, changes in hematocrit levels during pathology have been reported [44,45], which would influence the assumed value of the constant α in equation (10.4) [38]. Therefore, the absolute CBF value measured using method 2 could contain errors. In a similar way, the validity of a single conversion factor under various physiological conditions remains to be shown [40,41,46]. Therefore, absolute CBF measurements in the presence of pathology should be interpreted with caution. Work is currently under way to address many of these issues, and accurate absolute measurements of CBF may be possible in the near future.

Perfusion Quantification: Measurement of the AIF

On the basis of the methodology described above, an essential step for CBF quantification is measurement of the AIF. Although this may initially appear simple, it is in practice one of the major potential sources of error in perfusion quantification (e.g., see Ref. 47). In general terms (see Figure 10.6) [48], the AIF should be measured

1. In a voxel with *pure intravascular signal*, so that it gives a true reflection of the arterial signal.
2. *As close as possible to the tissue of interest*, so that it provides an accurate characterization of the input to that tissue.

In practice, the main problem is that these two conditions are incompatible; while the former requires measuring the AIF from the signal changes in voxels in large arteries (such as the internal carotid artery; see location 3 in Figure 10.6) to avoid partial volume effects [49], the latter requires measuring it from the very small arterial branch that supplies the particular tissue of interest (see location 1 in Figure 10.6) [50]. Therefore, if one favors option 1, the AIF measurement will be subject to the potential presence of bolus delay and dispersion between the artery and the tissue of interest, which can introduce errors in CBF quantification (see "Measurement of the AIF: Bolus Delay and Dispersion" section below). On the other hand, if option 2 is favored, significant partial-volume effects are likely to distort the shape of the true AIF, potentially also introducing CBF errors (see "Measurement of the AIF: Partial Volume Effect" section below). Given these limitations, the most commonly used approach to measuring the AIF is a compromise between these two conditions [31]; the AIF is generally measured from the signal changes in a major branch of the middle cerebral artery (usually the M_1 segment) (see location 2 in Figures 10.6 and 10.7). Therefore, it is important to recognize that errors related to partial-volume effects and bolus delay and dispersion can still be present when interpreting the calculated DSC-MRI maps.

Measurement of the AIF: Bolus Delay and Dispersion

As mentioned above, the AIF is commonly measured in a major artery (e.g., the internal carotid artery or the middle cerebral artery), which can lead to bolus delay and dispersion during the transit of the bolus from that artery to the input to the tissue of interest (see Figure 10.6). This can be particularly important in

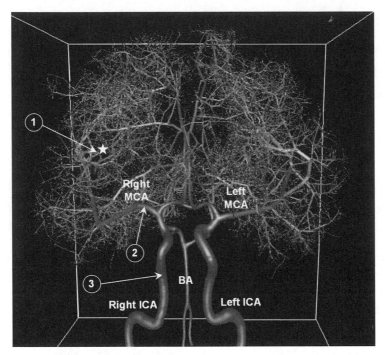

Figure 10.6. Schematic representation of location for AIF measurement. The figure shows the major cerebral arteries (MCA—middle cerebral artery; ICA—internal carotid artery; BA—basilar artery) and a model of the arterial tree. To calculate CBF using DSC-MRI in a voxel at the position indicated by the star, the AIF should (ideally) be measured from the small arteriole supplying the tissue in that voxel (labeled location 1 in the figure). However, to avoid partial volume effects, the AIF must be measured in a much larger artery, such as the ICA (location 3). In practice, a medium size artery (such as the MCA; see location 2) is commonly chosen as a compromise between partial volume effect and bolus delay/dispersion. (Modified from an image kindly provided by Dr. J. R. Cebral, and previously published in Ref. 48, © 2003, Kluwer Academic Publishers.)

patients with abnormal flow patterns, such as those with stenosis, occlusion, or collateral blood supply [38,51,52]. The presence of bolus delay and dispersion has been shown to introduce errors in CBF quantification (i.e., underestimation), which can be as much as 60–70% in patients with vascular abnormalities [53,54]; this CBF underestimation is accompanied by an overestimation in MTT, which can be up to 250% [53]. These errors can have very serious consequences for the management of acute stroke patients. In particular, the current state of the art in this context is the use of the so-called predictor models, in which all the available MRI information (e.g., structural imaging, diffusion MRI, and perfusion MRI) is combined to infer the most likely outcome for brain tissue in a given patient [55–57]. According to this prediction, these methods are aimed at aiding clinical management, in particular to identify acute stroke patients most likely to

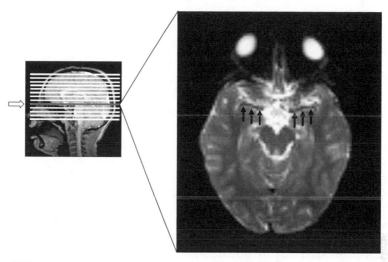

Figure 10.7. Commonly used site for AIF measurement. The sagittal image on the left illustrates the position of 13 axial slices (represented by the horizontal lines). One of these slices (highlighted in gray and marked by open arrows) is usually positioned to include the M_1 segments of the middle cerebral artery (see black arrows on axial image shown on right). The AIF is commonly estimated from the signal changes in this artery.

benefit from (potentially risky) reperfusion treatments, such as thrombolysis or via mechanical means. However, if the errors introduced by delay and dispersion give inaccurate CBF and MTT estimates, the outcome of the predictor model may lead to patients being treated inappropriately; this could have potentially serious clinical consequences, including increased risk of hemorrhagic infarctions [52].

Although some of the most commonly used deconvolution algorithms are prone to errors due to bolus delay (e.g., the SVD algorithm [16,53]), there are now many algorithms that have been shown to be delay-insensitive (e.g., see Refs. 21,22,25). Their use is therefore highly advisable, especially in patients with severe vascular abnormalities where bolus delay is likely to occur [54]. On the other hand, the errors due to bolus dispersion are not related to the particular deconvolution algorithm used, but they are a more fundamental limitation of the theory used to model the data. See equation (10.4), which assumes that the AIF measured represents the true AIF, and the unaccounted dispersion will therefore be assigned to occurring within the tissue of interest (i.e., interpreted as a prolonged MTT and decreased CBF [53]). Therefore, it should be noted that while the particular choice of deconvolution algorithm can avoid delay-related errors, it cannot eliminate those associated to bolus dispersion.

The bolus dispersion can be described mathematically by the *vascular transport function* VTF(*t*), which represents the probability density function of vascular transit time *t* between the location of the artery where the AIF was measured and the true input to the tissue of interest (Calamante et al. 2005 [50,58]):

$$AIF(t) = AIF_{meas}(t) \otimes VTF(t) \qquad (10.6)$$

where $AIF_{meas}(t)$ is the measured AIF. In practice, the presence of bolus dispersion therefore leads to a distortion of the calculated impulse response function; in other words, the deconvolution analysis will give an *effective* residue function

$$C(t) = CBF \cdot \left(AIF_{meas}(t) \otimes R_{eff}(t)\right) \qquad (10.7)$$

where the effective residue function, $[R_{eff}(t)]$ is the convolution of the true $R(t)$ with the vascular transport function [see equations (10.4) and (10.6)] [50].

One approach to correct for the effects of bolus dispersion requires modeling the vascular bed [i.e., $VTF(t)$]. The main problem with this approach is that the correct model is not known in practice. Various models have been proposed [53,58–60] and work is currently under way to determine the validity of some of these models [54,58]. In particular, a method that combines finite-element analysis and models of arterial blood flow from anatomic and physiologic MRI data has been proposed as a means to assess and optimize models [58]. This methodology was applied to obtain a better understanding of the dispersion process through stenosed arteries (one of the commonest source of dispersion). In brief, the method consists of the following steps [58]:

1. From MR anatomic images, a patient-specific geometric model of the arteries is constructed.
2. Using this geometric model and the physiologic data from the same subject (obtained from phase contrast MR flow velocity measurements), the pulsatile incompressible Navier–Stokes equations are solved using finite-element analysis.
3. The flow solution is then used to calculate the transport of the contrast agent by solving the advection–diffusion equation using finite-element analysis. By comparing the shape of the input bolus with the shape of the output of the geometric model, the degree of dispersion can be calculated (e.g., see Figure 10.8); the curves generated can then be used to assess and validate the use of simpler vascular models to describe the dispersion process [58].

Measurement of Global versus Local AIF

An alternative to address the problem of bolus dispersion is to avoid its presence altogether. As mentioned above (see section "Perfusion Quantification: Measurement of the AIF"), the main problem relates to the fact that the AIF is measured in a major artery, and this estimated function is used as a *global AIF* for the whole MRI dataset (see Figures 10.6 and 10.7). To minimize the errors related to bolus dispersion, it has been proposed that a *local AIF* be used instead [61]. In

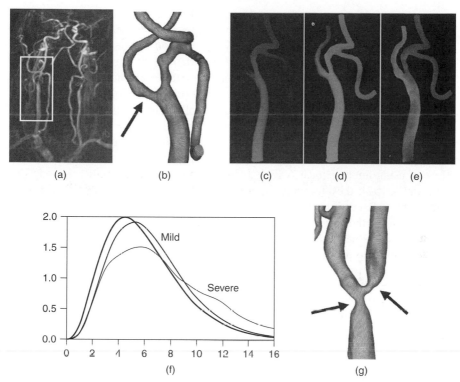

Figure 10.8. Finite-element analysis for modeling bolus dispersion. Contrast-enhanced MRA in the box shown in (a) indicates the part to be modeled. Finite-element mesh generated for the model in (b). There is a mild stenosis of the origin of the internal carotid artery in this model (arrow). The bolus passage calculated using finite-element analysis, visualized using maximum intensity projection (c–e). Arterial concentrations of contrast agent (f) for the simulated input to the common carotid artery (bold line) and for the calculated output at the outlet of the internal carotid artery for the mild stenosis case in (a–e) (gray line labeled "mild"). Model mesh (g) derived from a patient with severe stenosis of the distal common carotid artery and origin of the internal carotid artery (arrows). The calculated output of the internal carotid artery for this case is shown in (f) (gray line labeled "severe") for the same simulated input (bold line). (Image previously published in Ref. 50 with permission from Wiley-Liss, Inc, modified from figures previously published in Ref. 58, with permission from Elsevier.)

fact, by definition, the AIF should be calculated on a pixel-by-pixel basis because the input to the tissue can be potentially different for each voxel (depending on its blood supply). However, given the size of the smaller arteries required for measuring the local AIF, this approach is likely to be particularly sensitive to partial-volume effects [49]. This is an area of active research, and various methods to define a local AIF have now been proposed [61–63]. In particular, a method based in independent component analysis, a technique designed to identify independent spatiotemporal patterns, has been proposed as a means of defining the local AIF [62]. In brief, the methodology is based on the decomposition of the concentration–time course data into linearly independent components, followed by identification of those components that have arterial characteristics, which are then combined to define a local AIF. Using this methodology, the local AIF generated in patients with various cerebrovascular abnormalities was found to display regional heterogeneity, with some areas having delayed bolus arrival and wider peaks, which were consistent with the patients' vascular abnormalities [64] (see Figure 10.9). Furthermore, in a more recent study, Lorenz et al. assessed the effect of using another local AIF analysis in the outcome of predictor models of acute stroke [52]; they found an improved prediction as compared to the results from global AIF analysis (see Figure 10.10).

Although further work is required to validate these approaches (the main limitation is the lack of gold standard for local AIF measurement), they may prove to be a promising solution to minimizing the dispersion-related errors in certain group of patients, such as those with arterial stenosis or occlusion.

Measurement of the AIF: Partial Volume Effect

As discussed above (see section "Perfusion Quantification: Measurement of the AIF"), for the typical voxel resolution used in DSC-MRI studies (typical voxel size $\sim 2 \times 2 \times 5$ mm^3), partial-volume effects with the surrounding tissue will be often present when measuring the AIF. This effect leads to a distortion on the shape of the estimated AIF, which will affect the accuracy of CBF quantification [49]. Given the complex nature of the MRI signal, the relative contributions from the artery and tissue to the measured AIF can interfere constructively or destructively (depending, for example, on the orientation of the artery relative to the main magnetic field) [64]. It has been proposed that the magnitude and phase evolution of the MRI signal during the passage of the bolus can be used to correct for the partial-volume contamination [65]. However, this correction method has been shown to be valid for arteries that are approximately aligned with the main magnetic field (e.g., the internal carotid arteries), and will not correct for the partial-volume effect on arteries closer to the tissue of interest (where AIF measurement would be optimal for delay and dispersion minimization) [49].

Measurement of Contrast Agent Concentration: Nonlinearity

Although as mentioned above (see section "Perfusion Quantification: Indicator Dilution Theory"), a linear relationship between the concentration of the contrast agent and the changes in the relaxation time is usually used [see equation (10.1)], more recent studies have suggested that this linear relationship may not always be valid, particularly for high contrast concentration such as in large vessels [42,66,67] (see Figure 10.11). Therefore, although the assumption of a linear relationship may be valid for the concentration in the tissue, it may be a

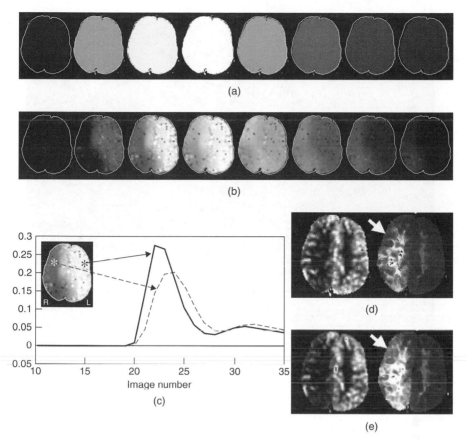

Figure 10.9. Comparison of global and local AIF results on a patient with vascular abnormality in the right major cerebral arteries (same patient as in Figure 10.1). The set of eight images are eight time samples of global (a) and local AIF (b) during passage of the bolus. As can be seen in the images, the local AIF data show heterogeneity throughout the slice, with delayed and dispersed regions on the right hemisphere. This is illustrated on the local AIF curves (c) obtained from the pixels indicated by asterisks. CBF and MTT maps calculated by deconvolution using the local AIF (d) or global AIF data (e). The local AIF methodology produced higher CBF and shorter MTT (compared to the global AIF case) in regions where the local AIF was distorted (e.g., see arrows). (Modified from figures previously published in Ref. 62, © 2004, Wiley-Liss, Inc.)

significant source of error in the measurement of the AIF, given the relatively high concentration inside the artery. As a solution to this problem, it has been suggested to exploit the phase information (usually discarded) of the MR images [66,68]. Empirical data have shown that the image phase changes during the passage of the bolus are linearly related to the contrast agent concentration, even at the large concentrations found in the arteries [66].

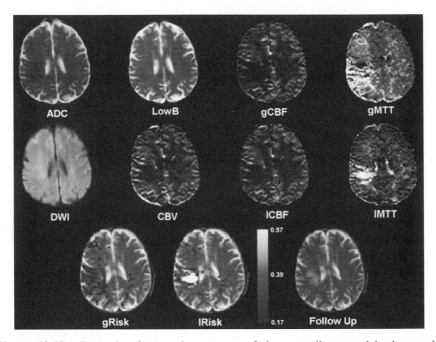

Figure 10.10. Example of errors in outcome of tissue predictor models due to the presence of bolus delay and dispersion. The data correspond to a patient scanned 90 min after acute onset of left-sided facial droop and left hemiparesis; the patient had a completely occluded right internal carotid artery (data not shown). This example shows the infarct predictions using the generalized linear model (GLM) [55], calculated using six parameters (LowB, ADC, DWI, CBV, CBF, and MTT). Two risk maps were calculated, analyzing the DSC-MRI data using either a global AIF (prefix letter "g" in the label) or a local AIF (prefix letter "l"). Because of minimization of the dispersion errors, the local AIF approach leads to increased flow estimates (lCBF) in the right hemisphere compared to the flow estimates produced by the global AIF (gCBF). This produced substantial changes in the GLM tissue outcome map (see gRisk and lRisk) because a higher risk of infarction was assigned to regions that eventually infracted (as seen on follow-up T_2 images 8 days after stroke onset), and a lower risk of infarction was assigned to regions that did not infarct. (*Key*: ADC—apparent diffusion coefficient; LowB—T_2-weighted image; DWI—diffusion-weighted image.) The risk of infarction in the maps (see gRisk and lRisk) is overlaid on a follow-up image; their values are given by the color bar (please refer to the original article for a color version of this figure). (Image kindly provided by Dr. A. G. Sorensen and previously published in Ref. 52, © 2006, Wiley-Liss, Inc.)

Perfusion Quantification: BBB Breakdown

The model used for DSC-MRI quantification described above [in particular, in equations (10.4) and (10.5)] is based on the assumption that the contrast agent remains intravascular. If this not the case (e.g., when the BBB is disrupted such as

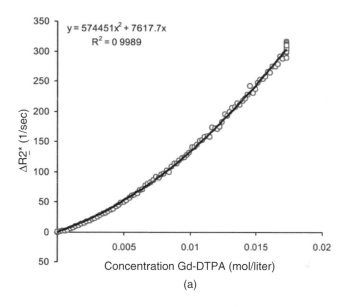

(a)

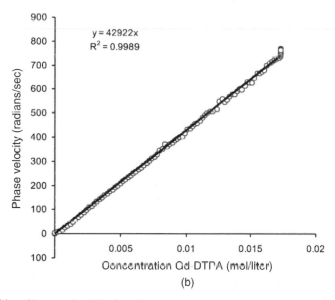

(b)

Figure 10.11. Changes in MR signal versus contrast agent concentration as measured in flowing, fully oxygenated blood at body temperature. Although the relationship is quadratic for $\Delta R2^*$ (a), the phase velocity ($\Delta\theta/\Delta TE$) is linear throughout the whole concentration range (b). (Image kindly provided by Dr. M. J. P. van Osch and adapted from a figure previously published in Ref. 66, © 2003, Wiley-Liss, Inc.)

in some brain tumors), the distribution of the contrast agent outside the vascular compartment decreases the T_2^* effects, as well as increases the T_1 effects (usually neglected) during passage of the bolus [see equations (10.2) and (10.3)]. If these effects are not minimized [69] or taken into account [70], large errors can be introduced in quantification of DSC-MRI data (see Ref. 17 for a more recent review on this issue). Various methods have been proposed to avoid the influence of T_1 contamination, such as the use of a dual-echo sequence (to calculate R_2^* directly) [70], or the use of a small predose injected before the DSC-MRI study to effectively saturate the T_1 enhancement [69]. However, these methods deal with part of the problem (the T_1 contamination), but do not address the distortions to the T_2^* effect. The latter require a modification of the kinetic model described in equations (10.4) and (10.5). To this end, various model modifications have been proposed, from relative simple modification to quantify only CBV [71,72], to more complex models to quantify also CBF [70,73]. In general terms, all these models are based on introducing a correction factor to account for leakage of the contrast agent. Therefore, they can be used not only to quantify perfusion but also to provide an estimation of vascular permeability or the extraction fraction, very important parameters on their own right (see Figure 10.12 [74]). Since all these models include the effects of contrast leakage, they should provide a more accurate estimation of perfusion when the BBB is disrupted. However, a full validation of these modified models remains to be done.

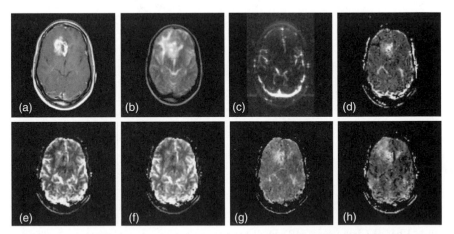

Figure 10.12.   MRI data on a patient with a gliobastoma multiforme. Shown are post-contrast T_1-weighted (a) and T_2-weighted (b) images, angiogram (c), apparent diffusion coefficient (d), CBV (e), CBF (f), MTT (g), and extraction fraction (h). This figure illustrates the wealth of information that can be obtained during an MRI examination of brain tumors: MRI allows assessment of many factors, including BBB leakage, edema, blood flow, and volume. (Image kindly provided by Dr. E. P. A Vonken and adapted from a figure previously published in Ref. 74, © 2000, Springer-Verlag.)

DSC-MRI Quantification: Bolus Recirculation Effects

After the initial passage of the contrast agent (the "first passage"), the measured changes in signal intensity include a second (overlapping) smaller, delayed signal drop, commonly referred to as *bolus recirculation* (see Figure 10.1). One of the implicit assumptions of the original kinetic model for DSC-MRI quantification is that the contrast agent does not reenter the tissue of interest once it leaves after the first passage [75]. Therefore, the contribution of recirculation must be eliminated (or at least minimized) to avoid errors in CBF and CBV quantification [76]. The most commonly used method to achieve this aim is to fit the first pass of the contrast agent concentration to an assumed bolus shape and to extend the resulting function to longer times; the most popular model is the so-called gamma-variate function [77]:

$$C(t) = A \cdot (t - B)^C e^{-(t-B)/D} \tag{10.8}$$

where the parameter B is the BAT (see section "DSC-MRI Quantification: Further Information Available"), A is a scaling factor, and the parameters C and D determine the shape of the function. This function is also commonly used for the quantification of summary parameters (e.g., TTP$= B + C \cdot D$). However, it should be noted that this method can give erroneous measures if the assumed model is inaccurate, such as when the recirculation peak is relatively large [78,79].

10.4. DSC-MRI IMAGING SEQUENCE

Ideally, the MRI sequence used for DSC-MRI should provide good spatial coverage (to include in the image volume as much brain tissue as possible), good temporal resolution (to fully characterize the concentration–time course changes during passage of the bolus), good spatial resolution (to minimize partial volume effects between different tissue types), and good signal-to-noise ratio (to help the inversion problem required for CBF quantification). However, many of these requirements are incompatible, and a compromise based on the particular MR system specifications and application of interest must be done. Currently, EPI [7] is by far the most commonly used MRI sequence for DSC-MRI studies; this fast imaging technique can acquire 15–20 slices with $2 \times 2 \times 5$ mm^3 voxel resolution, 1.5 s time resolution, and relatively good signal-to-noise ratio.

A further issue that must be decided when selecting the MRI sequence is the contrast mechanism that will be exploited for DSC-MRI quantification. The presence of the contrast agent affects both T_2^* and T_2 and, therefore, a gradient–echo or a spin-echo-type image acquisition can be used. Both sequence types are sensitive to the susceptibility gradients induced by the contrast agent, but their vascular specificities are very different [11,64]; while gradient–echo is sensitive to the total vasculature, spin echo is sensitive primarily to the microvasculature. Therefore, a spin-echo-based acquisition is more likely to reflect true perfusion

(*Note*: It should be remembered that perfusion is related to blood flow at the capillary level.) In practice, however, a gradient–echo sequence is more commonly used given its increased contrast-to-noise ratio.

10.5. CONCLUSION

The technical advances achieved during since the mid-1990s have transformed DSC-MRI into a very powerful technique, which provides unique information regarding cerebral hemodynamics. It has been extensively used for the assessment and management of patients, as well as being an invaluable tool in experimental studies. Many of the initial technical limitations have now been circumvented, and the remaining issues are currently a very active area of research in the field. The lack of ionizing radiation, combined with the good spatial resolution and extra information available within an MR examination make DSC-MRI one of the techniques of choice for the in vivo investigation of cerebral perfusion.

REFERENCES

1. Calamante F, Thomas DL, Pell GS, Wiersma J, Turner R: Measuring cerebral blood flow using magnetic resonance techniques, *J Cereb Blood Flow Metab* **19**:701–735 (1999).

2. Barbier EL, Lamalle L, Décorps M: Methodology of brain perfusion imaging, *J Magn Reson Imag* **13**:496–520 (2001).

3. Petersen ET, Zimine I, Ho Y-CL, Golay X: Non-invasive measurements of perfusion: A critical review of arterial spin labelling techniques, *Br J Radiol* **79**:688–701 (2006).

4. Conturo TE, Calamante F: Special section: ISMRM Perfusion Workshop Invited Papers, *J Magn Reson Imag* **22**:692 (2005).

5. Rosen BR, Belliveau JW, Vevea JM, Brady TJ: Perfusion imaging with NMR contrast agents, *Magn Reson Med* **14**:249–265 (1990).

6. Villringer A, Rosen BR, Belliveau JW, Ackerman JL, Lauffer RB, Buxton RB, Chao YS, Wedeen VJ, Brady TJ: Dynamic imaging with lanthanide chelates in normal brain: Contrast due to magnetic-susceptibility effects, *Magn Reson Med* **6**:164–174 (1988).

7. Stehling MK, Turner R, Masfield P: Echo-planar imaging: Magnetic resonance imaging in a fraction of a second, *Science* **254**:43–50 (1991).

8. Klarhöfer M, Dilharreguy B, van Gelderen P, Moonen CTW: A PRESTO-SENSE sequence with alternating partial-Fourier encoding for rapid susceptibility-weighted 3D MRI time series, *Magn Reson Med* **50**:830–838 (2003).

9. Koshimoto Y, Yamada H, Kimura H, Maeda M, Tsuchida C, Kawamura Y, Ishii Y: Quantitative analysis of cerebral microvascular hemodynamics with T2-weighted dynamic MR imaging, *J Magn Reson Imag* **9**:462–467 (1999).

10. Stollberger R, Fazekas F: Improved perfusion and tracer kinetic imaging using parallel imaging, *Top Magn Reson Imag* **15**:245–254 (2004).

11. Weisskoff RM, Zuo CS, Boxerman JL, Rosen BR: Microscopic susceptibility variation and transverse relaxation. Theory and experiment, *Magn Reson Med* **31**:601–610 (1994).

12. Weisskoff RM, Chesler D, Boxerman JL, Rosen BR: Pitfalls in MR measurement of tissue blood flow with intravascular tracers: Which mean transit-time? *Magn Reson Med* **29**:553–559 (1993).

13. Perthen JE, Calamante F, Gadian DG, Connelly A: Is quantification of bolus tracking MRI reliable without deconvolution? *Magn Reson Med* **47**:61–67 (2002).

14. Zierler KL: Theoretical basis of indicator-dilution methods for measuring flow and volume, *Circ Res* **10**:393–407 (1962).

15. Axel L: Cerebral blood flow determination by rapid sequence computed tomography, *Radiology* **137**:679–686 (1980).

16. Østergaard L, Weisskoff RM, Chesler DA, Gyldensted C, Rosen BR: High resolution measurement of cerebral blood flow using intravascular tracer bolus passages. Part I. Mathematical approach and statistical analysis, *Magn Reson Med* **36**:715–725 (1996).

17. Calamante F: Quantification of dynamic susceptibility contrast T2* MRI in oncology, in Jackson A, Buckley DL, Parker GJM, eds, *Dynamic Contrast-Enhanced Magnetic Resonance Imaging in Oncology*, Medical Radiology–Diagnostic Imaging (series), Springer-Verlag, Heidelberg, 2005, pp 53–67.

18. Hansen PC: Regularization tools: A MATLAB package for analysis and solution of discrete ill-posed problems, *Num Algorithms* **6**:1 35 (1994).

19. Rempp KA, Brix G, Wenz F, Becker CR, Guckel F, Lorenz WJ: Quantification of regional cerebral blood flow and volume with dynamic susceptibility contrast-enhanced MR imaging, *Radiology* **193**:637–641 (1994).

20. Liu HL, Pu Y, Liu Y, Nickerson L, Andrews T, Fox PT, Gao JH: Cerebral blood flow measurement by dynamic contrast MRI using singular value decomposition with an adaptive threshold, *Magn Reson Med* **42**:167–172 (1999).

21. Wu O, Østergaard L, Weisskoff RM, Benner T, Rosen BR, Sorensen AG: Tracer arrival timing-insensitive technique for estimating flow in MR perfusion-weighted imaging using singular value decomposition with a block-circulant deconvolution matrix, *Magn Reson Med* **50**:164–174 (2003).

22. Smith MR, Lu H, Trochet S, Frayne R: Removing the effect of SVD algorithmic artifacts present in quantitative MR perfusion studies, *Magn Reson Med* **51**:631–634 (2004).

23. Calamante F, Gadian DG, Connelly A: Quantification of bolus tracking MRI: Improved characterization of the tissue residue function using Tikhonov regularization, *Magn Reson Med* **50**:1237–1247 (2003).

24. Vonken EP, Beckman FJ, Bakker CJ, Viergever MA: Maximum likelihood estimation of cerebral blood flow in dynamic susceptibility contrast MRI, *Magn Reson Med* **41**:343–350 (1999).

25. Willats L, Connelly A, Calamante F: Improved deconvolution of perfusion MRI data in the presence of bolus delay and dispersion, *Magn Reson Med* **56**:146–156 (2006).

26. Schreiber WG, Guckel F, Stritzke P, Schmiedek P, Schwartz A, Brix G: Cerebral blood flow and cerebrovascular reserve capacity: Estimation by dynamic magnetic resonance imaging, *J Cereb Blood Flow Metab* **18**:1143–1156 (1998).

27. Andersen IK, Szymkowiak A, Rasmussen CE, Hanson L, Marstrand JR, Larsson HBW, Hansen LK: Perfusion quantification using Gaussian process deconvolution, *Magn Reson Med* **48**:351–361 (2002).

28. Stewart GN: Researches on the circulation time in organs and on the influences which affect it. Part I–III, *J Physiol* **15**:1–89 (1894).

29. Sorensen AG, Copen WA, Østergaard L, Buonanno FS, Gonzalez RG, Rordorf G, Rosen BR, Schwamm LH, Weisskoff RM, Koroshetz WJ: Hyperacute stroke: Simultaneous measurement of relative cerebral blood volume, relative cerebral blood flow, and mean tissue transit time, *Radiology* **210**:519–527 (1999).

30. Leenders KL, Perani D, Lammertsma AA, Heather JD, Buckingham P, Healy MJ, Gibbs JM, Wise RJ, Hatazawa J, Herold S, Beaney RP, Brooks DJ, Spinks T, Rhodes C, Frackowiak RSJ, Jones T: Cerebral blood flow, blood volume and oxygen utilization. Normal values and effect of age, *Brain* **113**:27–47 (1990).

31. Østergaard L, Sorensen AG, Kwong KK, Weisskoff RM, Gyldensted C, Rosen BR: High resolution measurement of cerebral blood flow using intravascular tracer bolus passages. Part II. Experimental comparison and preliminary results, *Magn Reson Med* **36**:726–736 (1996).

32. Vonken EPA, van Osch MJP, Baker CJG, Viergever MA: Measurement of cerebral perfusion with dual-echo multi-slice quantitative dynamic susceptibility contrast MRI, *J Magn Reson Imag* **10**:109–117 (1999).

33. Smith AM, Grandin CB, Duprez T, Mataigne F, Cosnar G: Whole brain quantitative CBF and CBV measurements using MRI bolus tracking: Comparison of methodolgies, *Magn Reson Med* **43**:559–654 (2000).

34. Grandin CB, Duprez TP, Smith AM, Mataigne F, Peeters A, Oppenheim C, Cosnard G: Usefulness of magnetic resonance-derived quantitative measurements of cerebral blood flow and volume in prediction of infarct growth in hyperacute stroke, *Stroke* **32**:1147–1153 (2001).

35. Østergaard L, Johannsen P, Poulsen PH, Vestergaard-Poulsen P, Asboe H, Gee AD, Hansen SB, Cold GE, Gjedde A, Gyldensted C: Cerebral blood flow measurements by magnetic resonance imaging bolus tracking: Comparison with [O-15] H_2O positron emission tomography in humans, *J Cereb Blood Flow Metab* **18**:935–940 (1998).

36. Østergaard L, Smith DF, Vestergaard-Poulsen P, Hansen SB, Gee AD, Gjedde A, Gyldensted C: Absolute cerebral blood flow and blood volume measured by magnetic resonance imaging bolus tracking: Comparison with positron emission tomography values, *J Cereb Blood Flow Metab* **18**:425–432 (1998).

37. Sorensen AG: What is the meaning of quantitative CBF? *Am J Neuroradiol* **22**:235–236 (2001).

38. Calamante F, Gadian DG, Connelly A: Quantification of perfusion using bolus tracking MRI in stroke. Assumptions, limitations, and potential implications for clinical use, *Stroke* **33**:1146–1151 (2002).

39. Calamante F: Artifacts and pitfalls in perfusion MR imaging, in Gillard J, Waldman A, Barker P, eds, *Clinical MR Neuroimaging: Diffusion, Perfusion and Spectroscopy*, Cambridge Univ Press, 2005, pp 141–160.

40. Lin W, Celik A, Derdeyn C, An H, Lee Y, Videen T, Østergaard L, Powers WJ: Quantitative measurements of cerebral blood flow in patients with unilateral carotid artery occlusion: A PET and MR study, *J Magn Reson Imag* **14**:659–667 (2001).

41. Mukherjee P, Kang HC, Videen TO, McKinstry RC, Powers WJ, Derdeyn CP: Measurement of cerebral blood flow in chronic carotid occlusive disease: Comparison of dynamic susceptibility contrast perfusion MR imaging with positron emission tomography, *Am J Neuroradiol* **24**:862–871 (2003).

42. Kiselev VG: On the theoretical basis of perfusion measurements by dynamic susceptibility contrast MRI, *Magn Reson Med* **46**:1113–1122 (2001).

43. Johnson KM, Tao JZT, Kennan RP, Gore JC: Intravascular susceptibility agent effects on tissue transverse relaxation rates in vivo, *Magn Reson Med* **44**:909–914 (2000).

44. Loufti I, Frackowiak RS, Myers MJ, Lavender JP: Regional brain hematocrit in stroke by single photon emission computer tomography imaging, *Am J Physiol Imag* **2**:10–16 (1987).

45. Yamamuchi H, Fukuyama H, Nagahama Y, Katsumi Y, Okazawa H: Cerebral hematocrit decreases with hemodynamic compromise in carotid artery occlusion: A PET study, *Stroke* **29**:98–103 (1998).

46. Grandin C, Bol A, Smith A, Michel C, Cosnard G: Absolute CBF and CBV measurements by MRI bolus tracking before and after acetazolamide challenge: Repeatability and comparison with PET in humans, *NeuroImage* **26**:525–535 (2005).

47. Conturo TE, Akbudak E, Kotys MS, Chen ML, Chun SJ, Hsu RM, Sweeney CC, Markham J: Arterial input functions for dynamic susceptibility contrast MRI: Requirements and signal options, *J Magn Reson Imag* **22**:697–703 (2005).

48. Cebral JR, Castro MA, Soto O, Löhner R, Alperin N: Blood-flow models of the circle of Willis from magnetic resonance data, *J Eng Math* **47**:369–386 (2003).

49. van Osch MJP, van der Grond J, Bakker CJG: Partial volume effects on arterial input functions: Shape and amplitude distortions and their correction, *J Magn Reson Imag* **22**:704–709 (2005).

50. Calamante F: Bolus dispersion issues related to the quantification of perfusion MRI data, *J Magn Reson Imag* **22**:718–722 (2005).

51. Calamante F, Ganesan V, Kirkham FJ, Jan W, Chong WK, Gadian DG, Connelly A: MR perfusion imaging in moyamoya syndrome. Potential implications for clinical evaluation of occlusive cerebrovascular disease, *Stroke* **32**:2810–2816 (2001).

52. Lorenz C, Benner T, Chen PJ, Lopez CJ, Ay H, Zhu MW, Menezes NM, Aronen H, Karonen J, Liu Y, Nuutinen J, Sorensen AG: Automated perfusion-weighted MRI using localized arterial input functions, *J Magn Reson Imag* **24**:1133–1139 (2006).

53. Calamante F, Gadian DG, Connelly A: Delay and dispersion effects in dynamic susceptibility contrast MRI: Simulations using singular value decomposition, *Magn Reson Med* **44**:466–473 (2000).

54. Calamante F, Willats L, Gadian DG, Connelly A: Bolus delay and dispersion in perfusion MRI: Implications for tissue predictor models in stroke. *Magn Reson Med* **55**:1180–1185 (2006).

55. Wu O, Koroshetz WJ, Østergaard L, Buonanno FS, Copen WA, Gonzalez RG, Rordorf G, Rosen BR, Schwamm LH, Weisskoff RM, Sorensen AG: Predicting tissue outcome in acute human cerebral ischemia using combined diffusion- and perfusion-weighted MR imaging, *Stroke* **32**:933–942 (2001).

56. Rose SE, Chalk JB, Griffin MP, Janke AL, Chen F, McLachan GJ, Peel D, Zelaya FO, Markus HS, Jones DK, Simmons A, O'Sullivan M, Jarosz JM, Strugnell W, Doddrell DM, Semple J: MRI based diffusion and perfusion predictive model to estimate stroke evolution, *Magn Reson Imag* **19**:1043–1053 (2001).

57. Gottrup C, Thomsen K, Locht P, Wu O, Sorensen AG, Koroshetz WJ, Østergaard L: Applying instance-based techniques to prediction of final outcome in acute stroke, *Artif Intell Med* **33**:223–236 (2005).

58. Calamante F, Yim PJ, Cebral JR: Estimation of bolus dispersion effects in perfusion MRI using image-based computational fluid dynamics, *NeuroImage* **19**:341–353 (2003).

59. King RB, Deussen A, Raymond GM, Bassingthwaighte JB: A vascular transport operator, *Am J Physiol Heart Circ Physiol* **265**:H2196–H2208 (1993).

60. Østergaard L, Chesler DA, Weisskoff RM, Sorensen AG, Rosen BR: Modeling cerebral blood flow and flow heterogeneity from magnetic resonance residue data, *J Cereb Blood Flow Metab* **19**:690–699 (1999).

61. Alsop DC, Wedmid A, Schlaug G: Defining a local input function for perfusion quantification with bolus contrast MRI, *Proc 10th Annual Meeting Int Soc Magn Reson Med*, Honolulu, May 18–24, 2002, p 659.

62. Calamante F, Mørup M, Hansen LK: Defining a local arterial input function for perfusion MRI using independent component analysis, *Magn Reson Med* **52**:789–797 (2004).

63. Grüner R, Bjørnarå B, Moen G, Taxt T: Magnetic resonance brain perfusion imaging with voxel-specific arterial input functions, *Magn Reson Med* **23**:273–284 (2006).

64. Boxerman JL, Hamberg LM, Rosen BR, Weisskoff RM: MR contrast due to intravascular magnetic-susceptibility perturbations, *Magn Reson Med* **34**:555–566 (1995).

65. van Osch MJP, Vonken EPA, Bakker CJG, Viergever MA: Correcting partial volume artifacts of the arterial input function in quantitative cerebral perfusion MRI, *Magn Reson Med* **45**:477–485 (2001).

66. van Osch MJP, Vonken EPA, Viergever MA, van der Grond J, Bakker CJG: Measuring the arterial input function with gradient echo sequences, *Magn Reson Med* **49**:1067–1076 (2003).

67. Kjolby BF, Østergaard L, Kiselev VG: Theoretical model of intravascular paramagnetic tracers effect on tissue relaxation, *Magn Reson Med* **56**:187–197 (2006).

68. Akbudak E, Conturo TE: Arterial input functions from MR phase imaging, *Magn Reson Med* **36**:809–815 (1996).

69. Sorensen AG, Reimer P: *Cerebral MR Perfusion Imaging. Principles and Current Applications*, Georg Thieme Verlag, Stuttgart, Germany, 2000.

70. Vonken EPA, van Osch MJP, Baker CJG, Viergever MA: Simultaneous qualitative cerebral perfusion and Gd-DTPA extravasation measurements with dual-echo dynamic susceptibility contrast MRI, *Magn Reson Med* **43**:820–827 (2000).

71. Weisskoff RM, Boxerman JL, Sorensen AG, Kulke SM, Campbell TA, Rosen BR: Simultaneous blood volume and permeability mapping using a single Gd-based contrast injection, *Proc 2nd Annual Meeting Soc Mag Reson Med*, San Francisco, 1994, p 279.

72. Donahue KM, Krouwer HGJ, Rand SD, Pathak AP, Marszalkowski CS, Censky SC, Prost RW: Utility of simultaneously acquired gradient-echo and spin-echo cerebral blood volume and morphology maps in brain tumor patients, *Magn Reson Med* **43**:845–853 (2000).

73. Quarles CC, Ward BD, Schmainda KM: Improving the reliability of obtaining tumor hemodynamic parameters in the presence of contrast agent extravasation, *Magn Reson Med* **53**:1307–1316 (2005).

74. Vonken EPA, van Osch MJP, Willems PWA, van der Zwan A, Bakker CJG, Viergever MA, Mali WPTM: Repeated quantitative perfusion and contrast permeability measurement in the MRI examination of a CNS tumor, *Eur Radiol* **10**:1447–1451 (2000).

75. Zierler KL: Equations for measuring blood flow by external monitoring of radioisotopes, *Circ Res* **16**:309–321 (1965).

76. Perkiö J, Aronen HJ, Kangasmaki A, Liu Y, Karonen J, Savolainen S, Østergaard L: Evaluation of four postprocessing methods for determination of cerebral blood volume and mean transit time by dynamic susceptibility contrast imaging, *Magn Reson Med* **47**:973–981 (2002).

77. Thompson HK, Starmer F, Whalen RE, McIntosh HD: Indicator transit time considered as a gamma variate, *Circ Res* **14**:502–515 (1964).

78. Levin JM, Kaufman MJ, Ross MJ, Mendelson JH, Maas LC, Cohen M, Renshaw PF: Sequential dynamic susceptibility contrast MR experiments in human brain: Residual contrast agent effect, steady state, and hemodynamic perturbation, *Magn Reson Med* **34**:655–663 (1995).

79. Kassner A, Annesley DJ, Zhu XP, Li KL, Kamaly-Asl ID, Watson Y, Jackson A: Abnormalities of the contrast re-circulation phase in cerebral tumors demonstrated using dynamic susceptibility contrast-enhanced imaging: A possible marker of vascular tortuosity, *J Magn Reson Imag* **11**:103–113 (2000).

CHAPTER 11

Cerebral Perfusion Computed Tomography in Stroke

MAX WINTERMARK

Department of Radiology, Neuroradiology Section, University of California, San Francisco, California

Abstract.   The role of neuroimaging in the evaluation of acute stroke has changed dramatically since the mid-1990s. Previously, neuroimaging was used in this setting to provide anatomic imaging that indicated the presence or absence of acute cerebral ischemia and excluded lesions that produce symptoms or signs mimicking those of stroke, such as hemorrhage and neoplasms. More recently, the introduction of thrombolysis has changed the goals of neuroimaging from providing solely anatomic information to providing physiologic information that could help to determine which patients might benefit from therapy. In particular, significant emphasis has been placed on the delineation of the ischemic penumbra, also called "tissue at risk." Modern CT survey, consisting of three indissociable elements—noncontrast CT (NCT), of course, perfusion CT (PCT), and CT angiography (CTA)—fulfills all the requirements for hyperacute stroke imaging. CTA can define the occlusion site, depict arterial dissection, grade collateral blood flow, and characterize atherosclerotic disease, whereas PCT accurately delineates the infarct core and the ischemic penumbra. CT offers a number of practical advantages over other cerebral perfusion imaging methods, including its wide availability. Using PCT and CTA to define new individualized strategies for acute reperfusion will allow more acute stroke patients to benefit from thrombolytic therapy.

11.1. THE BURDEN OF STROKE

Stroke is a major health issue in every industrialized country, and there is growing evidence that this issue also affects the developing countries. In the industrialized countries, stroke is the third cause of death, after cardiovascular diseases and

Vascular Hemodynamics: Bioengineering and Clinical Perspectives, Edited by Peter J. Yim
Copyright © 2008 John Wiley & Sons, Inc.

cancers. Of all patients who survive a stroke, 50% are left with a permanent handicap, generating a huge burden on healthcare and social services, with an estimated annual cost ranging between US $6.5 and $11.2 billion [1].

The positive National Institute of Neurological Disorders and Stroke (NINDS) trial of tissue plasminogen activator for acute ischemic stroke heralded the start of a new era in stroke management. This trial showed that tissue plasminogen activator given within 3 h of stroke onset increased independent survival by 30% and the absolute number of patients with no disability, by 12% [2]. Subsequent large trials confirmed these initial results [3,4], but, as a result of the significant associated risk of cerebral hemorrhage (6.4–20%) [5], thrombolysis is not yet a universally accepted routine treatment for stroke and remains the subject of intense debate and research. Current thrombolysis guidelines are based on a rigid time clock (less than 3 h) with imaging used only to rule out hemorrhage or risk of hemorrhage [6]. The 3-h time window is restrictive, and very few stroke patients (less than 2%) receive thrombolytic treatment [7].

11.2. REASONS FOR IMAGING ACUTE STROKE PATIENTS

The central premise of acute stroke thrombolysis is to rescue the ischemic penumbra.

When a cerebral artery is occluded, a core of brain tissue dies rapidly. Surrounding this infarct core is an area of brain that is hypoperfused but does not die quickly, thanks to collateral blood flow. This area is called the *ischemic* penumbra [8–10]. The fate of penumbra depends on reperfusion of the ischemic brain. In case of persistent arterial occlusion, the infarct core will grow and progressively replace penumbra. In case of early recanalization, either spontaneous or resulting from thrombolysis, penumbra will be salvaged from infarction [11,12].

The presence and extent of the ischemic penumbra is time-dependent, but especially patient-dependent. Indeed, from patient to patient, survival of the penumbra can vary from less than 3 h to well beyond 48 h. Of all patients with supratentorial arterial occlusion, 90–100% manifest ischemic penumbra in the first 3 h of a stroke, but, interestingly enough, 75–80% of patients still have penumbral tissue at 6 h after stroke onset [11–13].

The relatively negative results to date of thrombolysis trials between 3 and 6 h [3,4,13], despite the high percentage of patients with penumbra within this time window, reflects the fact that these trials did not use any method of penumbral imaging to select patients for therapy, although penumbra was the target for treatment.

Thus, a "tissue clock," where the extents of both infarct and penumbra are determined, would seem an ideal guide to patient selection for thrombolysis, rather than a rigid time window as in the current thrombolysis guidelines [14,15].

Extension of the therapeutic window beyond 3 h could substantially increase the number of patients able to receive thrombolysis. However, for this to occur with improved outcomes, a rapid and accessible neuroimaging technique able to assess the ischemic penumbra is required [16–20].

11.3. PERFUSION-COMPUTED TOMOGRAPHY (PCT) AND COMPUTED TOMOGRAPHY–ANGIOGRAPHY (CTA)

Modern CT survey includes noncontrast CT (NCT), of course, perfusion CT (PCT), and CT angiography (CTA) [21–25]. NCT has classically been used as the standard initial imaging examination for acute stroke patients because of its convenience and high sensitivity for the detection of intracranial hemorrhage, which represents an absolute contraindication to thrombolytic therapy. Occasionally, NCT can provide information supportive of the diagnosis of evolving infarction (e.g., the hyperdense artery sign, indicating arterial thrombus), even when ischemic changes in the brain parenchyma, such as hypodensity, are not visible. Unfortunately, NCT provides solely anatomic, and not physiologic, information and thus has very low sensitivity for acute stroke detection [26,27].

Then there comes sensitive—and specific—functional CT imaging, encompassing CTA and PCT, which provides complementary information about vessel patency and the hemodynamic repercussions of a possible vessel occlusion, respectively. PCT and CTA can be obtained immediately after NCT, during the same CT examination, obviating the need to move the patient to another imaging device for physiologic information needed for making treatment decisions. The total duration of a NCT, two series of PCT and a CTA, averages around 10 min [21,28].

Computed tomography–angiography (CTA) provides multiplanar two- and three-dimensional reformatted vascular images similar to angiography, affording a complete evaluation of the cerebral arteries, including the great vessel origins, the carotid bifurcations, and the circle of Willis, with excellent vascular anatomy. It can define the occlusion site, depict arterial dissection, grade collateral blood flow, and characterize atherosclerotic disease. The overall accuracy of CTA for detecting thromboses and stenoses of large intracranial and extracranial vessels is within the range of 95–99% [29–38]. Consequently, obtaining a CTA on admission may obviate the need for other tests, such as carotid sonography, MR angiography, or conventional catheter arteriography, traditionally ordered later during the hospital admission [39].

Perfusion computed tomography (PCT) imaging, using standard nonionic iodinated contrast, relies on the speed of modern helical CT scanners, that can sequentially trace the entry and washout of a bolus of contrast injected into an arm vein through an intravenous (IV) line [28]. The relationship between contrast concentration and signal intensity of CT data is linear. Therefore, analysis of the signal intensity increasing then decreasing during the passage of the contrast provides information about brain perfusion. More specifically, PCT description of brain perfusion consists of three types of parametric maps, relating to regional cerebral blood volume (rCBV), mean transit time (MTT), and regional cerebral blood flow (rCBF), respectively. Regional CBV reflects the blood content of each pixel. MTT designates the average time required by a bolus of blood to cross the capillary network in each pixel. Finally, rCBF relates to the amount of blood flowing through each pixel during a time interval of 1 min [28,40]. More recently, CBF values from PCT imaging have been shown to be highly accurate in humans when compared to the gold standard, position emission tomography (PET) [41].

By combining rCBF and rCBV results, PCT has the ability to reliably identify the ischemic reversible penumbra and the irretrievable infarct core in acute stroke patients, as soon as on hospital admission. In the infarct core, both rCBF and rCBV values are lowered, whereas in the penumbra, cerebral vascular autoregulation attempts to compensate for decreased rCBV by a local vasodilatation, resulting in increased rCBV values [42,43]. Commercial PCT software programs currently afford real-time automatic calculation of infarct and penumbra maps according to the abovementioned principles (Figure 11.1).

11.4. AVAILABILITY OF PCT

The PCT technique is easily accessible and available. It can be performed using an equipment routinely available in most hospitals, including a CT scanner and a power injector. The only element to be acquired is a postprocessing PCT software program.

Since a temporal resolution of 2 s is acceptable for the PCT data acquisition [44], it is technically possible to perform perfusion CT using nonhelical CT scanners. However, helical CT scanners equipped with cine mode, and especially multidetector-row CT scanners, definitely represent an advantage, because of the more extensive spatial coverage they afford.

The PCT technique uses standard nonionic iodinated contrast material, to be administered through a standard IV line; however, a power injection is mandatory in order to achieve the required injection rate (4 mL/s).

11.5. PCT/CTA VERSUS MRI

Computed tomography (CT) and magnetic resonance imaging (MRI) provide similar information. As a reminder, the diffusion-weighted imaging (DWI) lesion corresponds to the infarct core, whereas the DWI/perfusion-weighted imaging (PWI) mismatch is representative of the ischemic penumbra [12,45–47]. The infarct core and the ischemic penumbra as demonstrated by DWI/PWI and by PCT, respectively, are comparable [42,43,48–51]. Similarly, CTA and MRA results are very similar.

Besides the similarity of their results, both CT and MRI techniques show respective advantages and drawbacks to be considered in the special settings of acute stroke.

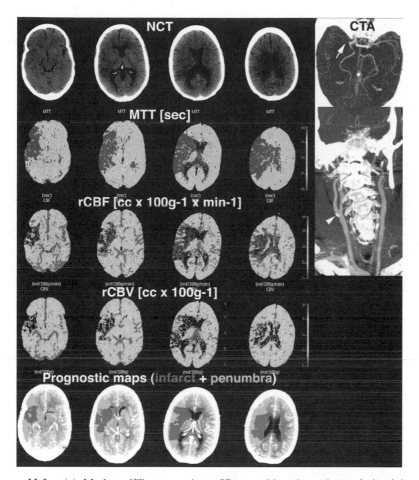

Figure 11.1. (a) Modern CT survey in a 57-year-old male patient admitted in our emergency room with a left hemisyndrome, including a noncontrast CT (first line), a perfusion-CT (lines 2–5), and a CT-angiography (column on the right). The noncontrast CT ruled out a cerebral hemorrhage. From the perfusion CT raw data, three parametric maps were extracted, relating to mean transit time (MTT, line 2), regional cerebral blood flow (rCBF, line 3), and regional cerebral blood volume (rCBV, line 4), respectively. Application of the concept of cerebral vascular autoregulation led to a prognostic map (line 5), describing the infarct in red and the penumbra in green; the latter is the target of thrombolytic drugs. CT angiography, identified an occlusion at the right M_1–M_2 junction (arrow) as the origin of the hemodynamic disturbance demonstrated by perfusion CT. Finally, CTA revealed a calcified atheromatous plaque at the right carotid bifurcation (arrowhead). (b) These findings were confirmed by an MR examination obtained 3 days later. The DWI images and the ADC maps showed that the whole MCA is now infarcted. The evolution of infarct over penumbra compared to the admission perfusion CT results from a persistent occlusion of the right M_1–M_2 junction, as shown on the MR angiography (arrow). The MR-angiographic view of the cervical vessels is very similar to the CT-angiographic one.

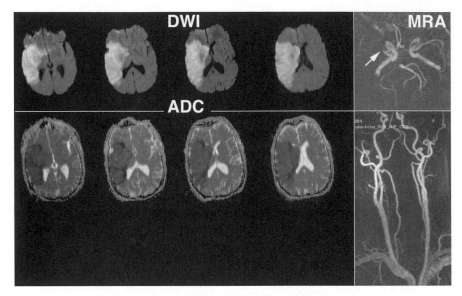

Figure 11.1.   (*Continued*)

Because of its use of X rays and iodinated contrast material, CT is seldom the method of choice. However, the radiation dose involved in PCT imaging is less than, that of a conventional cerebral CT examination [52], and no renal failure has yet been reported following a PCT examination [53]. Because of a limited spatial resolution, PCT cannot detect small lacunas, whereas NCT is not as sensitive to microbleeds as is gradient–echo MRI. PCT has a limited spatial coverage (20–48 mm thickness). However, the issue of spatial coverage will be addressed in the near future through the development of larger multidetector CT scanners with greater arrays of elements and, even at present, PCT has demonstrated 95% accurate in the delineation of the extent of supratentorial strokes despite its limited spatial coverage [54]. PCT has also demonstrated use in the evaluation of vertebrobasilar ischemia [55].

Hyperacute stroke MRI has also limitations. One limitation is the time required for MR scanning. Even a streamlined acute stroke MRI protocol takes 30 min (as opposed to 10 min for PCT/CTA), producing a substantial time delay in initiating acute reperfusion therapy in a situation where "time is brain." Other criticisms of MRI include its cost and limited availability in the emergency setting, in and outside metropolitan hospitals, both conditions that are unlikely to change in the near future. Even in the centers where MRI is available 24/7 (around the clock, 7 days per week), there is no MRI scanner, without an outpatient schedule, dedicated to emergency cases.

The relatively few requirements for performing PCT/CTA technology, and its wide availability, bode well for its eventual replacement of MRI in the imaging of acute stroke patients. Indeed, because of their relatively low cost and utility in other areas of medicine, particularly emergency medicine and trauma, CT scanners are becoming widely available, and, as opposed to MRI, it is foreseeable that every major emergency center will eventually be able to complete this form of imaging within minutes of the patient presenting to the emergency department. Another major advantage of PCT over MRI relates to its quantitative accuracy, whereas MRI perfusion imaging affords only semiquantitative comparison of one hemisphere to the other [56]. Quantitative accuracy of PCT makes it a potential surrogate marker to monitor the efficiency of acute reperfusion therapy, which is a decisive element when it comes to finding and validating new individualized therapeutic strategies for acute stroke patients. Similarly, PCT might demonstrate a benefit from neuroprotective drugs, which have been shown to preserve the penumbra from infarction in animal stroke models, but have failed many times to translate into positive human studies, probably because the latter did not use any method of penumbral imaging to select the patients for treatment [57,58].

11.6. INTEGRATION OF PCT/CTA RESULTS IN MANAGEMENT OF ACUTE STROKE PATIENTS

The new therapeutical strategies for acute reperfusion therapy remain to be defined. As mentioned earlier, the rigid time window of the first 3 h should be replaced by a "tissue clock" taking into account the extents of infarct and penumbra. This tissue clock should balance the benefits that can be expected in case of arterial recanalization and the risk of hemorrhagic transformation. The latter is most likely related to the size of the infarct core, which has been demonstrated to vary dramatically between patients in the first 6 h after stroke onset, and as the strongest predictor of outcome [59]. The potential clinical benefit of arterial recanalization is directly related to the relative extent of penumbra and infarct; the more extensive the penumbra compared to the infarct core, the better the clinical outcome that can be expected in case of early recanalization [43].

By using as new selection criteria the extent of the infarct core, and the relative extent of penumbra and infarct, both types of information provided by PCT, it could be possible to extend the time window and thus to enlarge the target population for acute thrombolysis. It might also help to exclude those patients who have nothing to gain from acute reperfusion therapy, even in the 0–3-h time window [16] (Figure 11.2).

11.7. CONCLUSION

Modern CT, including NCT, PCT, and CTA, fulfills all the requirements for hyperacute stroke imaging. CTA can define the occlusion site, depict arterial dissection, grade collateral blood flow, and characterize atherosclerotic disease. PCT accurately delineates the infarct core and the ischemic penumbra. Hopefully, using PCT and CTA to define new individualized strategies for acute reperfusion

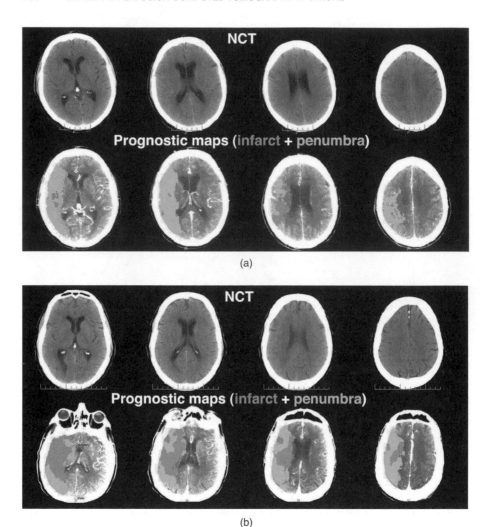

Figure 11.2.   These two sets of images feature two cases of acute stroke patients admitted within the first 6 h of symptomatology onset [5 h for patient represented in (a) and 4.5 h for patient represented in (b)]. In both cases, the noncontrast CT is normal. The perfusion CT prognostic map obtained on admission in the patient represented in (a) displays an extensive penumbra (green) and a very limited infarct (red). This first patient would be eligible for intravenous thrombolysis, according to the new criteria developed in our institution, despite a time interval of 5 h since onset. On the other hand, despite identical clinical and conventional noncontrast CT characteristics, the patient represented in (b) shows an extensive infarct extending to more than one-third of the MCA territory. This second patient would not be an adequate candidate for delayed therapy.

will lead to a significant increase in the number of acute stroke patients benefiting from thrombolytic therapy.

REFERENCES

1. Kaste M, Fogelholm R, Rissanen A: Economic burden of stroke and the evaluation of new therapies, *Public Health* **112**:103–112 (1998).
2. The National Institute of Neurological Disorders and Stroke; rt-PA Stroke Study Group: Tissue plasminogen activator for acute ischemic stroke, *N Engl J Med* **333**:1581–1587 (1995).
3. Hacke W, Kaste M, Fieschi C et al: Intravenous thrombolysis with recombinant tissue plasminogen activator for acute hemispheric stroke. The European Cooperative Acute Stroke Study (ECASS), *JAMA* **274**:1017–1025 (1995).
4. Hacke W, Kaste M, Fieschi C et al: Randomised double-blind placebo-controlled trial of thrombolytic therapy with intravenous alteplase in acute ischaemic stroke (ECASS II). Second European-Australasian Acute Stroke Study Investigators, *Lancet* **352**:1245–1251 (1998).
5. Patel SC, Mody A: Cerebral hemorrhagic complications of thrombolytic therapy, *Progr Cardiovasc Dis* **42**:217–233 (1999).
6. Kaste M, Thomassen L, Grond M et al, on behalf of the participants of the 3rd Karolinska Stroke Update, October 30–31, 2000. Thrombolysis for acute ischemic stroke. A consensus statement of the 3rd Karolinska Stroke Update, October 30–31, 2000, *Stroke* **32**:2717–2718 (2001).
7. Schellinger PD, Fiebach JB, Mohr A, Ringleb PA, Jansen O, Hacke W: Thrombolytic therapy for ischemic stroke—a review. Part I—Intravenous thrombolysis. *Crit Care Med* **29**:1812–1818 (2001).
8. Astrup J, Siesjo BK, Symon L: Thresholds in cerebral ischemia: The ischemic penumbra, *Stroke* **12**:723–725 (1981).
9. Hossmann KA: Neuronal survival and revival during and after cerebral ischemia, *Am J Emerg Med* **1**:191–197 (1983).
10. Hossmann KA: Viability thresholds and the penumbra of focal ischemia, *Ann Neurol* **36**:557–565 (1994).
11. Read SJ, Hirano T, Abbott DF, Markus R et al: The fate of hypoxic tissue on 18F-fluoromisonidazole positron emission tomography after ischemic stroke, *Ann Neurol* **48**:228–235 (2000).
12. Darby DG, Barber PA, Gerraty RP et al: Pathophysiological topography of acute ischemia by combined diffusion-weighted and perfusion MRI, *Stroke* **30**:2043–2052 (1999).
13. Hacke W, Donnan G, Fieschi C et al; ATLANTIS Trials Investigators; ECASS Trials Investigators; NINDS rt-PA Study Group Investigators: Association of outcome with early stroke treatment: Pooled analysis of ATLANTIS, ECASS, and NINDS rt PA stroke trials, *Lancet* **363**:768–774 (2004).
14. Donnan GA, Howells DW, Markus R, Toni D, Davis SM: Can the time window for administration of thrombolytics in stroke be increased? *CNS Drugs* **17**:995–1011 (2003).

15. Donnan GA, Davis SM: Neuroimaging, the ischaemic penumbra, and selection of patients for acute stroke therapy, *Lancet Neurol* **1**:417–25 (2002).

16. Kaste M: Reborn workhorse, CT, pulls the wagon toward thrombolysis beyond 3 hours, *Stroke* **35**:357–359 (2004).

17. Moonis M, Fisher M. Imaging of acute stroke, *Cerebrovasc Dis* **11**:143–150 (2001).

18. Heiss WD, Forsting M, Diener HC: Imaging in cerebrovascular disease, *Curr Opin Neurol* **14**:67–75 (2001).

19. Kidwell CS, Villablanca JP, Saver JL: Advances in neuroimaging of acute stroke, *Curr Atheroscler Rep* **2**:126–135 (2000).

20. Jager HR: Diagnosis of stroke with advanced CT and MR imaging, *Br Med Bull* **56**:318–333 (2000).

21. Wintermark M, Bogousslavsky J: Imaging of acute ischemic brain injury: The return of computed tomography, *Curr Opin Neurol* **16**:59–63 (2003).

22. Tomandl BF, Klotz E, Handschu R et al: Comprehensive imaging of ischemic stroke with multisection CT, *Radiographics* **23**:565–592 (2003).

23. Nabavi DG, Kloska SP, Nam EM et al: MOSAIC: Multimodal Stroke Assessment Using Computed Tomography: Novel diagnostic approach for the prediction of infarction size and clinical outcome, *Stroke* **33**:2819–26 (2002).

24. Konig M: Brain perfusion CT in acute stroke: Current status, *Eur J Radiol* (45 Suppl 1): S11–S22 (2003).

25. Latchaw RE, Yonas H, Hunter GJ et al; Council on Cardiovascular Radiology of the American Heart Association. Guidelines and recommendations for perfusion imaging in cerebral ischemia: A scientific statement for healthcare professionals by the writing group on perfusion imaging, from the Council on Cardiovascular Radiology of the American Heart Association, *Stroke* **34**:1084–1104 (2003).

26. Barber PA, Darby DG, Desmond PM et al: Identification of major ischemic change. Diffusion-weighted imaging versus computed tomography, *Stroke* **30**:2059–2065 (1999).

27. Symons SP, Cullen SP, Buonanno F, Gonzalez RG, Lev MH: Noncontrast conventional computed tomography in the evaluation of acute stroke, *Semin Roentgenol* **37**:185–191 (2002).

28. Eastwood JD, Lev MH, Provenzale JM: Perfusion CT with iodinated contrast material, *Am J Roentgenol* **180**:3–12 (2003).

29. Lev MH, Nichols SJ: Computed tomographic angiography and computed tomographic perfusion imaging of hyperacute stroke, *Top Magn Reson Imag* **11**:273–287 (2000).

30. Prokop M, Waaijer A, Kreuzer S: CT angiography of the carotid arteries, *JBR-BTR* **87**:23–29 (2004).

31. Lev MH, Farkas J, Rodriguez VR et al: CT angiography in the rapid triage of patients with hyperacute stroke to intraarterial thrombolysis: Accuracy in the detection of large vessel thrombus, *J Comput Assist Tomogr* **25**:520–528 (2001).

32. Wildermuth S, Knauth M, Brandt T, Winter R, Sartor K, Hacke W: Role of CT angiography in patient selection for thrombolytic therapy in acute hemispheric stroke, *Stroke* **29**:935–938 (1998).

33. Shrier D, Tanaka H, Numaguchi Y, Konno S, Patel U, Shibata D: CT angiography in the evaluation of acute stroke, *Am J Neuroradiol* **18**:1011–1020 (1997).

34. Cumming MJ, Morrow IM: Carotid artery stenosis: A prospective comparison of CT angiography and conventional angiography, *Am J Roentgenol* **163**:517–523 (1994).

35. Ezzeddine MA, Lev MH, McDonald CT et al: CT angiography with whole brain perfused blood volume imaging: Added clinical value in the assessment of acute stroke, *Stroke* **33**:959–966 (2002).

36. Hunter GJ, Hamberg LM, Ponzo JA et al: Assessment of cerebral perfusion and arterial anatomy in hyperacute stroke with three-dimensional functional CT: Early clinical results, *Am J Neuroradiol* **19**:29–37 (1998).

37. Lee KH, Cho SJ, Byun HS et al: Triphasic perfusion computed tomography in acute middle cerebral artery stroke: A correlation with angiographic findings, *Arch Neurol* **57**:990–999 (2000).

38. Grond M, Rudolf J, Schneweis S et al: Feasibility of source images of computed tomographic angiography to detect the extent of ischemia in hyperacute stroke, *Cerebrovasc Dis* **13**:251–256 (2002).

39. Gleason S, Furie KL, Lev MH et al: Potential influence of acute CT on inpatient costs in patients with ischemic stroke, *Acad Radiol* **8**:955–964 (2001).

40. Wintermark M, Maeder P, Thiran JP, Schnyder P, Meuli R: Quantitative assessment of regional cerebral blood flows by perfusion CT studies at low injection rates: A critical review of the underlying theoretical models, *Eur Radiol* **11**:1220–1230 (2001).

41. Kudo K, Terae S, Katoh C, Oka M, Shiga T, Tamaki N, Miyasaka K: Quantitative cerebral blood flow measurement with dynamic perfusion CT using the vascular-pixel elimination method: Comparison with H2(15)O positron emission tomography, *Am J Neuroradiol* **24**:419–426 (2003).

42. Wintermark M, Reichhart M, Cuisenaire O et al: Comparison of admission perfusion computed tomography and qualitative diffusion- and perfusion-weighted magnetic resonance imaging in acute stroke patients, *Stroke* **33**:2025–2031 (2002).

43. Wintermark M, Reichhart M, Thiran JP et al: Prognostic accuracy of cerebral blood flow measurement by perfusion computed tomography, at the time of emergency room admission, in acute stroke patients, *Ann Neurol* **51**:417–432 (2002).

44. Wintermark M, Smith WS, Ko NU, Quist M, Schnyder P, Dillon WP: Dynamic Perfusion CT: Optimizing the Temporal Resolution and Contrast Volume for Calculation of Perfusion CT Parameters in Stroke Patients. *Am J Neuroradiol* **25**:720–729 (2004).

45. Parsons MW, Yang Q, Barber PA et al: Perfusion magnetic resonance imaging maps in hyperacute stroke: Relative cerebral blood flow most accurately identifies tissue destined to infarct, *Stroke* **32**:1581–1587 (2001).

46. Rordorf G, Koroshetz WJ, Copen WA et al: Regional ischemia and ischemic injury in patients with acute middle cerebral artery stroke as defined by early diffusion weighted and perfusion-weighted MRI, *Stroke* **29**:939–943 (1998).

47. Sunshine JL, Bambakidis N, Tarr RW et al: Benefits of perfusion MR imaging relative to diffusion MR imaging in the diagnosis and treatment of hyperacute stroke, *Am J Neuroradiol* **22**:915–921 (2001).

48. Eastwood JD, Lev MH, Wintermark M et al: Correlation of early dynamic CT perfusion imaging with whole-brain MR diffusion and perfusion imaging in acute hemispheric stroke, *Am J Neuroradiol* **24**:1869–1875 (2003).

49. Eastwood JD, Lev MH, Azhari T et al: CT perfusion scanning with deconvolution analysis: Pilot study in patients with acute middle cerebral artery stroke, *Radiology* **222**:227–236 (2002).

50. Lev MH, Segal AZ, Farkas J et al: Utility of perfusion-weighted CT imaging in acute middle cerebral artery stroke treated with intra-arterial thrombolysis: Prediction of final infarct volume and clinical outcome, *Stroke* **32**:2021–2028 (2001).

51. Na DG, Ryoo JW, Lee KH et al: Multiphasic perfusion computed tomography in hyperacute ischemic stroke: Comparison with diffusion and perfusion magnetic resonance imaging, *J Comput Assist Tomogr* **27**:194–206 (2003).

52. Wintermark M, Maeder P, Verdun FR, Thiran JP, Valley JF, Schnyder P, Meuli R: Using 80 kVp versus 120 kVp in perfusion CT measurement of regional cerebral blood flow, *Am J Neuroradiol* **21**:1881–1884 (2000).

53. Smith WS, Roberts HC, Chuang NA et al: Safety and feasibility of a CT protocol for acute stroke: Combined CT, CT angiography, and CT perfusion imaging in 53 consecutive patients, *Am J Neuroradiol* **24**:688–690 (2003).

54. Wintermark M, Fischbein NJ, Smith WS, Ko NU, Quist M, Dillon WP: Accuracy of dynamic perfusion-CT with deconvolution in detecting acute hemispheric stroke, *Am J Neuroradiol* (in press).

55. Nagahori T, Hirashima Y, Umemura K et al: Supratentorial dynamic computed tomography for the diagnosis of vertebrobasilar ischemic stroke, *Neurol Med Chir (Tokyo)* **44**:105–110 (2004).

56. Sorensen AG, Reimer B: *Cerebral MR Perfusion Imaging. Principles and Current Applications*, Thieme, Stuttgart, Germany, 2001.

57. Davis SM, Donnan GA: Neuroprotection: Establishing proof of concept in human stroke, *Stroke* **33**:309–310 (2002).

58. Warach S: New imaging strategies for patient selection for thrombolytic and neuroprotective therapies, *Neurology* **57**(5 Suppl 2): S48–S52 (2001).

59. Jovin TG, Yonas H, Gebel JM, Kanal E, Chang YF, Grahovac SZ, Goldstein S, Wechsler LR: The cortical ischemic core and not the consistently present penumbra is a determinant of clinical outcome in acute middle cerebral artery occlusion, *Stroke* **34**:2426–2433 (2003).

■■■■■■ **CHAPTER 12**

Cerebrovascular Reactivity Changes in Symptomatic Carotid Stenosis

NATAN M. BORNSTEIN and ALEXANDER Y. GUR

Stroke Unit, Department of Neurology, Tel Aviv Sourasky Medical Center, Sackler Faculty of Medicine, Tel Aviv University, Tel Aviv, Israel

Abstract. Hemodynamic factors may play a key role in the occurrence, prediction of severity, progression, and outcome of ischemic stroke. One way of determining cerebral hemodynamic status is by assessing cerebral reactivity, also known as cerebral vasomotor reactivity (VMR), which provides information on cerebral autoregulation and collateral circulation. VMR is defined as a shift in cerebral blood flow or cerebral blood flow velocity before and after the administration of a potent vasodilatory stimulus test. VMR can be assessed by using transcranial Doppler and various vasodilatory tests (the breath-holding or apnea test, CO_2 inhalation, the Diamox (acetazolamide) test, and the L-arginine test). There are several practical applications of the combined transcranial Doppler and the vasodilatory tests in assessing VMR. VMR of the middle cerebral artery has frequently been assessed in patients with extracranial carotid occlusive disease, and several studies showed that high-grade stenosis or occlusion of the internal carotid artery can significantly reduce VMR of the ipsilateral cerebral middle artery. Moreover, the predictive value of impaired VMR for ischemic stroke occurrence was convincingly confirmed in subjects with carotid occlusive disease. Evaluation of VMR in patients with symptomatic carotid stenosis before and after carotid revascularization, patients with bilateral severe carotid stenosis, and patients with total carotid artery occlusion will be discussed.

12.1. INTRODUCTION

The cerebral vasculature has a unique ability to dilate during hypercapnia and to constrict during hypocapnia. These effects of carbon dioxide (CO_2) on the cerebral circulation are demonstrated mostly in resistance brain arterioles and play an

Vascular Hemodynamics: Bioengineering and Clinical Perspectives, Edited by Peter J. Yim
Copyright © 2008 John Wiley & Sons, Inc.

important role in cerebral autoregulation, which enables relatively constant cerebral blood flow (CBF) during variations of cerebral perfusion pressure. Thus, the differences between CBF at rest and after the induction of hypercapnia reflect the state of cerebral vasomotor reactivity (VMR) and, hence, cerebrovascular reserve capacity. VMR is defined as the vasodilation capacity of cerebral arterioles to external stimuli, such as increasing extracellular p_{CO_2} and decreasing extracellular pH. Indeed, VMR can be considered a shift in CBF and cerebral blood flow velocity (BFV) before and after the administration of a potent vasodilatory stimulus test. As an indirect parameter of cerebral autoregulation and collateral circulation, VMR provides important information about the cerebral hemodynamic status. VMR can be assessed by measuring regional CBF using single photon emission computer tomography (SPECT) or positron emission tomography (PET), and by measuring BFV using transcranial Doppler ultrasonography (TCD). At least four vasodilatory tests are currently used for VMR assessment: the breath-holding or apnea test, CO_2 inhalation, the Diamox (acetazolamide) test, and the L-arginine test. The breath-holding maneuver enables the assessment of VMR by means of calculating the breath-holding index (BHI) [1]. The apnea test can be replaced by inhalation of 5% CO_2. During the measurement of CO_2 reactivity, hypercapnia is induced by inhaling a mixture of 2–5% CO_2 in 95–98% oxygen. Measurement of CBF can be performed after stabilization of the end-tidal CO_2 concentration (as determined by capnograph) [2,3]. Diamox (acetazolamide), a potent, reversible inhibitor of carbonic anhydrase, is widely used as a vasodilatory stimulus for evaluating VMR. The enzyme catalyzes the following reaction:

$$CO_2 + H_2O = H_2CO_3 = H^+ + HCO_3^-$$ (12.1)

Although the exact mechanisms by which Diamox acts as a vasodilatory agent and increases the CBF remain controversial, it is most probable that these effects are stimulated by metabolic acidosis and by the direct effect of intravenous administration of 1000 mg acetazolamide on cerebral vessels. Dahl et al. [4] noted that a dose of at least 15 mg/kg body weight (corresponding to 1200 mg in a patient weighing 80 kg) is needed to obtain the maximal vasodilatory effect. Micieli et al. [5] used L-arginine as a vasodilatory agent for pre- and postsurgical evaluations of VMR in patients with severe carotid stenosis undergoing carotid endarterectomy (CEA). L-Arginine induces the vasodilation of resistance vessels, a process that is mediated by nitric oxide (NO) at the endothelial level. Intravenous infusion of L-arginine at a dose of 500 mg/kg per 30 min significantly increases BFV as measured by TCD. Vasodilatory response can be calculated as

$$\frac{\text{BFV after} - \text{BFV before}}{\text{BFV before}} \times 100 = \text{VMR}\%$$ (12.2)

where "BFV after" refers to BFV after the administration of a vasodilatory agent and "BFV before" refers to BFV before the administration of a vasodilatory agent.

Although BFV does not reflect CBF quantitatively, a direct proportion between these two values has been established, assuming that the diameter of the artery remains unchanged [6]. This is due to the fact that volume flow (Q) in a vessel is related to BFV according to the equation

$$Q = \text{BFV} \cdot \pi R^2 \tag{12.3}$$

where R is the vessel radius. Thus, BFV measurements can theoretically provide information regarding changes in volume flow in a supply artery and its perfusion territory if both the diameter of the artery and the size of the perfusion territory remain constant after a vasodilatory stimulus [7,8]. Several studies were performed to compare the relationship between CBF alterations after vasodilatory tests measured by SPECT and PET and changes in BFV after the same stimulus using the TCD technique [8–11]. A good correlation between the methods was found, and this opened a new era of cerebral hemodynamic investigations without requiring invasive and expensive procedures, such as SPECT or PET. The disadvantages of TCD-based methods are that they lack the regional specificity of other methods of CBF measurement, and are not possible in individuals who have no acoustic window.

Comparative investigations have also shown a good correlation when comparing CO_2 inhalation and acetazolamide test results, indicating a strong similarity between the vasodilatative effects of CO_2 and acetazolamide on cerebral arteries [3,8]. The advantages and disadvantages of the two tests are as follows: CO_2 is a more physiologic stimulus and allows CBF measurements using different concentrations. On the other hand, CO_2 inhalation methods require patient cooperation during the investigation ("respiratory work"). CO_2 inhalation is not performed in patients suffering from obstructive respiratory diseases. CO_2 inhalation may cause gasping and fear of death. As for acetazolamide, intravenous administration of 1000 mg achieves a supramaximal dilative effect on resistance arteries, and permits investigation of the time course of the vasodilatory response. Moreover, a 20-min vasodilatory effect of acetazolamide is ideal for hemodynamic studies, and no patient cooperation is required during the investigation. Some contraindications of acetazolamide administration are sulfonamid allergy, raised intracranial pressure, and severe hepatic or renal failure. The side effects of acetazolamide are mild (paresthesias of the extremities and of the face—especially around the mouth and tongue—lightheadedness, and a short-lasting, mild diuretic effect), transient and well tolerated by the majority of patients [12]. VMR can be rated as being either good or impaired. An approximately 40% increase in BFV in the cerebral arteries and a 20–30% increase in CBF after the administration of acetazolamide is indicative of good VMR, based on studies in healthy subjects [13]. Ringelstein [14] found an average of a 50% increase in BFV in normal volunteers after CO_2 inhalation. Markus and Cullinane [15] used a predetermined cutoff value of 20% for 8% CO_2 VMR. Silvestrini et al. [16] suggested a cutoff value of 0.69 for the BHI for distinguishing between an impaired and a normal VMR. Although, these thresholds have not been validated and only approximately demonstrate the exact state of VMR, this demarcation appears to adequately describe the extent of impairment.

12.2. VMR APPLICATIONS

VMR and Carotid Stenosis

The majority of the published VMR studies were performed in patients with carotid occlusive disease. Carotid bifurcation is an important site of the developing atherosclerotic lesion, and the landmark clinical trials, the North American Symptomatic Carotid Endarterectomy Trial (NASCET) Collaboration [17], the European Carotid Surgery Trialist's Collaborative Group [18], and the Asymptomatic Carotid Atherosclerosis Study (ACAS) [19], have conclusively demonstrated the etiologic importance of carotid atherosclerosis in ischemic stroke. In the Harvard stroke registry, 24% of ischemic strokes were due to carotid artery disease [20]. Ischemic stroke is assumed to be caused by several mechanisms, either embolic or hemodynamic. This is especially applicable in patients with severe carotid stenosis, for whom both mechanisms should be considered as being potential etiologies for focal cerebral ischemia. Although the majority of cerebral ischemic events are thromboembolic, hemodynamic factors may play a significant role, and recognition of a hemodynamic high-risk subgroup has important implications for evaluation and management [23]. Impairment of brain hemisphere perfusion begins with an approximately 60% diameter stenosis of the carotid artery [24]. Thus, in certain situations (e.g., carotid occlusive disease), the presence and the state of intracranial collateral blood supply and cerebral autoregulation are clearly very important, and intracranial hemodynamic features might have prognostic value for the symptomatic or asymptomatic course of carotid occlusive disease and stroke recurrence [25]. Significantly reduced VMR has been demonstrated in patients with high-grade stenosis or occlusion of the internal carotid artery (ICA) [26–29]. Only Nighoghossian et al. [30] failed to show any significant difference in postacetazolamide CBF between the patients with ICA high-grade stenosis and control subjects. Fujioka [31] suggested that dilatation of the cerebral resistance vessels occurs in an attempt to maintain stable levels of CBF in these two conditions. This can ultimately lead to the abolition or reduction in the extent to which the cerebral resistance vessels can further dilate in response to additional reduction in flow, whereby VMR is reduced. In spite of unilateral or even bilateral ICA stenosis or occlusion, however, some patients maintain a well-preserved VMR, and this may indicate a sufficient collateral capacity of the circle of Willis and satisfactory cerebral autoregulation. Thus, the intracerebral hemodynamic status of patients with carotid stenosis plays a significant role in stroke incidence and outcome.

Several authors reported higher stroke risk in patients with an impaired VMR in carotid occlusive disease. Kleiser and Widder [2] investigated 85 patients with CO_2 inhalation and found a 55% risk for cerebral ischemic events during a follow-up of 38 ± 15 months in the group with an impaired VMR. Powers et al. [32] found a 29% stroke rate in a one-year follow-up of patients with ICA occlusion revealed by a PET study. Acetazolamide tests assessing VMR provided similar results: 27% of the patients with impaired and 3% with normal VMR suffered from stroke during an 18-month follow-up [33]. Yonas et al. [34] found a 36% stroke risk in an impaired VMR group. The Yonas et al. study [34] was conducted on symptomatic patients, and the authors reported that a compromised VMR increased their risk of recurrent stroke. There is an important difference between asymptomatic and symptomatic patients in terms of their natural history; therefore, the only conclusion that can be drawn from that study is that VMR can serve as a predictor for stroke recurrence but not the relative likelihood of stroke occurrence in asymptomatic patients. Kleiser and Widder [2] performed their cerebral hemodynamic investigations in a combined group of symptomatic and asymptomatic patients. Although they also found a positive relationship between stroke incidence and diminished or impaired cerebrovascular reserve capacity, these results are not necessarily applicable when symptomatic or asymptomatic patients are considered as independent groups. In asymptomatic patients the following studies strongly support the value of the impaired VMR in stroke occurrence. We assessed the VMR in 44 asymptomatic patients with severe unilateral carotid stenosis and followed them in order to evaluate its role in stroke occurrence [35]. During the follow-up period, the overall annual rate was 7.9% for all ischemic cerebral events and 2.3% for ipsilateral stokes. No strokes or transient ischemic attacks (TIAs) occurred in the group with a good VMR, but there were seven cerebral ischemic events (two strokes, one of which was fatal, and five TIAs) in the impaired VMR group. There was a statistically significant association between cerebral ischemic events and impaired VMR ($p < .09$). These findings were confirmed in two subsequent larger prospective, blinded longitudinal studies. In the first, Silvestrini et al. [16] investigated 94 asymptomatic patients with ICA stenosis of at least 70%. They used BHI values and found an annual ipsilateral ischemic event risk of 4.1% in patients with normal BHI values and 13.9% in those with impaired BHI values ($p = .001$; hazard ratio, 0.009; 95% confidence interval 0.02–0.38). Markus and Cullinane [15] studied and followed 107 asymptomatic patients with carotid stenosis and occlusion using TCD and 8% CO_2 inhalation for VMR assessment. There were 11 ipsilateral ischemic events during follow-up (six strokes and five TIAs), and the authors concluded that impaired VMRs of the ipsilateral middle cerebral artery (MCA) predicted ipsilateral stroke and TIA risk. Moreover, impaired VMR remained an independent predictor of ipsilateral stroke or TIA after adjustment for age, gender, hypertension, diabetes, smoking, ipsilateral infarct, and degree of contralateral stenosis. Nicolaides [36] suggested that a high-risk subgroup of asymptomatic patients could be arbitrarily defined as a group that has an annual rate of at least 4% of ipsilateral ischemic cerebrovascular events. Identification of a high-risk group was the main goal of the Asymptomatic Carotid Stenosis and Risk of Stroke Study (ACSRS), with special attention paid to parameters such as plaque morphology, vascular risk factors, silent brain infarcts, progression of stenosis, and VMR [37]. The results of the ACSRS have not yet been published, but those of the other above-cited studies strongly support the value of VMR assessment for identifying patients with carotid stenosis who belong to a high-risk subgroup for whom carotid surgery is justified to prevent ischemic cerebrovascular events.

VMR and Carotid Surgery

The measurements of VMR parameters before and after vascular or endovascular surgery are valuable for examining the effects of revascularization procedures on cerebral hemodynamics in patients with carotid occlusive disease. Several studies confirmed that a revascularization procedure leads to improve VMR in patients with severe carotid stenosis [38–42]. In our study [42], we assessed and compared the effect of CEA on VMR in symptomatic and asymptomatic patients. TCD and the Diamox test were performed before and 3 months after CEA in 42 patients (21 symptomatic, 21 asymptomatic) with severe (70–99%) carotid stenosis. Our data suggested that CEA improves cerebral hemodynamics solely in asymptomatic patients. Others found contradictory results. For instance, Russel et al. [38] used SPECT to evaluate VMR in a symptomatic study cohort and showed that impaired VMR may be improved by surgery on patients with severe carotid stenosis. The same results were achieved by Hartl et al. [40], who used TCD and CO_2 inhalation, but they did not differentiate between asymptomatic and symptomatic patients. Barzó et al. [41] demonstrated normalized VMR following CEA even in the early postoperative period in both asymptomatic and symptomatic patients. Soinne et al. [43] found improved VMR using BHI after CEA only in the symptomatic carotid stenosis patients. Baracchini et al. [44] sought to investigate whether CEA can achieve long-term cerebral hemodynamic improvement and reduce recurrence of cerebral ischemic events in symptomatic and asymptomatic patients with severe (>70%) carotid artery stenosis contralateral to carotid occlusion. Thirty-nine patients with severe carotid lesion contralateral to carotid occlusion were studied before (1 day) and after CEA (at 7 days, 1, 3, and 6 months, and then yearly thereafter). Collateral flow and VMR were assessed by TCD. A total of 32 nonsurgical patients with severe carotid lesion contralateral to carotid occlusion who were comparable with respect to age and sex served as a control group. The average period of TCD follow-up was 10 years and was obtained in all patients; during this period, major clinical events (stroke, acute myocardial infarction, and death) were also recorded. The proportion of patients with collateral flow via the anterior communicating artery increased significantly from 61.5% before to 89.7% after CEA. Cerebral VMR ipsilateral to carotid occlusion improved in 85.7% of patients (30 of 35) within 30 days of CEA, and in all patients within 90 days. No significant spontaneous VMR recovery was recorded in the control group. After the initial recovery, no significant change in VMR was observed in the surgical group or the control group during the follow-up. In conclusion, in patients with severe carotid stenosis, CEA contralateral to symptomatic and asymptomatic carotid occlusion determines a durable cerebral hemodynamic improvement not only on the side of the CEA but also on the contralateral side, with no difference between symptomatic and asymptomatic patients.

In contrast to the important selective role played by VMR assessment in association with carotid surgery, the attempts to use TCD prior to CEA in order to prevent complications during surgery or to assist presurgical planning (e.g., performing CEA with or without a shunt) were less successful. Lucertini et al. [45] evaluated VMR using TCD and the Diamox test as a preoperative tool in predicting cerebral tolerance to carotid clamping in a consecutive series of 115 CEAs. There was no significant difference between the VMR in the shunted subgroup and the nonshunted one. The positive results of prediction of cerebral ischemia during CEA and the indications for clamping were obtained only in one preoperative TCD and CO_2-reactivity study by Lam et al. [46]. The study by Sfyroeras et al. [47] was conducted to determine the effect of carotid angioplasty and stenting on the hemodynamic parameters and VMR of the ipsilateral middle cerebral artery (MCA) and examine the relation between pre-procedural exhausted VMR and perioperative neurological events. The study included 29 (13 symptomatic) patients with severe extracranial carotid stenosis undergoing endovascular procedures. TCD and the breath-holding test were performed before the procedure, 2 days, and 2–4 months postoperatively. When stimulated by breath holding, preoperative mean flow velocity did not increase significantly compared with the resting values; however, it did increase significantly during breath holding in both studies after stenting. The BHI improved significantly from -0.35 (from -0.71 to 0.55) to 0.38 (0.12–0.61) at 2 days and 0.44 (0.31–0.92) at 2–4 months. Exhausted VMR of the MCA preoperatively was associated with increased risk of neurological complications during or after the procedure.

VMR and Total Carotid Occlusion

In symptomatic patients at least two studies failed to demonstrate a major role of reduced vasodilatory capacity in stroke recurrence. Yokota et al. [48] performed a prospective follow-up study in ischemic stroke patients with occlusive carotid disease to determine whether stroke recurrence is related to reduced vasodilatory capacity. They followed 105 consecutive stroke patients with severe internal carotid artery stenosis (>75%) or occlusion for 8 years after examination of their VMR with SPECT and acetazolamide challenge. All patients were divided into either the reduced or normal vasodilatory capacity groups according to the percentage of radioisotope activity changes of a region of interest in the MCA after acetazolamide challenge. After observation period there was no significant difference in stroke recurrence and death between the groups. Moreover, the same authors reported that CBF of the affected hemisphere increased spontaneously within 40 months of stroke [49]. Widder et al. [50] reported that improvement in CO_2 VMR occurs primarily during the first few months after ICA occlusions and in 64% of patients over 5 years. Spontaneous improvement in reduced vasodilator capacity has been demonstrated in medically treated symptomatic patients with carotid occlusion or severe stenosis in the study by Cao et al. [51]. A spontaneous return to normal was observed in 40% of patients with initially abnormal vasodilatory capacity, while 17.6% of patients with initially normal capacity showed an abnormality 1–2 years after the acetazolamide challenge. In the study by Zbornikova [52], the long-term (mean 4.3 ± 1.8 years) follow-up of 27 symptomatic patients with unilateral occlusion of the ICA including repeated tests of VMR by TCD with the Diamox test was not found significant relationship between impaired VMR and new strokes. During the follow-up, seven patients had new strokes (five minor and two major ones), two ipsilateral and four contralateral to the ICA occlusion, and one in the posterior circulation. Four patients died. VMR in the anterior cerebral artery decreased slightly on both the nonoccluded and occluded sides, while impaired VMR $<$ or $= 11\%$ was not significantly connected with new strokes. The opposite results were obtained in the study by Kuroda et al. [53]; 77 symptomatic patients with ICA or MCA occlusion were enrolled in this prospective, longitudinal cohort study. CBF and VMR to acetazolamide were quantitatively determined by the ^{133}Xe SPECT. During an average follow-up period of 42.7 months, 16 total and seven ischemic strokes occurred. When strokes were categorized by patients with and without decreased CBF and VMR, Kaplan–Meier analysis revealed that the annual risks of total and ipsilateral strokes in patients with decreased CBF and VMR were 35.6% and 23.7%, respectively, risks that are higher than those in other types of patients. Provinciali et al. [29] studied a group of 30 patients with symptomatic ICA occlusion and different computed tomography patterns of cerebral ischemia (14 borderzone and/or terminal, 16 territorial) by means of TCD to determine the relationship between VMR and topography of the infarct on computed tomography. The VMR was evaluated by assessing the mean BFV changes observed in the MCA after apnea and Diamox tests. An impairment in the VMR was found in 13 out of 14 patients with borderzone and/or territorial ischemia but in only 1 out 16 patients with complete territorial ischemia. VMR impairment correlated well with the occurrence of borderzone or terminal brain infarcts, which are assumed to have a hemodynamic basis. The annual risk of stroke in patients with symptomatic carotid artery total occlusion and impaired VMR is reportedly ~10–14% versus 4–6% in those with preserved VMR [54,55]. Occlusion of the ICA is associated with a high mortality rate and frequent disability in survivors. In the past, extracranial to intracranial (EC/IC) arterial anastomosis was performed in this category of patients with carotid occlusive disease. The international randomized EC/IC Bypass Study [56] however, failed to confirm the benefit of this treatment when compared to appropriate medical care, and the EC/IC bypass operation has been largely abandoned worldwide since then. The EC/IC bypass results were more recently reevaluated subsequent to the significant progress of surgical techniques and the availability of more advanced tools to identify patients with carotid occlusion and hemodynamic compromise. Karnik et al. [57] and Neff et al. [58] found that EC/IC bypass surgery improves VMR and total brain blood supply in selected patients with unilateral ICA occlusion and insufficient collateralization. In a review on this issue, Herzig et al. [59] analyzed related data and suggested further studies on the subject of VMR testing in patients with ICA occlusion for possible selection of those who would benefit from EC/IC bypass.

VMR and Bilateral Carotid Occlusive Disease

The importance of intracranial hemodynamics increases significantly among subjects with bilateral high-grade ICA stenosis. Bilateral severe ICA stenosis accounts for approximately 10% of carotid occlusive disease [60,61]. This group represents a high-risk population for ischemic stroke as well as for any perioperative vascular complications after heart, carotid, and general surgery [62,63]. Bilateral severe carotid stenosis can result in persistent low-flow states in the cerebral vasculature due to the loss of cerebral autoregulatory mechanisms in chronically dilated intracerebral vessels [64,65]. The data on the intracranial hemodynamic features of bilateral severe carotid stenosis are still scanty. Liu et al. [66] investigated VMR using xenon-CBF measurements and an acetazolamide challenge test in patients with bilateral high-grade ICA stenosis and found no significant differences in the VMR measurements between the territories of bilateral high-grade ICA stenosis. Only four asymptomatic patients with bilateral severe stenosis were studied, and a significant increase of CBF after acetazolamide was found in one of them. Six other patients in this study were diagnosed as having unilateral ICA occlusion with high-grade stenosis on the contralateral side. On the basis of these limited data, the authors did not recommend performing the acetazolamide test to assess VMR.

Vernieri et al. [67] measured cerebral hemodynamics in patients with carotid artery occlusion and contralateral moderate or severe ICA stenosis. VMR in the MCA was evaluated by calculating the BHI. Their data demonstrated that the cerebral hemodynamic status of patients with occlusive ICA disease is influenced by individual anatomic and functional characteristics, with particular focus on collateral pathways. Matteis et al. [68] used TCD and BHI to evaluate patterns of VMR in asymptomatic and symptomatic patients with carotid occlusion and severe contralateral stenosis. A significant decrease of VMR on the occluded side was observed in symptomatic patients compared to asymptomatic ones. Moreover, VMR on the stenotic side was significantly higher in the asymptomatic but not in the symptomatic patients. In that study, the patterns of VMR in patients with severe bilateral carotid occlusive disease were strictly dependent on the presence of previous symptoms. Similar results were obtained by Reinhard et al. [69], who assessed VMR as a part of the analysis of dynamic cerebral autoregulation and collateral flow patterns in patients with bilateral severe carotid artery stenosis or occlusion. We evaluated the cerebral hemodynamic features of patients with severe bilateral carotid stenosis by assessing and comparing VMR in the MCA and vertebral arteries by TCD and the Diamox test [70]. We found that VMR of the MCA in symptomatic patients with bilateral severe carotid stenosis is significantly lower than in asymptomatic ones and, in contrast, that VMR of the posterior circulation remains similar in patients with an either symptomatic or asymptomatic course of bilateral carotid stenosis. These data are in accordance with our previous study, in which we assessed VMR of the posterior circulation in patients with carotid occlusive disease [71]. Our findings suggest an independent cerebrovascular reserve capacity of posterior circulation in the presence of carotid occlusive disease, and a key role of the circle of Willis in the intracerebral hemodynamics.

12.3. CONCLUSIONS

In summary, VMR assessment is useful for detecting the altered cerebral hemodynamics in the different categories of symptomatic carotid occlusive disease and selecting candidates for revascularization procedures. The implementation of VMR testing in routine clinical practice might be of vital importance, and we believe that this method will be an indispensable tool of vascular neurology in the future.

REFERENCES

1. Silvestrini M, Troisi E, Matteis M et al: Transcranial Doppler assessment of cerebrovascular reactivity in symptomatic and asymptomatic severe carotid stenosis, *Stroke* **27**:1970–1973 (1996).
2. Kleiser B, Widder B: Course of carotid artery occlusions with impaired cerebrovascular reactivity, *Stroke* **23**:171–174 (1992).
3. Ringelstein EB, Van-Eyck S, Mertens I: Evaluation of cerebral vasomotor reactivity by various vasodilating stimuli: Comparison of CO_2 to acetazolamide, *J Cereb Blood Flow Metab* **12**:162–168 (1992).
4. Dahl A, Russell D, Rootwelt K et al: Cerebral vasoreactivity assessed with transcranial Doppler and regional cerebral blood flow measurements: Dose, serum concentration, and time of the response to acetazolamide, *Stroke* **26**:2302–2306 (1995).
5. Micieli G, Bosone D, Zappoli F et al: Vasomotor response to CO_2 and L-arginine in patients with severe internal carotid artery stenosis; pre- and post-surgical evaluation with transcranial Doppler, *J Neurol Sci* **163**:153–158 (1999).
6. Aaslid R, Lindegaard K-F, Sorteberg W et al: Cerebral autoregulation dynamics in humans, *Stroke* **20**:45–52 (1989).
7. Giller CA, Bowman G, Dyer H et al: Cerebral arterial diameters during changes in blood pressure and carbon dioxide during craniotomy, *Neurosurgery* **32**:737–741 (1993).
8. Dahl A, Russel D, Nyberg-Hansen R et al: Cerebral vasoreactivity in unilateral carotid artery disease. A comparison of blood flow velocity and regional cerebral blood flow measurements, *Stroke* **25**:621–626 (1994).
9. Dahl A, Lindegaard K-F, Russel D et al: A comparison of transcranial Doppler and cerebral blood flow studies to assess cerebral vasoreactivity, *Stroke* **23**:15–19 (1992).
10. Rosenkranz K, Hierholzer J, Langer R et al: Acetazolamide stimulation test in patients with unilateral internal carotid artery obstructions using transcranial Doppler and 99mTc-HMPAO-SPECT, *Neurol Res* **14**:135–138 (1992).
11. Vorstrup S, Brun B, Lassen NA: Evaluation by the acetazolamide test before EC-IC bypass surgery in patients with occlusion of the internal carotid artery, *Stroke* **17**:1291–1298 (1986).

12. Settakis G, Molnar C, Kerenyi L et al: Acetazolamide as a vasodilatory stimulus in cerebrovascular diseases and in conditions affecting the cerebral vasculature, *Eur J Neurol* **10**:609–620 (2003).

13. Sorteberg W, Lindegaard KF, Rootwelt K et al: Effect of acetazolamide on cerebral artery blood velocity and regional cerebral blood flow in normal subjects, *Acta Neurochir* (Wien) **97**:139–145 (1989).

14. Ringelstein EB: CO_2-reactivity: Dependence from collateral circulation and significance in symptomatic and asymptomatic patients, in Caplan LR, Shifrin EG, Nicolaides AN, Moore WS, eds, *Cerebrovascular Ischemia. Investigation and Management*, Med-Orion Publishing, Nicosia, 1996, pp 149–154.

15. Markus H, Cullinane M: Severely impaired cerebrovascular reactivity predicts stroke and TIA risk in patients with carotid artery stenosis and occlusion, *Brain* **124**:457–467 (2001).

16. Silvestrini M, Vernieri F, Pasqualetti P et al: Impaired cerebral vasoreactivity and risk of stroke in patients with asymptomatic carotid artery stenosis, *JAMA* **283**:2122–2127 (2000).

17. North American Symptomatic Carotid Endarterectomy Trial (NASCET) Collaboration: Beneficial effect of carotid endarterectomy in asymptomatic patients with high-grade carotid stenosis, *N Engl J Med* **325**:445–453 (1991).

18. European Carotid Surgery Trialist's Collaborative Group: MRC European Carotid Surgery Trial: Interim results for symptomatic patients with severe (70–99%) or mild (0–29%) carotid stenosis, *Lancet* **337**:1235–1243 (1991).

19. Asymptomatic Carotid Atherosclerosis Study (ACAS); Executive Committee for the Asymptomatic Carotid Atherosclerosis Study: Endarterectomy for asymptomatic carotid stenosis, *JAMA* **273**:1421–1428 (1995).

20. Mohr JR, Caplan LR, Melski JW et al: The Harvard Cooperative Stroke Registry: A prospective registry, *Neurology* **28**:754–762 (1978).

21. Piepgras A, Schmiedek P, Leinsinger G et al: A simple test to assess cerebrovascular reserve capacity using transcranial Doppler sonography and acetazolamide, *Stroke* **21**:1306–1311 (1990).

22. Chimowitz MB, Furlan AJ, Jones SC et al: Transcranial Doppler assessment of cerebral perfusion reserve in patients with carotid occlusive disease and no evidence of cerebral infarction, *Neurology* **43**:353–357 (1993).

23. Bladin CF, Chambers BR: Frequency and pathogenesis of hemodynamic stroke, *Stroke* **25**:2179–2182 (1994).

24. Archie JP, Feldman RW: Critical stenosis of the internal carotid artery, *Surgery* **89**:67–72 (1981).

25. Derdeyn CP, Grubb RL, Powers WJ: Cerebral hemodynamic impairment. Methods of measurement and association with stroke risk, *Neurology* **53**:251–259 (1999).

26. Bishop CCR, Powell S, Insall M et al: Effect of internal carotid artery occlusion on middle cerebral artery blood flow at rest and in response to hypercapnia, *Lancet* **29**:710–712 (1986).

27. Ringelstein EB, Sievers C, Ecker S et al: Noninvasive assessment of CO_2-induced cerebral vasomotor response in normal individuals and patients with internal carotid artery occlusions, *Stroke* **19**:963–969 (1988).

28. Norris JM, Krajewski A, Bornstein NM: The clinical role of the cerebral collateral circulation in carotid occlusion, *J Vasc Surg* **12**:113–118 (1990).

29. Provinciali L, Ceravolo MG, Minciotti P: A transcranial Doppler study of vasomotor reactivity in symptomatic carotid occlusion, *Cerebrovasc Dis* **3**:27–32 (1993).

30. Nighoghossian N, Trouillas P, Philippon B et al: Cerebral blood flow reserve assessment in symptomatic versus asymptomatic high-grade internal carotid artery stenosis, *Stroke* **25**:1010–1013 (1994).

31. Fujioka KA: Transcranial Doppler sonography in extracranial arterial occlusive disease, *Symposium and Tutorials on Cerebral Hemodynamics*, 1995, pp 57–60.

32. Powers WJ, Tempel LW, Grubb RL: Influence of cerebral hemodynamics on stroke risk: One-year follow-up of 30 medically treated patients, *Ann Neurol* **25**:325–331 (1989).

33. Durham SR, Smith HA, Rutigliano MJ: Assessment of cerebral vasoreactivity and stroke risk using Xe-CT acetazolamide challenge (abstract), *Stroke* **22**:138 (1991).

34. Yonas H, Smith HA, Durham SR et al: Increased stroke risk predicted by compromised cerebral blood flow reactivity, *J Neurosurg* **79**:483–489 (1993).

35. Gur AY, Bova I, Bornstein NM: Is impaired cerebral vasomotor reactivity a predictive factor of stroke in asymptomatic patients? *Stroke* **22**:2188–2190 (1996).

36. Nicolaides AN: Asymptomatic carotid stenosis. The "doctor's dilemma," *Int Angiol* **14**:1–4 (1995).

37. Nicolaides AN: Asymptomatic Carotid Stenosis and the Risk of Stroke (The ACSRS Study): Identification of a high risk group, in Caplan LR, Shifrin EG, Nicolaides AN, Moore WS, eds, *Cerebrovascular Ischemia. Investigation and Management*, Med-Orion Publishing, Nicosia, 1996, pp 435–441.

38. Russel D, Dybevold S, Kjartansson O et al: Cerebral vasoreactivity and blood flow before and 3 months after carotid endarterectomy, *Stroke* **21**:1029–1032 (1990).

39. Demarin V, Rundek T, Despot I et al: Importance of the evaluation of cerebral vasoreactive capacity in the indication for carotid endarterectomy, *Angiologia* **45**:10–15 (1993).

40. Hartl WH, Janssen I, Fürst H: Effect of carotid endarterectomy on patterns of cerebrovascular reactivity in patients with unilateral carotid artery stenosis, *Stroke* **25**:1952–1957 (1994).

41. Barzó P, Vörös E, Bodosi M: Use of transcranial Doppler sonography and acetazolamide test to demonstrate changes in cerebrovascular reserve capacity following carotid endarterectomy, *Eur J Vasc Endovasc Surg* **11**:83–89 (1996).

42. Bornstein N, Gur A, Shifrin E, Morag B: Does carotid endarterectomy modify cerebral vasomotor reactivity? *Cerebrovasc Dis* **7**:201–204 (1997).

43. Soinne L, Helenius J, Tatlisumak T et al: Cerebral hemodynamics in asymptomatic and symptomatic patients with high-grade carotid stenosis undergoing carotid endarterectomy, *Stroke* **34**:1655–1661 (2003).

44. Baracchini C, Meneghetti G, Manara R et al: Cerebral hemodynamics after contralateral carotid endarterectomy in patients with symptomatic and asymptomatic carotid occlusion: A 10-year follow-up. *J Cereb Blood Flow Metab* **26**:899–905 (2006).

45. Lucertini G, Cariati P, Ermirio D et al: Can cerebral vasoreactivity predict cerebral tolerance to carotid clamping during carotid endarterectomy? *Cardiovasc Surg* **10**:123–127 (2002).

46. Lam JM, Smielewski P, al-Rawi P et al: Prediction of cerebral ischaemia during carotid endarterectomy with preoperative CO_2-reactivity studies and angiography, *Br J Neurosurg* **14**:441–448 (2000).

47. Sfyroeras G, Karkos CD, Liasidis C et al: The impact of carotid stenting on the hemo-dynamic parameters and cerebrovascular reactivity of the ipsilateral middle cerebral artery, *J Vasc Surg* **44**:1016–1022 (2006).

48. Yokota C, Hasegawa Y, Minematsu K et al: Effect of acetazolamide reactivity on long-term outcome in patients with major cerebral artery occlusive diseases, *Stroke* **29**:640–644 (1998).

49. Toyoda K, Minematsu K, Yamaguchi T: Long-term changes in cerebral blood flow according to different types of ischemic stroke, *J Neurol Sci* **121**:222–228 (1994).

50. Widder B, Kleiser B, Krapf H: Course of cerebrovascular reactivity in patients with carotid artery occlusion, *Stroke* **25**:1963–1967 (1994).

51. Cao B, Haseqawa Y, Yokota C et al: Spontaneous improvement in reduced vasodila-tory capacity in major cerebral arterial occlusive disease, *Neuroradiology* **42**:19–25 (2000).

52. Zbornikova V: Long term follow-up of unilateral occlusion of the internal carotid artery including repeated tests of vasomotor reactivity by transcranial Doppler, *Neurol Res* **28**:220–224 (2006).

53. Kuroda S, Houkin K, Kamiyama H et al: Long-term prognosis of medically treated patients with internal carotid or middle cerebral artery occlusion: can acetazolamide test predict it? *Stroke* **32**:2110–2116 (2001).

54. Klijn CJ, Kappelle LJ, Tulleken CA et al: Symptomatic carotid artery occlusion. A reappraisal of hemodynamic factors, *Stroke* **28**:2084–2093 (1997).

55. Vernieri F, Pasqualetti P, Passarelli F et al: Outcome of carotid artery occlusion is predicted by cerebrovascular reactivity, *Stroke* **30**:593–598 (1999).

56. The EC-IC Bypass Study Group: Failure of extracranial intracranial bypass to reduce the risk of ischemic stroke, *N Engl J Med* **313**:1191–1200 (1985).

57. Karnik R, Valentin A, Ammerer H-P et al: Elevation of vasomotor reactivity by transcranial Doppler and acetazolamide test before and after extracranial-intracranial bypass in patients with internal carotid artery occlusion, *Stroke* **23**:812–817 (1992).

58. Neff KW, Horn P, Dinter D et al: Extracranial-intracranial arterial bypass surgery improves total brain blood supply in selected symptomatic patients with unilateral internal carotid artery occlusion and insufficient collateralization, *Neuroradiology* **46**:730–737 (2004).

59. Herzig R, Hlustik P, Urbanek K et al: Can we identify patients with carotid occlu-sion who would benefit from EC/IC bypass? (Review) *Biomed Papers* **148**:119–122 (2004).

60. Fraunhofer S, Kiossis D, Helmberger H, Von Sommoggy S, Maurer P: High-degree bilateral carotid stenoses, *Vasa* **23**:125–130 (1994).

61. Robless P, Emson M, Thomas D et al: Are we detecting and operating on high risk patients in the asymptomatic carotid surgery trial? The Asymptomatic Carotid Surgery Trial Collaborators, *Eur J Vasc Endovasc Surg* **16**:59–64 (1998).

62. Fraunhofer S, Kiossis D, Helmberger H, Von Sommoggy S, Maurer P: Severe bilateral carotid stenosis, *J Maladies Vasc* **18**:225–228 (1993).

63. Evans BA, Wijdicks EF: High-grade carotid stenosis detected before general surgery: Is endarterectomy indicated? *Neurology* **57**:1328–1330 (2001).

64. Furst H, Hartl WH, Janssen I: Patterns of cerebrovascular reactivity in patients with unilateral asymptomatic carotid artery stenosis, *Stroke* **25**:1193–1200 (1994).

65. White RP, Markus HS: Impaired dynamic cerebral autoregulation in carotid artery stenosis, *Stroke* **28**:1340–1344 (1997).

66. Liu H-M, Tu Y-K, Yip P-K, Su C-T: Cerebral blood flow and cerebrovascular reactivity capacity in patients with bilateral high-grade stenosis, *Acta Neurol Scand* **166**:90–92 (1996).

67. Vernieri F, Pasqualetti P, Diomedi M et al: Cerebral hemodynamics in patients with carotid artery occlusion and contralateral moderate or severe internal carotid artery stenosis, *J Neurosurg* **94**:559–564 (2001).

68. Matteis M, Vernieri F, Caltagirone C et al: Patterns of cerebrovascular reactivity in patients with carotid artery occlusion and severe contralateral stenosis, *J Neurol Sci* **168**:47–51 (1999).

69. Reinhard M, Muller T, Roth M et al: Bilateral severe carotid artery stenosis or occlusion—cerebral autoregulation dynamics and collateral flow patterns, *Acta Neirochir* (Wien) **145**:1053–1059 (2003).

70. Gur AY, Bornstein NM: Cerebral vasomotor reactivity of bilateral severe carotid stenosis: Is stroke unavoidable? *Eur J Neurol* **13**:183–186 (2006).

71. Gur AY, Bornstein NM: Cerebral vasomotor reactivity of the posterior circulation in patients with carotid occlusive disease, *Eur J Neurol* **10**:75–78 (2003).

■■■■■■■ CHAPTER 13

Essential Hypertension, Cerebrovascular Reactivity, and Risk of Stroke

CRISTINA SIERRA

Hypertension and Geriatrics Units, Department of Internal Medicine, Hospital Clinic of Barcelona, University of Barcelona, Spain

Abstract.   Stroke is the third most frequent cause of death after cancer and heart disease in developed countries and one of the most common reasons for developing cognitive impairment and vascular dementia. High blood pressure (BP) is a major risk factor for stroke, and a continuous relationship between BP and the occurrence of stroke has been well established. Hypertension may also predispose to the development of more subtle cerebral processes based on arteriolar narrowing or pathological microvascular changes. Indeed, high BP influences the cerebral circulation, causing adaptive vascular changes. It has been suggested that changes in cerebral hemodynamics may play a role in the development of these early cerebral changes related to high BP.

Transcranial Doppler sonography has been extensively used in various clinical situations, and since the mid-1980s has established its role in the management of patients with cerebrovascular disease and stroke. Transcranial Doppler provides continuous recordings of the instantaneous flow velocity in cerebral arteries and veins, and it has become widely used in assessing cerebral vasomotor reactivity that provides information regarding cerebral autoregulation and collateral circulation.

Hypertension influences the autoregulation of cerebral blood flow by shifting both the lower and upper limits of autoregulatory capacity toward higher BP, while hypertensive patients may be especially vulnerable to episodes of hypotension, which may play a role in the development of silent cerebrovascular damage, such as white matter lesions or lacunar infarct. The presence of silent cerebrovascular damage is an important prognostic factor for developing stroke.

Prospective studies are necessary to elucidate the role of a decreased cerebral vasomotor reactivity as a risk factor for first-ever and recurrent stroke.

Vascular Hemodynamics: Bioengineering and Clinical Perspectives, Edited by Peter J. Yim
Copyright © 2008 John Wiley & Sons, Inc.

13.1. INTRODUCTION

Stroke is the third most frequent cause of death after cancer and heart disease in developed countries and one of the most common reasons for developing cognitive impairment and vascular dementia [1]. High blood pressure (BP) is a major risk factor for stroke, and a lineal relationship between BP and the occurrence of stroke has been well established [2,3]. On the other hand, evidence from hypertension treatment trials has shown that relatively small reductions in BP (5–6 mmHg in diastolic BP, 10–12 mmHg in systolic BP over 3–5 years) reduce the risk of stroke by more than one-third [4]. The primary prevention of stroke through antihypertensive therapy and BP control is well established. Likewise, higher BP levels after stroke increase the risk of recurrent stroke [5], and more recent trials indicate that BP reduction with combined antihypertensive therapy is beneficial in reducing stroke recurrence [6].

Hypertension is known to be the most important factor for developing macrovascular cerebral complications such as stroke and, consequently, vascular dementia [2,3,7]. Hypertension may also predispose to the development of more subtle cerebral processes, based on arteriolar narrowing or pathological microvascular changes.

The brain is highly vulnerable to the deleterious effects of elevated BP. Systolic and diastolic hypertension in both men and women are well-established risk factors for the development of ischemic and hemorrhagic stroke. Hypertension is a major risk factor for two distinct kinds of vascular problems: (1) the complications of atherosclerosis, including cerebral infarction; and (2) the complications of hypertensive small-vessel disease, including intracerebral haemorrhage and lacunar infarctions, and cerebral white-matter lesions. In some cases, some of these lesions, such as lacunar infarcts and cerebral white-matter lesions (WMLs), may be silent and detectable only by radiological findings.

The presence of cerebral WML is an important prognostic factor for the development of stroke [8,9], cognitive impairment [10], and dementia [11]. Older age and hypertension are constantly reported to be the main risk factors for cerebral WML [12]. A hemodynamic contribution to WML has been found [13]. It has been suggested that changes in cerebral hemodynamics may play a role in the development of WML [13]. Cerebral hypoperfusion may be an early feature in the development of WML and, consequently, the development of stroke. Nevertheless, the question of whether hypoperfusion is a primary pathogenic mechanism or simply a secondary effect of damaged tissue remains unanswered.

Transcranial Doppler (TCD) has been extensively used in various clinical situations, and since the mid-1980s has established its role in the management of patients with cerebrovascular disease and stroke. According to the Doppler principle, it uses ultrasound waves to insonate the blood vessels supplying the brain to obtain hemodynamic information. Anatomic abnormalities of vascular occlusion, stenosis, and spasm can be indirectly derived. Intracranial arterial disease is an important cause of ischemic stroke, and TCD can detect these with a fair amount of sensitivity and specificity. In hemodynamically significant extracranial internal carotid artery disease, TCD shows significant abnormalities in flow dynamics of the anterior circulation and abnormalities of cerebral vasomotor reactivity. TCD ultrasonography is a noninvasive examination method, is relatively inexpensive, and can be performed at bedside.

13.2. EPIDEMIOLOGY OF VASCULAR CEREBRAL DAMAGE

Hypertension represents a relative risk of stroke up to 6 times [14], while stroke is the most frequent complication in hypertensives (Figure 13.1) [15]. As mentioned above, stroke is one of the leading causes of death worldwide and of disability in developed countries, and also a major economic burden with a considerable public health impact. In Western countries, ischemic stroke accounts for approximately 80% of all stroke and hemorrhagic stroke for the remaining 20%. Incidence rates, commonly quoted at 2 per 1000 population, rise steeply from less than 1 per 1000 among people aged <45 years, to more than 15 per 1000 among those aged ≥85 years, but vary widely [16]. In industrialized countries, approximately 75% of all strokes occur in people aged >65 years. Around 80% of people survive the first 4 weeks following stroke, and 70% survive for a year or more. Prevalence rates exceed 8 per 1000 adults with a similarly marked age gradient [16], suggesting future pressure on health services. Disabilities are common and sometimes severe among stroke survivors, requiring increased formal and informal care.

Prevalence of Cerebral White-Matter Lesions

Various studies have examined the prevalence of WML in both normotensive and hypertensive subjects. The ARIC study [17] reported a prevalence of WML of 24.6% in individuals aged 55–72 years, 49% of whom were hypertensive. The Cardiovascular Health Study [18] found a prevalence of 33.3% in individuals

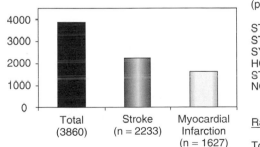

11 Trials
(published between 1991 and 2000):

STOP-1, SHEP,
STONE, SYST-EUR,
SYST-CHINA,
HOT, CAPPP,
STOP 2, NICS,
NORDIL, INSIGHT

Randomized Patients: 59.550

Total Stroke: 2.233
Total Myocardial Infarction: 1.627

Figure 13.1. Number of fatal and nonfatal cerebral strokes and fatal and nonfatal myocardial infarctions reported in large prospective hypertension trials published after 1990. (Adapted from Kjeldsen et al. [15].)

aged $\geq$65 years, 44% of whom were hypertensive. The prevalence was 27% in the Rotterdam Study [19], which included individuals aged 65–84 years, 39% of whom were hypertensive. Shimada et al. [20] studied 28 normotensives and 20 hypertensives aged 59–83 years and found a prevalence of advanced WML of 25% and 40%, respectively. Goldstein et al. [21] found a prevalence of WML of 54.9% in 144 normotensive individuals aged 55–79 years (10% with casual BP elevations). The differences in prevalence between studies may be due to subtle variations in WML assessment, but especially to the impact of risk factors, such as age and hypertension, which are influenced by study selection criteria. Most studies included both normotensive and hypertensive patients (untreated and treated), or subjects with a wide age ranges or only elderly people. Our group found a prevalence of WML of 40.9% in a cohort of 66 untreated hypertensives aged 50–60 years [22].

13.3. HIGH BLOOD PRESSURE AND RISK OF STROKE

Overviews of large-scale observational studies have demonstrated that usual levels of BP are positively and continuously associated with the risk of stroke in a loglinear fashion [23]. This relationship between BP and stroke holds over a wide BD range, from systolic levels as low as 115 mmHg and diastolic levels as low as 70 mmHg [23]. Data from prospective observational studies indicate that usual levels of BP are directly and continuously related to the risk of initial stroke and a prolonged difference in usual BP levels of just 9/5 mmHg is associated with an approximately one-third difference in stroke risk, with similar proportional effects in hypertensives and normotensives [3,4]. Each 5–6 mmHg reduction in usual diastolic BP is associated with a 38% lower risk of stroke [4]. Elevated BP is positively associated with both ischemic and hemorrhagic stroke, but the association appears to be steeper for hemorrhagic stroke. The relationship between BP and stroke risk remains virtually unchanged after adjustment for serum cholesterol levels, smoking, alcohol, or a history of previous cardiovascular disease [23]. Similar associations appear to exist between BP and the risk of recurrent stroke, although much of the evidence on recurrent stroke comes from smaller cohort and observational studies [23]. Data from the United Kingdom Transient Ischemic Attack (UK TIA) Collaborative Group showed that a 10 mmHg reduction in usual systolic BP was associated with a 28% reduction in the risk of recurrent stroke [24].

Although a continuous relationship between both systolic and diastolic BP and the occurrence of stroke has been well established, there is epidemiological evidence from the Multiple Risk Factor Intervention Trial (MRFIT) study that the systolic component of BP may exert a strong deleterious effect on cerebrovascular disease [25]. It is known that increased arterial stiffness results in increased characteristic impedance of the aorta and increased pulsed-wave velocity, which increases systolic and pulse pressures. Large-artery stiffness is the main determinant of pulse pressure. Data from the Systolic Hypertension Elderly Program

(SHEP) study show an 11% increase in stroke risk and a 16% increase in the risk of all-causes mortality for each 10-mmHg increase in pulse pressure [26]. Laurent et al. [27], in a longitudinal study, found that aortic stiffness, assessed by carotid–femoral pulsed-wave velocity, is an independent predictor of fatal stroke in patients with essential hypertension.

High Blood Pressure and White-Matter Lesions

The association between hypertension and WML has been established in cross-sectional [12,17–20] and longitudinal studies [28–30]. However, some reports have suggested that this relationship is evident only when 24-h ambulatory BP monitoring (ABPM) is used to assess BP. Goldstein et al. [21] found a correlation between WML and office systolic, but not diastolic, BP, in a group of elderly normotensive subjects. Conversely, the severity of WML correlated with both systolic and diastolic BP, measured by ABPM. In a group of mixed normotensives, "white coat" hypertensives and sustained hypertensives, Shimada et al. [20] also found a correlation between the number of lacunae and periventricular hyperintensities with 24-h BP, but not with office BP. Sierra et al. [22] found a correlation between WML and both clinic and 24-h ABPM in 66 untreated middle-aged hypertensive patients. This study also showed higher BP values (including office, 24-h, daytime, and nighttime estimates) in hypertensive patients with WML, compared with those without [22].

With respect to the circadian pattern of BP, Kario et al. [31] reported that both nondippers (nocturnal BP fall less than 10%) and extreme dippers (nocturnal BP fall more than 20%) had significantly more silent cerebrovascular damage (measuring both lacunar infarcts and WML) than did dippers (nocturnal BP fall within 10–20%). Although BP variability has been related to target organ damage in hypertension, its relationship with cerebral alterations has not been established. A report by Goldstein et al. [21] suggested a higher standard deviation of waking systolic BP in patients with more severe WML. In contrast, neither the circadian rhythm nor the long-term variability of BP were related to WML in a group of 66 middle-aged never-treated hypertensive patients [22].

13.4. TRANSCRANIAL DOPPLER AND CEREBRAL HEMODYNAMICS

Theoretical Background and Cerebral Blood Flow

The Doppler principle as we know it in physics is a wave theory that describes the relationship between velocity of objects and transmitted or received wave frequencies. Transcranial Doppler (TCD) provides continuous recordings of the instantaneous flow velocity in cerebral arteries and veins. The human brain receives blood through defined cerebral artery systems; each system consists of a cerebral artery with its branches extending down through the level of the capillaries. When investigating the cerebral circulation, we thus examine the behavior of the blood flow at certain points along these transmission lines. Transcranial

Doppler records the blood velocities in precerebral neck arteries as well as in the basal cerebral arteries and their branches. When relating cerebral artery blood velocity to hemispheric blood flow, velocity recordings from the mainstem middle cerebral artery (MCA) is the prime choice (insonating through the temporal bone).

The mechanics of flow in a vascular bed are usually simplified to three concepts: (1) perfusion pressure, the pressure differential between the inflow side and the outflow side; (2) the resistance to flow; and (3) the resultant flow volume.

In the cerebral circulation, the perfusion pressure is the difference between the arterial BP and the intracranial pressure (ICP) because the venous pressure inside the dura cannot possibly be lower than the ICP, due to the collapsible walls of the veins. The concept of cerebrovascular resistance (CVR) is sometimes assumed to have been borrowed from electrical theory (Ohm's law), but the basis for this concept is Poiseuille's law for steady laminar flow in long cylindrical tubes. According to this concept, cerebral blood flow (CBF) at any time should be given by

$$CBF = \frac{arterial\ BP - ICP}{CVR} = \frac{cerebral\ perfusion\ pressure}{CVR}$$

Assuming constant CVR (no autoregulation or other factors changing the caliber of the resistance vessels), flow and pressure would be perfectly proportional to flow, going to zero with zero perfusion pressure.

Central arteries and the aorta are elastic to buffer the intermittent ejection of the left ventricle. This effect serves to preserve the systolic energy release to maintain perfusion in diastole. The distance from the basal cerebral arteries to the vascular bed is short, and the cerebral conductance arteries are stiff. The compliance of the microcirculation itself is unknown, but some studies have indicated that cerebral vascular compliance introduces only small errors in the flow pulse waveform [32].

Pulsatility Index

The first attempts to use Doppler to estimate vascular resistance and tone employed so-called pulsatility indices. The development of a resistance index for Doppler recordings was originally based on the assumption of the interplay between the resistance and compliance c13s of the vascular bed. Pulsatility analysis, the investigation of the excursions of the blood velocity waveform during one cardiac cycle, is commonly used in clinical and scientific studies. The indices of pulsatility most frequently used is that based on work on peripheral arterial disease by Gosling et al. [33] and defined as the maximal vertical excursion of the waveform divided by its mean height. The pulsatility index (PI) is given by the following formula [33]:

$$PI = \frac{highest\ systolic\ velocity - velocity\ at\ end\ of\ diastole}{mean\ velocity}$$

The pulsatility index measured by TCD characterizes the shape of a spectral waveform. This index is postulated to reflect the degree of downstream vascular resistance [34]. An increase in cerebral vascular resistance could be due to narrowing of the small vessels by lipohialynosis and microatherosclerosis.

Cerebrovascular Reactivity

Critically reduced perfusion pressure in the cerebral arteries may lead to functional ischemic impairment or even ischemic tissue damage in certain vulnerable areas of the brain. The main reasons for a reduction of cerebral perfusion in humans are severe extracranial occlusive disease, and an unfavorable configuration of the circle of Willis. Such conditions may lead to borderzone infarctions of the cortex, infarctions in the terminal supply area of the long perforating arteries, and more diffuse selective ischemic neuronal damage in certain critical layers of the hippocampus and basal ganglia. The perfusion pressure of the brain cannot be measured directly in humans. Parameters indirectly reflecting cerebral perfusion pressure are (1) the regional CBF/regional cerebral blood volume ratio, evaluated by either positron emission tomography (PET) scan or single photon emission computed tomography (SPECT) or (b) the reactivity of the cerebral vasculature to various vasodilating stimuli (CO_2, acetazolamide), evaluated by either regional CBF techniques or TCD. As mentioned before, the measurement of cerebral hemodynamics by TCD is a noninvasive technique and simpler than other complex methods (SPECT, PET, xenon computed tomography) to investigate cerebral hemodynamics.

Transcranial Doppler sonography has become widely used in assessing cerebral vasomotor reactivity that provides information regarding cerebral autoregulation and collateral circulation. Cerebrovascular reactivity, also known as cerebral vasomotor reactivity (VMR), is defined as a shift between cerebral blood flow or cerebral blood velocity before and after administration of a potent vasodilatory stimulus test. Three such tests are currently used for this purpose: the apnea test (breath-holding index), CO_2 inhalation, and the Diamox test (IV acetazolamide), all of which are based on the dilatatory response of cerebral blood flow to hypercapnia. Certain advantages of the Diamox test were described, but each of the three tests has its strong and weak points. There are several practical applications of the combined TCD and the vasodilatory tests in assessing cerebral VMR (Table 13.1). However, further large-scale studies are needed in order to better support, with more scientific evidence, and to augment the applications of cerebral vasomotor reactivity assessment in the clinical setting.

Early investigators of cerebral VMR used CO_2 as cerebral vasodilating stimuli. However, patients with chronic lung disease, or those with coronary heart disease and congestive heart failure would not be able to perform this test. In contrast, acetazolamide testing is influenced less by the patient's cooperation. Acetazolamide is a selective inhibitor of carbonic anhydrase. One gram of this drug given intravenously increases CBF by more than 50%, in 10–20 min. Both techniques are comparable in their potential to identify patients with severely reduced cerebral perfusion pressure.

TABLE 13.1. Possible Applications of Combined Transcranial Doppler and Vasodilatory Tests in Assessing of Cerebral Vasomotor Reactivity

To evaluate the intracranial hemodynamic status in patients with carotid occlusive
   disease with the intent of predicting the occurrence of ischemic brain events.
To compare intracranial hemodynamics before and after carotid endarterectomy
To compare autoregulation and collateral circulation in the different parts of the circle
   of Willis
To investigate vascular impairment caused by hypertension and in follow-up of
   hypertensive patients, and the effectiveness of pharmacological therapy
To predict dementia after stroke

The cerebral VMR (or vasodilatory capacity, or cerebrovascular reserve capacity) of cerebral vessels is usually evaluated 10 min after the intravenous injection of 1 g of acetazolamide (Diamox test), and the response is calculated by the following formula:

$$\text{VMR} = \frac{\text{MCA velocity}_{\text{acetazolamide}} - \text{MCA velocity}_{\text{baseline}}}{\text{MCA velocity}_{\text{baseline}}} \times 100$$

The measurement of VMR by means of TCD has turned out to be a valuable noninvasive instrument for both practical clinical work and pathophysiological research in the field of stroke and cerebrovascular disease. Cerebral VMR reflects the compensatory dilatory capacity of cerebral arterioles to a dilatory stimulus. In the absence of major stenosis, an impaired cerebral VMR may reflect increased rigidity of the arteriolar walls. Decreased cerebral VMR has been observed in patients with hypertension and in patients with insulin-dependent diabetes mellitus. Moreover, impaired cerebral VMR in young hypertensive subjects appears to improve after the initiation of antihypertensive treatment, suggesting that hypertensive microangiopathic changes could be, at least initially, reversible [35].

13.5. CEREBRAL AUTOREGULATION

Cerebral autoregulation is defined as the (1) ability of the cerebral arterioles to compensate for a decrease in cerebral perfusion pressure by vasodilation, thus keeping CBF constant (a failure of this type of autoregulation would result in brain ischemia and infarction) and (2) the ability of the cerebral resistance vessels to protect the brain against increased BP by vasoconstriction (a failure of this type could lead to brain edema and herniation).

High Blood Pressure and Cerebral Blood Flow Autoregulation

High BP influences the cerebral circulation, causing adaptive vascular changes. Thus, hypertension influences the autoregulation of cerebral blood flow by shifting both the lower and upper limits of autoregulatory capacity toward higher blood pressure, while hypertensive patients may be especially vulnerable to episodes of hypotension [12,13], which may play a role in the development of silent cerebrovascular damage such as WML. In the development and progression of chronic high BP, hypertensive cerebral angiopathy occurs, as do secondary reparative changes and adaptive processes at all structural and functional levels of the cerebral vascular system (Tables 13.2 and 13.3). Hypertension causes marked adaptive changes in the cerebral circulation, including increased brain vessel resistance and loss of the physiological mechanism of autoregulation.

Increased cerebral vascular resistance could be due to narrowing of the small vessels by lipohyalinosis and microatherosclerosis. The effect of high BP on small vessels is well known, with vascular remodeling occurring in cerebral blood vessels during chronic hypertension. It has been suggested that this structural alteration impairs autoregulation, exposing the white matter to fluctuations in blood pressure. For this reason it has been hypothesized that changes in cerebral hemodynamics may play a role in the development of WML [13].

However, most studies have found no significant changes in resting cerebral blood flow in either normotensive and hypertensive individuals with silent WML, and, in fact, there are contradictory findings on the relationship between cerebral VMR (or vasodilatory capacity) and WML. Kuwabara et al. [36] reported a close

TABLE 13.2. Main Physiopathological Cerebrovascular Changes Associated with High Blood Pressure

Mechanical stress (endothelial lesion)
Endothelial dysfunction (loss of vasodilatory capacity)
Increased vascular permeability
Opened ionic channels
Hypertrophy of smooth muscle vascular vessels (reduced lumen)
Contraction of smooth muscle vascular vessels (increased vascular resistance)
Synthesis of collagen fiber (vascular stiffness)
Transudation of plasmatic products to the arterial wall

TABLE 13.3. Early Cerebrovascular Damage Associated with Hypertension

Functional abnormalities
  Reduced cerebral blood flow
  Increased cerebrovascular resistance
  Reduced cerebral vasomotor reactivity
  Incipient cognitive impairment
Structural abnormalities
  Vascular remodelling
  Lacunar infarct: small deep infarcts caused by penetrating arteriolar occlusive disease
  White-matter lesions: periventricular white-matter lesions caused by subcortical
    hypertensive small-vessel disease

relationship between cerebral hemodynamic reserve capacity, measured by PET, and the severity of WML in hypertensive patients. Bakker et al. [37] confirmed the association between decreased cerebral VMR and WML, measured by TCD in 73 elderly individuals, 56% of whom were hypertensives. Conversely, Chamorro et al. [38] showed preserved cerebral VMR in 41 patients (71% hypertensives) with silent WML and first-ever lacunar infarction, although they had increased cerebrovascular tone measured by TCD. We recently found an association between silent cerebral WML and increased cerebrovascular tone (increased PI measured by TCD) in middle-aged never-treated essential hypertensive patients, without affecting either cerebral blood flow velocity or the vasodilatory capacity of cerebral vessels [39]. Using exogenous contrast-based perfusion magnetic resonance imaging (MRI), O'Sullivan et al. [40] showed that elderly hypertensive patients with WML have a significant reduction in the cerebral blood flow of normal-appearing white matter compared with hypertensives without WML, suggesting that hypoperfusion may be an early feature of the development of WML. Nevertheless, it remains unclear whether hypoperfusion is a primary pathogenic mechanism or simply a secondary effect of damaged tissue.

13.6. CEREBROVASCULAR REACTIVITY AS A RISK MARKER FOR LACUNAR INFARCTION

There are contradictory findings on the relation between cerebral VMR and the presence of a lacunar infarction [41–43]. This may be due to methodological shortcomings (i.e., patients with other risk factors for a reduced VMR and/or with carotid stenosis).

A case–control study reported a significantly impaired cerebral VMR, measured by TCD (Diamox test), in patients with first-ever symptomatic lacunar infarction and without carotid stenosis, as compared with sex- and age-matched control subjects [41] (46 patients, 63% of whom were hypertensives and 15% diabetic patients), and 46 controls). These findings support the assumption that microangiopathic changes (arteriolosclerosis) may be an independent contributor to impaired reactivity unrelated to the presence of carotid stenosis [44]. It is known that hypertension is the strongest risk factor for first-ever and recurrent lacunar infarction. In the study previously mentioned, Molina et al. [41] observed that cerebral VMR was lower in untreated than in treated hypertensive patients, and that untreated hypertensives have a higher risk for first-ever lacunar infarction. These findings suggest that a more severe arteriolar damage exists in uncontrolled hypertension and that cerebral VMR allows estimation of the degree of diffuse arteriolosclerosis.

Cupini et al. [42] investigated the association between different kinds of ischemic lesions [(1) cortical infarction, (2) single subcortical infarction restricted to the basal ganglia and/or white matter, and (3) subcortical infarction with multiple silent subcortical infarctions], and cerebral VMR evaluated by TCD

(CO_2, breath-holding index) in 41 patients with first-ever schemic stroke (with no stenotic carotid disease; 56% of them were hypertensives, and 14.6% were diabetic patients) and in 15 controls. Results showed that cerebral VMR was significantly lower in the multiple subcortical infarctions group, than in control subjects, single subcortical infarctions group, and cortical infarctions group. In all groups, hypertension, regardless of whether hypertension was treated, correlated with low VMR. The authors suggest the role of hypoperfusion as possible patho genetic mechanisms of subcortical infarctions with multiple silent infarctions.

Chamorro et al. [43] found, in a group of 43 patients with symptomatic lacunes and patent extracranial vessels, that systolic and diastolic BP at stroke onset and diastolic BP and vascular resistance (PI) at stroke follow-up were higher when silent infarctions coexisted. However, cerebral blood flow at rest and after acetazolamide injection were unrelated to silent infarction. De Leeuw et al. [45] studied the cerebral VMR, by means of CO_2-enhanced TCD, in 12 patients with a single symptomatic lacunar infarction (41% were hypertensives) and in 12 controls. None of them were diabetic, and did not have carotid stenosis. Results showed that VMR was significantly lower among individuals with a lacunar infarction than in those without.

Owing to the cross-sectional design of the studies, it is still impossible to establish a causal relationship between cerebral VMR and the occurrence of a lacunar infarction. Prospective studies are necessary to elucidate the role of a decreased cerebral VMR as a risk factor for first-ever and recurrent lacunar infarction.

13.7. CEREBROVASCULAR REACTIVITY AND RISK OF STROKE AND TRANSIENT ISCHEMIC ATTACK IN PATIENTS WITH CAROTID STENOSIS

The management of patients with asymptomatic carotid stenosis is one of the most controversial topics in the cerebrovascular disease literature. Standards for treating patients with asymptomatic carotid stenosis have been difficult to establish because of the lack of evidence for factors influencing these patients' prognoses. Some studies have suggested that an alteration in cerebral hemodynamic function may play a relevant role in the occurrence of stroke.

Silvestrini et al. [46] investigated the relationship between cerebral VMR and cerebrovascular events in a prospective, blinded longitudinal study. Vaso motor reactivity was evaluated by the breath-holding index. The breath-holding index was obtained by dividing the percentage increase in mean flow velocity (measured by TCD in the MCA) occurring during breath holding by the length of time (seconds) that subjects hold their breath after a normal inspiration [(mean flow velocity at the end of breath holding minus mean flow velocity at rest divided by mean flow velocity at rest) multiplied by 100 divided by seconds of breath holding]. Ninety-four patients with asymptomatic carotid stenosis of at least 70% were included. The mean follow-up was 28.5 months. Seventeen patients developed ischemic events (transient ischemic attack or stroke). Results showed a link between impaired cerebral VMR and the risk of ischemic events ipsilateral to severe asymptomatic carotid stenosis.

Another longitudinal study was performed in 107 patients with either carotid occlusion ($n = 48$) or asymptomatic carotid $\geq 70\%$ ($n = 59$) by Markus et al. [47]. Subjects were followed prospectively until stroke, transient ischemic attack (TIA), death, or study end. The mean follow-up was 21.1 months. TCD was used to determine the reactivity of MCA to CO_2 administered in air. There were 11 ipsilateral ischemic events during follow-up. Results showed that severely reduced cerebral VMR predicts the risk of ipsilateral stroke or TIA in patients with carotid occlusion, and to a lesser extent in asymptomatic carotid stenosis.

All of these results support the role of hemodynamic factors in the pathogenesis of stroke in patients with carotid artery stenosis or occlusion. They suggest that the evaluation of cerebral hemodynamics using TCD may provide a method of identifying a subgroup of high-risk patients who may benefit from revascularization. However, this hypothesis requires further analyses in randomized controlled intervention studies.

13.8. PHARMACOLOGIC INTERVENTIONS

There is growing evidence that pharmacologic interference with the renin–angiotensin system may reduce risk of stroke [48], and stroke recurrence [6,49], although the mechanism is unclear, and is difficult to elucidate whether this beneficial effect was related to the degree of BP lowering achieved. Walters et al. [50] examined the effect of the angiotensin-converting enzyme (ACE) inhibitor perindopril on cerebral vasomotor reactivity to acetazolamide in a cohort of male patients between 3 and 12 months after lacunar infarction confirmed on computed tomography. Each patient received perindopril 4 mg daily or matching placebo for 2 weeks in a randomized, double-blind, placebo-controlled crossover fashion. Cerebral vasomotor reactivity (increase in middle cerebral artery mean flow velocity in response to intravenous injection of 15 mg/kg acetazolamide) was measured before and after each dosing period using TCD. Results showed a significant improvement in cerebral vasomotor reactivity induced by perindopril, beyond any effect on blood pressure.

On the other hand, in animal models it has been reported that cholesterol-lowering therapy with 3-hydroxy-3-methylglutaryl coenzyme-A reductase inhibitors (statins) may augment absolute CBF by enhancing nitric oxide synthase (eNOS) [51]. An observational study by Sterzer et al. [52] provided the first evidence for a significant improvement of cerebral vasomotor reactivity by using statins in patients with cerebral small-vessel disease. In this study, CBF velocity increase after bolus injection of 1 g acetazolamide was determined before and after 2-month treatment with pravastatin 20 mg. Although no control group was included, a significant CBF velocity increase was observed after pravastatin therapy. Pretnar-Oblak et al. [53] provide some insights into the pathophysiology of cerebral small-vessel disease and the mechanism of action of statins on cerebral vasomotor reactivity. The effect of atorvastatin treatment on cerebral endothelial function, as measured by the response to L-arginine reactivity on TCD, in 18 multiple lacunar stroke patients, 20 age- and gender-matched longstanding hypertension and hypercholesterolemia patients, and 19 gender-matched healthy control subjects was studied. As expected, baseline L-arginine reactivity was decreased in patients with lacunar stroke and vascular risk factors compared with healthy controls. After 3-month atorvastatin treatment, decreased L-arginine reactivity and flow-mediated dilatation significantly improved in both types of patients.

13.9. CONCLUSIONS

The results of these studies on the pathophysiological effects of statins on cerebral vasomotor reserve should be considered with caution. The expanding indications for statins in cerebral ischemia should be supported by evidence-based medical analysis. Further studies are required to determine whether chronic treatment with statins can improve white-matter lesions and cerebral vasomotor reactivity and prevent the risk of recurrence of lacunar infarctions.

REFERENCES

1. Ivan CS, Seshadri S, Beiser A et al: Dementia after stroke: The Framingham Study, *Stroke* **35**(6):1264–1268 (2004).

2. Multiple Risk Factor Intervention Trial: Mortality after 10 years for hypertensive participants in the Multiple Risk Factor Intervention Trial, *Circulation* **82**:1616–1628 (1990).

3. MacMahon S, Peto R, Cutler J et al: Blood pressure, stroke, and coronary heart disease, Part 1: Prolonged differences in blood pressure. Prospective observational studies corrected for the regression dilution bias, *Lancet* **355**:765–774 (1990).

4. Collins R, Peto R, MacMahon S et al: Blood pressure, stroke, and coronary heart disease, Part 2: Short-term reductions in blood pressure. Overview of randomised drug trials in their epidemiological context, *Lancet* **355**:827–838 (1990).

5. Rodgers A, MacMahon S, Gamble G, Slattery J, Sandercock P, Warlow C: Blood pressure and risk of stroke in patients with cerebrovascular disease: The United Kingdom Transient Ischaemic Attack Collaborative Group, *Br Med J* **313**:147–150 (1996).

6. PROGRESS Collaborative Group: Randomised trial of a perindopril-based blood-pressure-lowering regimen among 6105 individuals with previous stroke or transient ischaemic attack, *Lancet* **358**:1033–1041 (2001).

7. Kannel WB, Wolf PA, Verter MS, McNamara PM: Epidemiologic assessment of the role of blood pressure in stroke. The Framingham Study, *JAMA* **214**:301–310 (1970).

8. Vermeer SE, Hollander M, van Dijk EJ, Hofman A, Koudstaal PJ, Breteler MM; Rotterdam Scan Study: Silent brain infarcts and white matter lesions increase stroke risk in the general population: The Rotterdam Scan Study, *Stroke* **34**(5):1126–1129 (2003).

9. Kuller LH, Longstreth WT, Arnold AM, Bernick C, Bryan N, Beauchamp NJ, for the Cardiovascular Health Study Collaborative Research Group: White matter hyperintensity on cranial magnetic resonance imaging. A predictor of stroke, *Stroke* **35**:1821–1825 (2004).

10. De Groot JC, de Leeuw FE, Oudkerk M et al: Periventricular cerebral white matter lesions predict rate of cognitive decline, *Ann Neurol* **52**:335–341 (2002).

11. Prins ND, van Dijk EJ, den Heijer T et al: Cerebral white matter lesions and the risk of dementia, *Arch Neurol* **61**:1531–1534 (2004).

12. Pantoni L, Garcia JH: The significance of cerebral white matter abnormalities 100 years after Binswanger's report, *Stroke* **26**:1293–1301 (1995).

13. Pantoni L, Garcia JH: Pathogenesis of leukoaraiosis. A review, *Stroke* **28**:652–659 (1997).

14. National Stroke Association: Stroke prevention: The importance of risk factors, *Stroke* **1**:17–20 (1991).

15. Kjeldsen SE, Julius S, Hedner T, Hansson L: Stroke is more common than myocardial infarction in hypertension: Analysis based on 11 major randomized intervention trials, *Blood Press* **10**(4):190–192 (2001).

16. Kavanagh S, Knapp M, Patel A: Costs and disability among stroke patients, *J Publ Health Med* **21**:385–394 (1999).

17. Liao D, Cooper L, Cai J et al: Presence and severity of cerebral white matter lesions and hypertension, its treatment, and its control. The ARIC Study, *Stroke* **27**:2262–2270 (1996).

18. Longstreth WT, Manolio TA, Arnold A et al, for the Cardiovascular Health Study Collaborative Research Group: Clinical correlates of white matter findings on cranial magnetic resonance imaging of 3301 elderly people. The Cardiovascular Health Study, *Stroke* **27**:1274–1282 (1996).

19. Breteler MMB, van Swieten JC, Bots ML et al: Cerebral white matter lesions, vascular risk factors, and cognitive function in a population-based study: The Rotterdam Study, *Neurology* **44**:1246–1252 (1994).

20. Shimada K, Kawamoto A, Matsubayashi K, Ozawa T: Silent cerebrovascular disease in the elderly. Correlation with ambulatory pressure, *Hypertension* **16**:692–699 (1990).

21. Goldstein IB, Bartzokis G, Hance DB, Shapiro D: Relationship between blood pressure and subcortical lesions in healthy elderly people, *Stroke* **29**:765–772 (1998).

22. Sierra C, de la Sierra A, Mercader J, Gómez-Angelats E, Urbano-Márquez A, Coca A: Silent cerebral white matter lesions in middle-aged essential hypertensive patients, *J Hypertens* **20**:519–524 (2002).

23. International Society of Hypertension Writing Group: International Society of Hypertension (ISH): Statement on blood pressure lowering and stroke prevention, *J Hypertens* **21**:651–663 (2003).

24. Rodgers A, MacMahon S, Gamble G, Slattery J, Sandercock P, Warlow C, on behalf of the UKTIA Collaborative Group: Blood pressure and the risk of stroke in patients with cerebrovascular disease, *Br Med J* **313**:147 (1996).

25. Stamler J, Stamler R, Neaton JD: Blood pressure, systolic and diastolic, and cardiovascular risks, *Arch Intern Med* **153**:598–615 (1993).

26. Domanski MJ, Davis BR, Pfeffer MA, Kastantin M, Mitchell GF: Isolated systolic hypertension. Prognostic information provided by pulse pressure, *Hypertension* **34**:375–380 (1999).

27. Laurent S, Katsahian S, Fassot C et al: Aortic stiffness is an independent predictor of fatal stroke in essential hypertension, *Stroke* **34**:1203–1206 (2003).

28. Schmidt R, Fazekas F, Kapeller P, Schmidt H, Hartung HP: MRI white matter hyperintensities. Three-year follow-up of the Austrian Stroke Prevention Study, *Neurology* **53**:132–139 (1999).

29. Dufouil C, de Kersaint-Gilly A, Besancon V et al: Longitudinal study on blood pressure and white matter hyperintensities. The EVA MRI cohort, *Neurology* **56**:921–926 (2001).

30. De Leeuw FE, de Groot JC, Oudkerk M, Witteman JCM, Hofman A, van Gijn J et al: Hypertension and cerebral white matter lesions in a prospective cohort study, *Brain* **125**:765–772 (2002).

31. Kario K, Matsuo T, Kobayashi H, Imiya M, Matsuo M, Shimada K: Nocturnal fall of blood pressure and silent cerebrovascular damage in elderly hypertensive patients. Advanced silent cerebrovascular damage in extreme dippers, *Hypertension* **27**:130–135 (1996).

32. Aaslid R: Cerebral hemodynamics, in Newell DW, Aaslid R, eds, *Transcranial Doppler*, Raven Press, New York, 1992, pp 49–55.

33. Gosling RG, Dunbar G, King DH: The quantitative analysis of occlusive peripheral arterial disease by a non-invasive ultrasonic technique, *Angiology* **22**:52–55 (1971).

34. Lindegaard KF: Indices of pulsatility, in Newell DW, Aaslid R, eds, *Transcranial Doppler*, Raven Press, New York, 1992, pp 67–81.

35. Troisi E, Attanasio A, Matteis M, Bragoni M, Monaldo BC, Caltagirone C et al: Cerebral hemodynamics in young hypertensive subjects and effects of atenolol treatment, *J Neurol Sci* **159**:115–119 (1998).

36. Kuwabara Y, Ichiya Y, Sasaki M et al: Cerebral blood flow and vascular response to hypercapnia in hypertensive patients with leukoaraiosis, *Ann Nucl Med* **10**:293–298 (1996).

37. Bakker SLM, de Leeuw FE, de Groot JC, Hofman A, Koudstaal PJ, Breteler MMB: Cerebral vasomotor reactivity and cerebral white matter lesions in the elderly, *Neurology* **52**:578–583 (1999).

38. Chamorro A, Pujol J, Saiz A et al: Periventricular white matter lucencies in patients with lacunar stroke, *Arch Neurol* **54**:1284–1288 (1997).

39. Sierra C, de la Sierra A, Chamorro A, Larrousse M, Domenech M, Coca A: Cerebral hemodynamics and silent cerebral white matter lesions in middle-aged essential hypertensive patients, *Blood Press* **13**:304–309 (2004).

40. O'Sullivan M, Lythgoe DJ, Pereira AC et al: Patterns of cerebral blood flow reduction in patients with ischemic leukoaraiosis, *Neurology* **59**:321–326 (2002).

41. Molina C, Álvarez-Sabín J, Montaner J, Rovira A, Abilleira S, Codina A: Impaired cerebrovascular reactivity as a risk marker for first-ever lacunar infarction. A case-control study, *Stroke* **30**:2296–2301 (1999).

42. Cupini LM, Diomedi M, Placidi F, Silvestrini M, Giacomini P: Cerebrovascular reactivity and subcirtical infarctions, *Arch Neurol* **58**:577–581 (2001).

43. Chamorro A, Saiz A, Vila N, Ascaso C, Blanc R, Alday M et al: Contribution of arterial blood pressure to the clinical expression of lacunar infarction, *Stroke* **27**:388–392 (1996).

44. Maeda H, Matsumoto M, Handa N, Hougaku H, Ogawa S, Itoh T et al: Reactivity of cerebral blood flow to carbon dioxide in various type of ischemic cerebrovascular disease: Evaluation by the transcranial Doppler method, *Stroke* **24**:670–675 (1993).

45. de Leeuw FE, van Huffelen A, Kapelle J: Cerebrovascular reactivity in patients with a recent lacunar infarction, *J Neurol* **250**:232–233 (2003).

46. Silvestrini M, Vernieri F, Pasqualetti P, Matteis M, Passarelli F, Troisi E et al: Impaired cerebral vasoreactivity and risk of stroke in patients with asymptomatic carotid artery stenosis, *JAMA* **283**:2122–2127 (2000).

47. Markus H, Cullinane M: Severely impaired cerebrovascular reactivity predicts stroke and TIA risk in patients with carotid stenosis and occlusion, *Brain* **124**:457–467 (2001).

48. Dahlöf B, Devereux RB, Kjeldsen SE, Julius S, Beevers G, de Faire U et al: Cardiovascular morbidity and mortality in the Losartan Intervention for Endpoint reduction in hypertension study (LIFE): A randomised trial against atenolol, *Lancet* **359**:995–1003 (2002).

49. Schrader J, Lüders S, Kulchewski A, Hammersen F, Plate K, Berger J et al: Morbidity and mortality after stroke, eprosartan compared with nitrendipine for secondary prevention. Principal results of a prospective randomized controlled study (MOSES), *Stroke* **36**:1218–1224 (2005).

50. Walters M, Muir S, Shah I, Lees K: Effect of perindopril on cerebral vasomotor reactivity in patients with lacunar infarction, *Stroke* **35**:1899–1902 (2004).

51. Yamada M, Huang Z, Dalkara T, Endres M, Laufs U, Waeber C, Huang PL et al: Endothelial nitric oxide synthase-dependent cerebral blood flow augmentation by L-arginine after chronic statin treatment, *J Cereb Blood Flow Metab* **20**:709–717 (2000).

52. Sterzer P, Meintzschel F, Rosler A, Lanfermann H, Steinmetz H, Sitzer M: Pravastatin improves cerebral vasomotor reactivity in patients with subcortical small-vessel disease, *Stroke* **32**:2817–2820 (2001).

53. Pretnar-Oblak J, Sabovic M, Sebestjen M, Pogacnik T, Zaletel M: The influence of atorvastatin treatment on L-arginine cerebrovascular reactivity and flow-mediated dilatation in patients with lacunar infarction, *Stroke* **37**:2540–2545 (2006).

INDEX